Manual for the Homemaker/Home Health Aide

Manual for the
Homemaker/Home Health Aide

Elizabeth Hazen Willborn, R.N., B.A., B.S.N.
Home Health Consultant
Former Coordinator of the Nebraska Statewide
Homemaker/Home Health Aide Training Project

Photographs by Linda Story
Illustrations by Lynn Soloway

J.B. Lippincott Company
Philadelphia
London   Mexico City   New York   St. Louis   São Paulo   Sydney

Acquisition/Sponsoring Editor: Patricia Cleary
Coordinating Editorial Assistant: Diana Merritt
Manuscript Editor: Virginia Barishek
Indexer: Alexandra Weir
Design Coordinator: Anita Curry
Designer: Anne O'Donnell
Production Manager: Kathleen Dunn
Production Coordinator: Fred D. Wood IV
Compositor: Digitype
Printer/Binder: The Murray Printing Company

6 5 4 3

Library of Congress Cataloging in Publication Data

Willborn, Elizabeth Hazen.
    Manual for the homemaker/home health aide /
Elizabeth Hazen Willborn.
        p. cm.
    Includes index.
    ISBN 0-397-54635-1
    1. Home care services.   2. Home health aides.
        I. Title.
RA645.3.W54 1988
610.73'7—dc19   87-36871
                                                    CIP

Any procedure or practice described in this book should be
applied by the health-care practitioner under appropriate
supervision in accordance with professional standards of care
used with regard to the unique circumstances that apply in
each practice situation. Care has been taken to confirm the
accuracy of information presented and to describe generally
accepted practices. However, the authors, editors, and pub-
lisher cannot accept any responsibility for errors or omissions
or for consequences from application of the information in
this book and make no warranty, express or implied, with
respect to the contents of the book.

Every effort has been made to ensure drug selections and
dosages are in accordance with current recommendations
and practice. Because of ongoing research, changes in government regulations, and the constant flow of information
on drug therapy, reactions, and interactions, the reader is
cautioned to check the package insert for each drug for
indications, dosages, warnings, and precautions, particularly
if the drug is new or infrequently used.

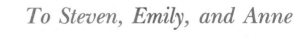

To Steven, Emily, and Anne

Preface

To the Student: How to Use This Book

Welcome to one of the fastest-growing industries in the country—home health care. This book on home health care can be used both for your homemaker/home health aide classes and as a reference book after your classes are over. Read this section carefully, because it will help you find information in the book quickly and easily.

Parts of the Book

Objectives. The objectives are the goals found at the beginning of each chapter. The objectives will tell you what you should know after reading the chapter. When you finish the chapter, go back and read the objectives again to see if you have met your goals. If not, you should reread the material.

New Terms and the Glossary. New words are defined and printed in *italics* to stand out. You can also look up new terms in the *glossary*. The glossary is at the back of the book and includes some of the new terms in the book and others that will be handy for you to know.

Homemaker/Home Health Aide Procedures. The homemaker/home health aide procedures provide easy-to-follow directions on tasks you will be asked to perform. Each procedure explains the purpose of the procedure, equipment that you will need to do the procedure, and safety precautions. The procedures are printed in two columns.

The left column has step-by-step directions and the right column explains why the step should be done in that manner.

Review Questions. At the end of each chapter you will find a number of *review questions*. The review questions allow you to test yourself on the material covered in each chapter. The answers can be found at the back of the book, but try to work out the review questions yourself without looking at the answers. The review section also includes some questions for class discussion.

The Homemaker/Home Health Aide Evaluation. This checklist can be found at the back of the book just before the glossary. It lists the skills and knowledge you will learn from this book. Your instructor or a professional member of your home health agency will complete the form. For your client's safety, do not perform any of the procedures in this book on a client until your supervisor has watched you demonstrate the skill and passed you on your ability.

How to Find Information in This Book

This book is intended to be used both in the classroom and as a reference book after you have completed your homemaker/home health aide training. Because it is a large book, I have tried to include several ways for you to find the information that you need quickly.

1. The *table of contents* is a detailed outline of the material in this book. It lists page

numbers for each chapter and for the main section in the chapter.

2. A *chapter outline* can be found on the first page of every chapter. It lists the main points covered in the chapter.

3. There is an *index* at the back of the book. When you look up a word in the index, it will tell you where you can find that term discussed in the book. If, for example, you would like to know more about bedsores, you would look up the word in the index. You will find a few different page numbers for "bedsores" because they are discussed in a few different places in the book.

To the Home Health Agency and Classroom Instructor

Manual for the Homemaker/Home Health Aide is a comprehensive book that gives students the background knowledge and skills needed to become a homemaker/home health aide. However, no book can replace the personal guidance that a competent instructor can provide. This book is intended to be used in a classroom with instructors who are qualified to teach home health care skills. Many states have homemaker/home health aide certification programs that require up to 120 hours of classroom training (theory and lab demonstrations) and training in the home setting under the supervision of a registered nurse. This book should be adequate as the primary text for any homemaker/home health aide course.

Training programs for homemaker/home health aides are very important and deserve careful thought. The homemaker/home health aide often sees clients more than any other member of the home care team, and may be valuable minutes away from professional assistance in emergencies. For these reasons the homemaker/home health aide needs thorough training and a good understanding of the skills and knowledge required for home care. The homemaker/home health aide must know how to give safe, responsible, effective care, and know when and how to call the supervisor for assistance. (Because it is difficult for many people to call a supervisor with questions, the supervisor, in turn, must be supportive and answer any questions the homemaker/home health aide has with understanding and compassion.) An effective homemaker/home health aide training program also provides higher job satisfaction and lower turnover rates. That translates into substantial savings for both the client and home health agency and better care for clients.

With the growing costs of hospital and institutional care and the growing population of older adults, it is clear that the home care industry is just beginning to blossom. With proper training and supervision, homemaker/home health aides will provide safe and effective care for their clients.

Elizabeth Hazen Willborn, R.N., B.A., B.S.N.

Acknowledgments

My most sincere thanks go to Steven L. Willborn, who reviewed drafts and gave me a tremendous amount of support and encouragement throughout the course of this project, and to Emily who slept through the night since the day she was born. I would also like to thank those who carefully reviewed the manuscript, especially Evonne Rodriguez-Sierra, R.N., M.S., M.S.N.; Nola Aalberts, Administrative Director of the National Association of Home Care, Washington, D.C.; Karen Bogenschneider, B.A., M.S., home economist, Spring Green, Wisconsin; Susan Vaughn Williams, League of Human Dignity, Lincoln, Nebraska; Becky Mojica, R.N., B.S.N., Pacific Grove, California; and the staff at J.B. Lippincott Company.

I'd also like to thank Linda Story, photographer, and Lynn Soloway, illustrator, for their prompt work and attention to detail. More thanks go to the models, homemaker/home health aides, and clients who posed for the photographs: Karen Tearston; Jane Weber; Evonne and Jorge Rodriguez-Sierra; Janice M. Genthe; Pippa Lawson; Nancy and Grant Buckley; Lione Griesemer; De-Lora Nubo; Suzanne Kalish; Barb Johnson Frank; Grace, Cameron, and Kenneth Shum; Rachel Frank; Gregory Lawson; Grant Story; Ruth Jackson; Heidi Sitzman; Sean Story; Martha L. McKown; Beryl F. Bristow; and Emily Love Willborn.

My appreciation also goes to the American Heart Association, the National Dairy Council, the Nebraska State Department of Health; the Nebraska State Department of Aging; and the libraries and staffs of the Royal College of Nursing Library in London, the University of Nebraska Libraries, and the Lincoln Public Library System. I would also like to thank Mary Munter, Director of Community Health Nursing for the Nebraska State Department of Health; my colleagues from the Nebraska State Department of Health who encouraged me to begin and complete this project; and all the homemaker/home health aides who have participated in the Nebraska Statewide Homemaker/Home Health Aide Training Project. Finally, I'd like to thank all of my friends and family who gave me support along the way.

Chapter Titles

Contents

Contents

Contents

Part Six

Personal Care and Medical Procedures 155

Contents

Homemaker/Home Health Aide Procedures

Manual for the Homemaker/Home Health Aide

Part One

Homemaker/Home Health Aide Services

Chapter 1
Introduction to Home Health Care

Objectives

At the conclusion of this chapter, the homemaker/home health aide will:

1. Be able to define home care and understand how the home health agency provides services.

2. Be able to explain several professions that may be included on the home care team, what they do, and how the homemaker/home health aide works with the team.

3. Understand the role of the supervisor and how the homemaker/home health aide and supervisor work together.

4. Understand the homemaker/home health aide's job and responsibilities when working with the client and family.

Home Health Care and the Home Care Team

Most Americans are too young to remember a time when health care was regularly provided in the home. A family doctor visiting homes with his black bag of supplies is rarely seen today, but at one time that was the most common way of receiving health care. There is a growing movement to provide health care and support services to people in their homes once again. But today, instead of the doctor making the home visits himself, it is done by the home health agency and the home care team. Home health services allow people, who otherwise might have to live in a nursing home or a long-term care facility, to stay in their own homes. Being cared for at home in familiar surroundings frequently makes the recovery period short.

This chapter will explain the responsibilities of the home health agency and the members of the home care team. One of the most important members of the home care team is you: The homemaker/home health aide (HM/HHA). Your job will be explained thoroughly later in this chapter.

The Home Health Agency

The home health agency is the company that employs most members of the home care team and organizes their work. If home care is needed, the client, family, or doctor will contact the home health agency. The home health agency will then arrange the care. Home care services are often recommended to a family by a physician, a hospital discharge planner when a patient leaves the hospital, a social services agency, or friends.

The home health agency usually begins the process by assigning a nurse to visit the client at home. The nurse interviews the client, and may do a physical examination if one is needed. Based on this information, the nurse writes a *care plan*. The care plan is a written record of the services and treatments that will be provided. It also lists the goals of care. If home care services have been ordered by a doctor, the care plan is sent to the physician for approval. After the physician approves the care plan, the *supervisor*, or home care professional who is overseeing the care of that particular client, may assign a HM/HHA to the client. The supervisor then monitors the progress of the client and updates the care plan as needed. You, the HM/HHA, will receive instructions about when to visit the client and what to do for the client based on information from the written care plan and your supervisor. The set of written instructions that your supervisor provides for you is called *the assignment sheet* (Figure 1-1). Later, in Chapter 11, you will learn how to report information on the client's progress to your supervisor.

The Home Care Team

The *home care team* is the group of people who provide health-related services in the home. The people on the team are listed in the box, Members of the Home Care Team. These services range from helping with medical treatments to assisting with activities of daily living such as bathing, dressing, preparing meals, and light housekeeping. The person who needs care is called the *client*. We use the word client because it reminds us that the person who receives home care has hired the home health agency to provide this service. Generally a home care client takes a more active role in his plan of treatment than does a hospital patient.

The home care team consists of several people or just a few, depending on the client's needs. Not every client uses every member of an agency's home care team. Each member has an important role. Each member of the home care team is like a link of a chain that supports the client. If one

Homemaker/Home Health Aide Assignment Sheet

Client's name _____

Address _____

Supervisor's name _____

Service covered
from _____ to _____
Phone _____

Take vital signs (T, P, R, BP)
Directions _____

☐ Check mental status
Directions _____

☐ Weigh client
Directions _____

☐ With shoes ☐ Without shoes

☐ Special procedures _____

Skin care
☐ Backrub
☐ Shave
☐ Reposition client ____ times
☐ Report on skin condition _____
☐ Other _____

Foot/Nail care
☐ Soak feet ☐ Soak hands
☐ File toenails ☐ File fingernails
Directions _____

Hair care
☐ Shampoo ☐ Assist ☐ Alone
☐ Shampoo in bed
☐ Comb/brush hair

Activity/Exercise
Encourage ☐ Cane ☐ Walker
☐ Crutches ☐ Wheelchair
☐ Bedrest orders _____
☐ Walks ☐ With assistance
　　　　 ☐ Without assistance
☐ Transfers ☐ With assistance
　　　　　 ☐ Without assistance
☐ Range of motion exercises _____

☐ Other exercises _____

Home Management
☐ Laundry _____

☐ Change linens _____

☐ Clean
Bathroom _____
Kitchen _____
Bedroom _____
Other _____

☐ Other _____

Mouth care
☐ Brush teeth ☐ Dentures
☐ Floss teeth ☐ Assist

Bath
☐ Bed bath ☐ Tub bath
☐ Shower ☐ At sink
☐ Use tub stool
☐ Assist with _____

Dress
☐ Bed clothes ☐ Street clothes
☐ Alone ☐ Assist

Elimination/toilet care
☐ Toilet ☐ Bedside commode
☐ Bedpan ☐ Urinal
☐ Assist ☐ Alone
☐ Empty catheter bag at (time) _____
☐ Urine test directions _____

☐ Measure fluid output
☐ Observe urine ☐ Observe BM
Directions _____

Meals/Nutrition
Make ☐ Breakfast
☐ Lunch ☐ Supper
Directions _____

Eats ☐ Alone ☐ With assistance
☐ Meals on wheels

☐ Restrict fluids
☐ Force fluids
☐ Measure fluid intake
Other Directions _____

Special Directions
_____
_____
_____

In case of emergency notify:
Fire department # _____　　　Police _____　　　Relative/responsible adult _____
Emergency services # _____　　　Home health agency _____

Figure 1-1

This is an example of a homemaker/home health aide assignment sheet. Your supervisor will fill it out to let you and the family know what you are to do for your client. One basic rule of being a homemaker/home health aide is that you should not perform any tasks that have not been written on the assignment sheet by your supervisor.

Members of the Home Care Team

All members of the home care team are equally important. The following members of the home care team are listed alphabetically.

Dietician has special training in the way food affects health, and teaches clients about special diets.

Home Economist teaches domestic skills such as cleaning, cooking, and laundry. May have training in family counseling.

Home Health Administrator directs and organizes the budget and other activities for the home health agency.

Homemaker/Home Health Aide (HM/HHA) may also be called Homemaker, Home Care Aide, Home Health Aide, Personal Care Aide, or Home Nursing Assistant. Employed by a home health agency and supervised by professional staff members. Provides home care based on a care plan. Duties may include personal care, meal planning and preparation, and light housekeeping. The job description will vary among home health agencies, and the job title may reflect various skill and training levels. Needs to be sensitive and able to work effectively with a variety of people.

Licensed Practical Nurse (LPN) or Licensed Vocational Nurse (LVN) provides nursing care under the direction of a registered nurse.

Medical Social Worker has been trained to treat or counsel individuals, families, and groups. Assists with problems that are related to physical, emotional, and psychological health. May arrange financial assistance for families in need.

Occupational Therapist (OT) has been trained to assist people to maintain, improve, or regain practical skills that have been affected by a disease or injury. The focus is on retraining people to care for themselves in their own homes. For example, a person with a hand injury may have to learn a new way to use a knife, fork, and spoon for eating.

Physical Therapist (PT) has been trained to help people maintain, improve, or regain the ability to use a body part that has been affected by a disease or injury. The focus is on improving function and preventing disability.

Physician (MD) diagnoses the client's medical problems and participates in planning the client's care. The physician also prescribes medications and treatments.

Public Health Nurse (PHN) may be called a Community Health Nurse (CHN). Registered nurse who provides nursing care to promote and preserve health in the community. Usually plans and supervises the medical care provided by the HM/HHA.

Registered Nurse (RN) has been trained to provide skilled nursing care. Usually plans and supervises the medical care provided by the HM/HHA.

Respiratory Therapist provides care for clients who have difficulty breathing. May go to the client's home to administer treatments or assist in planning treatments.

Speech Therapist provides treatment for clients with speech disorders. Speech can be affected by disease or injury.

---

member is not doing his part, the whole chain is weakened and the client is the one who suffers.

The primary *goal* or purpose of the home care team is to help the client to lead as normal and productive a life as possible. The home health agencies often provides two kinds of services: health services and support services.

Health Services

- homemaker/home health aide
- nutritional counseling
- skilled nursing care
- physical therapy
- occupational therapy
- speech therapy
- respiratory therapy

Support Services

- meals on wheels—hot meals are delivered to a client's home
- respite care—care that is provided to give family members some time off
- chore service—help with daily chores that may be too difficult for a client to do. This allows him to live in his home.
- money management
- parenting skills

The Role of the Homemaker/ Home Health Aide

What Is a Homemaker/Home Health Aide?

A HM/HHA is a person who works in someone's home while that person is injured, ill, disabled, or cannot care for himself. The HM/HHA helps with light housekeeping and personal care tasks, which allows the client to live as normal and independent a life as possible until he is able to take care of himself again.

A HM/HHA may be assigned several different duties. She may provide personal care, such as helping a client with bathing and dressing. Or the HM/HHA may prepare meals and do light housekeeping. She may even perform basic medical procedures such as taking the client's pulse, blood pressure, or temperature. Sometimes clients live alone and need assistance during a time of illness or injury. Other clients may have family members who help them most of the time, but who need a HM/HHA to help with certain procedures or to let those family members have some time off. A family may need help caring for children while a parent is ill, or a HM/HHA may help care for children who are ill.

The job of a HM/HHA is quite different from that of a regular housekeeper. A HM/HHA has been trained to work with clients with health problems and can do things that an ordinary housekeeper would not know how to do. Also, a HM/HHA is part of a home care team. The team is available for advice and guidance and, if an emergency occurs, the HM/HHA can quickly contact another member of the team (a nurse or a doctor, for example) for help.

In addition to helping individual clients who need assistance, the HM/HHA also provides an important community service. Home care services allow people to remain at home while receiving health care, which is often less expensive than hospital care. Home care also allows clients to recover in comfortable and familiar surroundings.

The job of the HM/HHA is very important and not easy. It requires training, intelligence, patience, and a willingness to help others. A cheerful disposition is also important when working with people who are ill. Although it may not be obvious each day with every client, the HM/HHA usually learns quickly that she can make a difference in someone's life, and that is very rewarding.

The Supervisor and the Homemaker/ Home Health Aide

When you work for a home health agency, you will never work alone. You will always have a supervisor to answer your questions and assist you. The supervisor is experienced in home care, works closely with the physician and other members of the team, and has helped plan the client's treatment or care plan. Usually your supervisor will be a registered nurse.

Before you meet a new client, your supervisor will give you information about the client (Figure 1-2). This information will help you to understand

1. why the client needs home care;
2. the agency's goals for that client;
3. when you are expected to make home visits;
4. what you are expected to do for the client; and
5. the kind of information the home health agency will want you to report about the client's progress.

Your supervisor may go with you to meet a new client, and she may make periodic visits to check on the client's progress. If you do not understand what you are to do or if you need assistance with an assigned procedure, your supervisor will help you. Never go to a client's house without

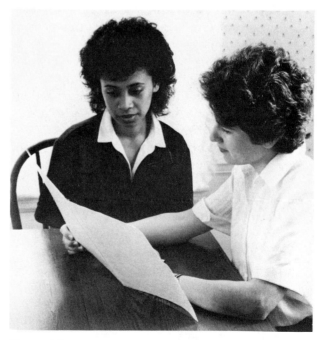

Figure 1-2

The nurse and homemaker/home health aide are reviewing the assignment sheet for a new client. Whenever you have a question about a client or a procedure, ask your supervisor.

knowing how you can reach your supervisor. Include the home health agency's phone number on a list of emergency phone numbers and always carry that list with you. (See Figure 12-1 later in the book.)

Responsibilities of the Homemaker/ Home Health Aide

As a HM/HHA, you will have responsibilities to your clients and their families, to the home health agency, and to yourself. *Ethics* are the moral codes or standards of behavior that you are expected to follow when working in a client's home. You must be honest, do your job to the best of your ability, and keep information about the client and his family confidential. *Confidentiality* means that certain information is kept private and not discussed with others. Following the ethical standards your home health agency sets and keeping information about your clients confidential are important responsibilities of the HM/HHA. The list below includes other policies that most home health agencies ask each HM/HHA to follow.

1. Appearance and grooming
   - Before you start your workday, make sure you are clean and well groomed. Daily bathing is recommended.
   - Brush your teeth after meals.
   - Keep your hair clean, combed, and away from your face.
   - Wear a freshly laundered uniform every day.
   - Make-up can be worn, but it should be light. Perfume or cologne can be irritating to some people, especially those who are ill, so do not wear it while working.
   - Fingernails should be kept short and clean.
   - Large rings and jewelery should not be worn. They can scratch a client's skin and can also carry germs from one house to another.
   - Do not smoke in the client's home. It does not look professional. In addition, many people who need home care should not be around smoke. If the client or other family members smoke, that is their decision, but it is still inappropriate for you to smoke in a client's home.
   - Most important, wash your hands after using the toilet, before and after giving care to your client, and before and after preparing food.

2. Working with your supervisor and the home care team.
   - Follow the care plan carefully and do only the tasks assigned by the supervisor.
   - Talk to your supervisor if you are not sure how to do a procedure. Phone if there is an accident or an error, even if you are not sure it is significant.
   - Occasionally you may come across an incident or situation that you think is affecting the client's health, but you are not sure how to record it in the client's written progress note. Talk to your supervisor for advice.
   - Keep accurate written reports and give them to the agency in a timely manner according to the agency's guidelines. You will learn to keep records in Chapter 11.
   - Work as a team member. Accept guidance from your supervisor and the other professional members of the home care team. Share your observations with others on the team.

3. Working with the client and family.
   - Arrive on time. Show consideration by phoning if you are going to be even 15 minutes late.
   - Respect the client's and family's right to privacy. Never discuss a client's family situation or health problems with anyone who is not working for the home health agency on that particular client's case. If anyone asks you about your client's health, have that person talk with the client, his family, his doctor, or his nurse.
   - Do not give clients your home phone number. Clients should be encouraged to call the home health agency with questions. The agency will have an appropriate health professional deal with emergencies, answer questions, or arrange for home care services.
   - Accept other lifestyles. When you work in another person's home, you will notice differences from the way you do things in your home. The other person's standards of cleanliness, eating habits, religious practices, and child-rearing techniques may be different from yours. Try not to judge the person, but instead realize that these differences make us unique individuals. One of the rewards of being a HM/HHA is learning about how other people live.

- Respect the client's right to be treated with dignity. Every client is a human being with feelings.
- Keep your conversation light and cheerful. People who are in need of home care generally have enough to worry about. Usually clients are interested in hearing about your family, but try not to discuss your personal problems.
- Realize that you are in the home to take care of the client for health reasons. If the family or client wants you to do extra work around the house, tell them you can only do assigned tasks. Your supervisor can work with the family if they do not accept that answer. Do let your supervisor know if you feel the client requires more care than is written in the care plan.
- Do not accept gifts. The giver may assume you will do extra work. Or if Client B hears that you do favors for Client A, he may wonder why he is not getting the same special treatment. Or a client may give you a prized possession that was really meant for one of his children. Any of these situations could get very difficult.
- Do not use the client's telephone to make personal phone calls. You may use the client's phone to call your agency or your supervisor.
- Never forget that you are a guest in the client's home. Be careful with the client's personal items.

4. Know your limits.
- Laws vary among states regarding what tasks a HM/HHA is permitted to do. You will not overstep your legal bounds if you do only the assigned tasks on the care plan written by your supervisor.
- If a client asks you to do something you are not qualified to do, simply tell the client you are not qualified. Then call the home care agency so the problem can be solved.
- Your supervisor is the best person to help you understand what you are and are not allowed to do. For example, the HM/HHA is not permitted to provide "skilled nursing care," because she is not trained or licensed as a nurse. Here are some examples of nursing services that HM/HHAs are not permitted to perform in any state. The HM/HHA may *not*

change the written care plan for a client;

administer or give the client medications of any kind;

insert, remove, or irrigate a catheter;

refer a client to another health care service; or

discuss information about a client's medical condition or family situation with anyone who is not working with that client on the home care team.

Review Questions

1. The written record of services and treatments that will be provided for the client is called a
_____ _____.

2. If you ever have questions about the care of a client you should ask _____.

3. Name six professional members of the home health team and explain what they do.

4. Briefly explain the job of the HM/HHA.

5. If you needed to be cared for at home, what qualities would you want your HM/HHA to have?

6. Explain the following terms in your own words:
- Confidentiality
- Care plan
- Ethics

Part Two
The Helping Relationship

Chapter 2
Communication Skills

Objectives

At the conclusion of this chapter, the homemaker/ home health aide will:

1. Understand how communication takes place and the need for good communication skills.

2. Be able to give examples of verbal and nonverbal communication and explain the importance of nonverbal communication.

3. Describe ways to encourage communication and ways to block communication.

4. Explain how to communicate with a client who speaks a foreign language.

5. Understand when it is appropriate for the HM/HHA to teach clients and discuss how to teach.

Introduction to Communication

Communication is the exchange of information between two people. This may seem to be a simple idea, but communication can be complicated. The game where a simple message is whispered from one person to the next is a good example of how difficult communication can be. When the last person gets the message, it is often not even close to the original message. People are communicating all the time, even when they do not realize it. When working with clients, your communication skills need to be sharp so you can understand your clients and so they can understand you.

How Communication Takes Place

Communication begins when one person (the sender) has a message to send to another person (the receiver). The sender chooses his idea, puts it into words, and then makes a statement. The receiver hears the statement, and if communication has been good, understands the sender's idea. The receiver should respond to the message to let the sender know that he has been understood (Figure 2-1).

Verbal and Nonverbal Communication

When we talk, we use words to express our ideas. This is *verbal* communication. Communication can also be *nonverbal*. These are the messages you get from someone by observing him. You can learn many things about a person from his smiles, frowns, and gestures. A person's body posture, hairstyle, and clothes also reveal something about that person even before he has said a word.

Sometimes verbal and nonverbal messages conflict. For example, the HM/HHA tells a client who had just spilled food all over the bed, "Let me change your sheets so you'll be more comfortable," but then shakes her head and sighs as she changes the linens. She is sending two messages. The first message is, "I understand that food sometimes gets spilled; let me help." The second message is, "What a clumsy oaf you are." Which message will the client believe? Or, how would you

THE GREAT COMMUNICATORS

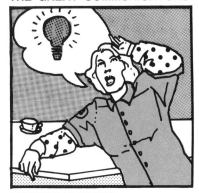
SENDER HAS AN IDEA.

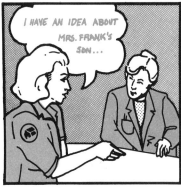
SENDER SENDS MESSAGE.

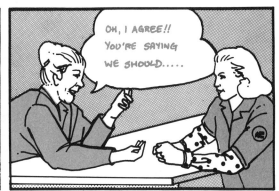
RECEIVER RESPONDS.

Figure 2-1
How verbal communication takes place.

respond to a client who says "I feel great today" and smiles, compared to one who says the same thing but growls and frowns as he says it. The HM/HHA must be sensitive to both the verbal and nonverbal ways of communicating. A perceptive HM/HHA might say to the growler, "I know you said you feel great, but you don't sound as though you do. Is there something I can do to help?"

Techniques for Better Communication

Communication is a skill that can be learned and will improve with practice. The techniques covered are not meant to make you feel that you are qualified to counsel a client. Your agency either has professional counselors on staff or can refer the client if it is necessary. If your client discusses matters that you do not feel you can handle, discuss the situation with your supervisor. The cornerstones of effective communication are listening and responding.

Listening

Listening is hard work and it takes concentration. How many times have you been introduced to someone and within five minutes realize you don't know the person's name? Actually, you heard the words, but you weren't listening to what was being said. Instead you were probably concentrating on how you looked or what you would talk about.

Listening may be one of the most useful and most difficult skills you will learn as a HM/HHA. Good listening helps you gather useful information. When you listen carefully, you are letting the speaker know that you care about his ideas and feelings. Good listening will help you communicate better with your supervisor, your clients, and your own family and friends.

Guidelines for Good Listening

1. *Concentrate on what the speaker is saying, instead of letting your mind wander.* Look at the speaker and maintain eye contact while he is talking. Think about questions that might clarify what the person is saying. Pay attention to nonverbal cues such as his facial expression and tone of voice.

2. *Do not interrupt the speaker.* You cannot talk and listen to someone else at the same time!
3. *Keep an open mind.* We often stop listening to someone when we think we don't agree with them. A good listener does not make judgments about the speaker before he has completed his thought.
4. *How do you know if you have listened well?* If you can restate the client's message and describe what you think the person was feeling when he was talking, you probably were listening effectively.

Responding

Your response to a person's message can be verbal or nonverbal.

Nonverbal Responses

1. *Body language.* The nonverbal message you send in response to what you hear includes the way you sit or stand. In most situations, the best way to listen to someone is by looking directly at them and leaning towards them a bit.
2. *Touch.* Touch is another nonverbal response. It is one of the best ways to communicate caring or tenderness. A touch on the arm or hand can often be more effective than words when you are trying to reassure or show that you care (Figure 2-2).

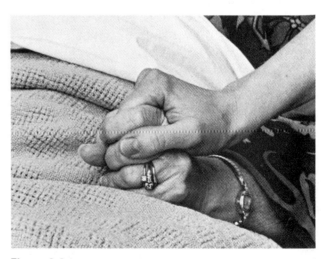

Figure 2-2
Touch may be one of the best ways of letting a client know you care. (Wolff L, Weitzel MH, Zornow RA et al: Fundamentals of Nursing, 7th ed, p 231. Philadelphia, JB Lippincott, 1983)

How to Encourage Communication With Your Client

1. Ask open-ended questions.
   - *How are you feeling today?*
   - *What are you thinking about?*
   - *Tell me how your leg feels.*
2. Use silence. After you have asked a broad opening question, count to 10 slowly in your head. This will give the client time to respond to your question.
3. Restate what the client has just told you to make sure you understand exactly what he means. This encourages the client to add more to make his message clear.

Mr. S:	I feel horrible. My leg has been bothering me since Friday.
HM/HHA:	Your leg has been hurting you since Friday.
Mr. S:	Well, no. I bumped it Friday, but it didn't start hurting until Saturday morning.

4. Ask for more information.

Mrs. T:	I don't feel well.
HM/HHA:	Tell me what is wrong. Can you describe how you feel?
Mrs. T:	Well, yes . . .

Barriers to Good Communication

1. Do not reassure client with pat answers.
   - *You will be fine.*
   - *There is nothing to worry about.*
2. Do not ask for explanations. This may make the client defensive if he thinks you're probing or frustrated if he cannot answer the question.
   - *Why don't you feel well?*
   - *What makes you say that?*
   - *Why do you think that?*
3. Do not give advice when you haven't been asked. Giving advice can also be dangerous if that advice conflicts with either the home health agency's or doctor's policies.
   - *In my house, we do it this way . . .*
   - *If I were you . . .*
   - *Why don't you . . .*
4. Use your own words instead of medical terms or terms the client does not understand. People in the medical profession often forget that medical jargon is almost like another language. Do not get into that bad habit.

Compare:
- Mrs. Smith, we need to monitor your vital signs today.
- Mrs. Smith, I'm going to take your temperature, pulse, and blood pressure.

Special Areas of Communication

Communicating With Clients Who Are Hard of Hearing

Being hard of hearing can be extremely frustrating, especially since most people assume that everyone can hear. Here are some suggestions for communicating with people who are hard of hearing.

1. *Sit down and let the client know you have time to listen and talk with him,* even if it is just for a few minutes.
2. *Make sure the client can see your face clearly as you talk.* This allows the client to read your facial expressions, your gestures, and your lips.
3. *Use simple words and short sentences.* Check to see if your message has been understood. If your client is lipreading, he will probably not be able to read half of the words you use. Rephrasing the statement using other words may make the message more clear.
4. *Speak clearly, use a normal volume, or talk slightly louder.* Shouting is not necessary and may make the client who is hard of hearing feel embarrassed or ashamed. For most people, a voice with a low pitch is easier to hear than one with a high pitch.
5. *Eliminate background noises such as radio or television.* Extra sounds make it difficult for your client to hear your voice.
6. *Learn how to work your client's hearing aid if your client has one.* Know how to make sure that it is clean and that the batteries are working. Always check to see that it is on and that the volume is adjusted properly. If the volume is on too high, the sound might become distorted, just as it does when you turn on a radio too loudly.
7. See Guidelines for Working With Clients Who Have a Sensory Loss in Chapter 5 for more suggestions.

Communicating With Clients Who Speak a Foreign Language

You may work for clients who do not speak English or who do not speak English very well. This can be a challenge, but it can also be a rewarding experience when you do communicate. You can use pictures, gestures, facial expressions, and all the other nonverbal types of communication that have been discussed. A family member or friend may serve as an interpreter. Even with a translator, use short simple phrases. Avoid using slang because it may be hard for the translator to understand. Your agency or your local library may also provide you with a phrase book in the client's language to help communication.

How the Homemaker/Home Health Aide Communicates as a Teacher

Every doctor has particular ideas about the information taught to his clients. The doctor and nurse will always do the initial teaching for clients who have medical problems or health concerns. Clients and family members are usually under so much stress when the doctor or nurse first teaches them about the health problem that they often need to have the information repeated. This is normal and understandable. The HM/HHA may be asked to reinforce some of the teaching that has already been done. Before you do any client teaching,

- Make sure your supervisor knows what you are about to teach. This will ensure that you are not going against the doctor's orders.
- Find out how much the client knows about what you are going to review with him.

Guidelines for Teaching

1. *Break the information you will be teaching into steps.* Your supervisor will help with this.
2. *Limit the amount of material you cover in one session.* Most people find it easier to learn one or two things at a time, instead of a long list of ideas.
3. *Give encouragement.* Praise the positive effort a client makes, even if the result is not perfect.
4. *Don't be afraid to say "I don't know."* When a client asks you a question that you can't answer, simply say "I don't know, but I'll try to find out for you." Make a note to yourself right away so you don't forget

about it, or call your supervisor. When a client has a question for the doctor, let your supervisor phone the doctor.

5. For a variety of reasons, some clients will not follow the instructions given by the doctor, the nurse, or the HM/HHA. If you notice that a client is not following the instructions given by the doctor, let your supervisor know. Your supervisor may be better able to explain the reasons for the treatment plan. Ultimately, the client has a right to decide if he wants to follow the care plan.
6. Remember that you are a role model. Even though you may not be trying to teach anything, the family may learn how to do many things just by watching you. For example, a person may learn how to handle an unexpected situation calmly after seeing you smile and cheerfully clean up a spilled glass of juice without blaming the client.
7. For more information on teaching, see Chapter 5.

Homemade Communication Tools

The Homemade Call Bell

1. Put pennies in an empty margarine or sour cream tub.
2. String small jingle bells on a ribbon and tie it within reach of the client. This call bell may be easier for the client who has a paralyzed or weak arm.

The Message Ring

For the client who cannot talk, write often-used phrases on small index cards. Punch a hole in the cards and put the messages on a key ring (Figure 2-3). You could make two message rings, one for general use and one for meals. If the client cannot read, or if he speaks a foreign language, use pictures on the cards.

The Communication Board

The communication board has letters, pictures, and phrases the client may want to use. The client who has had a stroke and is not able to write or

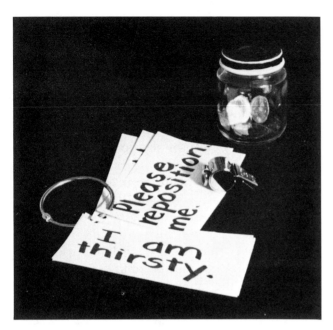

Figure 2-3
A whistle, a call bell made from coins in a jar, and a message ring are ways that help your client communicate his needs.

talk may be able to point to letters and pictures to let you know his needs. Keep a pencil and notepad handy so you can write the letters down as he points them out.

Review Questions

True or False

1. ___ You are not doing your job if you sit down for a few minutes and listen to a client.

2. ___ Nonverbal communication can be as important as verbal communication.

3. ___ If you ever work with a client who speaks another language, it will be impossible to communicate.

Multiple Choice

4. Your client wears a hearing aid, but is still having trouble hearing. What would you do to make it easier for him to hear you?
   a. Speak very loudly in a high-pitched voice.
   b. Turn the radio off, look directly at him while speaking, and speak up a little.
   c. Leave the radio on and talk louder.
   d. Ask the client if his hearing aid is working, and offer to adjust it if it is not (if you know how the hearing aid works).
   e. *b* and *d*

5. Your client asks you a question about his illness and you do not know the answer. What would you do?
   a. Give him an answer that you think is right.
   b. Tell him that you do not know the answer, but you will find out by calling your supervisor.
   c. Pretend you didn't hear the question.
   d. Call the doctor to find out the answer.

6. Your client says he doesn't feel well. Which response will encourage the client to tell the HM/HHA more about how he feels?
   a. "Well, no wonder—you had that window open all night last night. I'll bet you'll get a cold now."
   b. "If I were you, I'd call the doctor right away."
   c. "Tell me about it. Are you in pain?"
   d. "You're not feeling well today."
   e. *c* and *d*

Questions for Discussion

7. Why are listening skills so important? List three things that you can do to improve your listening skills.

8. Sometimes clients need to be retaught information that the doctor, nurse, or therapist has already given them. Why does this happen? Have you ever seen this happen?

9. Briefly explain how the HM/HHA uses verbal and nonverbal communication when working in a client's home.

Chapter 3

Basic Human Needs, the Family, and Cultural Practices

Objectives

At the conclusion of this chapter, the homemaker/home health aide will:

1. Be able to explain what a basic human need is and list three physical needs and three psychological needs.

2. Understand how basic human needs are met and what happens if they are not met.

3. Be able to describe several different kinds of families and what purpose the family serves.

4. Understand and explain the role of the HM/HHA in relation to a client's family.

5. Explain the kinds of differences you might see when working for a client from another culture.

6. Understand how to work for people who come from a different background.

Basic Human Needs

Understanding What Every Human Being Needs

All people, regardless of age, race, sex, religion, skin color, education, or economic situation, share *basic human needs*. These are needs that all humans must have fulfilled in order to survive and maintain a sense of well-being. Needs can be divided into physical needs and psychological (social and emotional) needs.

Physical Needs

air

water/food

shelter/warmth

exercise/activity

rest/sleep

safety

cleanliness

removal of body wastes

avoidance of pain

Psychological Needs

to give and accept affection and love

to trust and be trusted

to accept strengths and weaknesses in self and others

independence and self-confidence

spiritual needs

to be creative

to be useful

socialization

What Happens When Basic Human Needs Are Not Met?

Everyone reacts in different ways when basic human needs are not met. Here are some common reactions.

- Anger
- Depression
- Irritability
- Inability to think about the feelings of others or about things that need to be done

Think about how *you* react when your needs are not met. Have you ever skipped lunch when you were busy and then found you were not able to eat dinner until late at night? Or have you ever had a restless night and had to go to work the next day knowing that you had not slept more than 3 or 4 hours? How did you feel? You were feeling what people feel when their basic human needs are not met.

If one of your clients is irritable or depressed, try to think about whether he might have an unmet need. Instead of taking a grouchy remark personally, try to understand the client's position in terms of unmet needs.

How Are Basic Human Needs Met?

Basic human needs are met in many ways. Children depend on adults and family members to help them meet their survival needs. In our society, adults are expected to meet their own needs through family and community activities, and work. Work allows people to earn money for physical needs such as food, shelter, and clothing. It also meets some of the social needs such as building self-confidence, affording pride in a job well done, and providing a place to meet people with similar interests. A client who can no longer work may feel frustrated because many of these needs are not being met. It is normal for adults who have led independent lives to find it hard to accept care from others.

You will help clients meet some of their physical needs when you assist with personal care and home management. But also be aware of the psychological needs of the client. Imagine yourself in Mr. Miller's place:

> Mr. Miller is a 56-year-old high school teacher. He is not married, and his family lives out of state. He must stay home for 6 weeks to recover from a car accident. After the accident, several friends visited the hospital, but no one visited him after he got home. Jeff, the HM/ HHA, comes in once a day to assist with Mr. Miller's bath and meals. Mr. Miller welcomes Jeff's visits for the company as well as the care. The supervisor and Jeff recognized Mr. Miller's need for contact with other people early. They discussed the importance of talking and being a companion in addition to doing the assigned physical care and home management tasks.

Working With the Family

What Is a Family?

The *nuclear family* consists of a married couple with children living in one household (Figure 3-1). It may surprise you to know that most Americans do not live in such a family situation. In our society, any of the following groups can be considered a family.

- A nuclear family (mother, father, and children)
- An extended family (may include relatives and friends)
- An unmarried couple (with or without children)
- Two roommates or a couple of the same sex
- A single-parent family (mother or father and children)
- A blended family (both partners have children from former marriages)

It helps to know who the client considers family, because in most cases, the family helps the client make decisions about his health care. For example, if a neighbor has more influence with the client than anyone in the immediate family

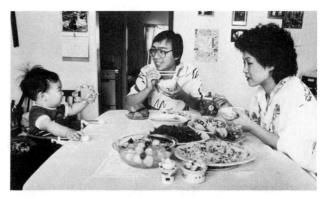

Figure 3-1
This family is enjoying a traditional Chinese meal.

does, it might be important for the nurse or doctor to include the neighbor in the client/family conferences. The neighbor could then learn about the goals of the treatment and how he could help support the client.

What Are the Jobs of the Family?

1. To provide a home where physical needs are met (food, warmth, shelter, safety, and health care)
2. To meet emotional needs (love, encouragement, self-esteem)
3. To raise children and teach cultural practices

Guidelines for Working With the Family

Nearly every time you care for a client in his home, you will also have the chance to meet and work with the family. The following are some suggestions for working with families.

1. Every family is unique. Each family will have its own ideas about religion, how to spend money, what foods to eat, and even health care. You must be sensitive to the family, and not make judgments about those whose lifestyle differs from your own.
2. People in the family often want to help, but may not know what they can or should do. Talk to your supervisor for ideas on how they can assist. For example, you might teach a man good body mechanics so he can help his wife out of a chair without straining his back. The family will appreciate having you teach them how to care for the client

when the HM/HHA service is no longer available.

3. The family is often under tremendous stress. It pays to spend a few minutes listening to their suggestions, questions, and complaints. The family will probably have some valuable suggestions that can help you and the home care team. If someone asks a question you cannot answer, tell him you do not know the answer, but will try to find out soon. If there is a complaint, ask questions to find out as much as you can about the problem. Let the family know you will work with your supervisor to find out the answers to their questions, complaints, and suggestions.

4. Families do have disagreements, and they could happen when you are in the house. Do not interfere or take sides in an argument. Your only interest should be the safety and well-being of your client. If a family discussion starts to get heated and you are uncomfortable, leave the house and phone your agency right away to let them know why you left.

5. Let the family know what your responsibilities are. Occasionally, someone in the family feels the HM/HHA is there to clean the house from last night's party or to walk the dog. Tell the family you can only do the assigned tasks on the written assignment sheet or care plan. If that doesn't work, discuss the matter with your supervisor. Do not argue with the family. This is a good reason why a written care plan and assignment sheet should always be kept in the client's house.

6. During a crisis such as illness or problems with finances, the stability of the family may be threatened. In some cases, people may not be able to cope. Promptly report situations that seem unusual to your supervisor, such as any of the following.
   • There is not enough food, clothing, or medical supplies.
   • Someone in the family goes into the hospital.
   • The children are not attending school.
   • Any signs of neglect or abuse to any member of the household.

7. Remember, anything that happens within a client's home is confidential and should never be discussed with anyone other than your supervisor.

Understanding People From Other Cultures

Understanding Differences Between People

In your job as a HM/HHA you will have the opportunity to work with people from different backgrounds. Some of your clients may come from another country. Some may eat foods you've never tried or prepare foods in a way you've never seen before. Even the way some clients spend their money may puzzle you. You may have clients who live in large, fine homes and others who have very little money and live in small trailers. In any case, home is a special place. Never forget that when you work in a client's home you are a guest.

Cultural Practices

Culture is the set of values, beliefs, and way of life held by a particular group of people. Cultural practices are passed from generation to generation. We learn our own culture from our family when they teach religious beliefs, how to spend money, how to raise children, how to express our feelings, how to spend free time, what foods to eat, and how to care for our health (Figure 3-2).

Part of your success in working with clients from other cultures depends upon your willingness to understand and accept cultural differences. One culture is not better than others. Each one is different and each has its strengths and weaknesses.

When you *stereotype*, you are assuming all people who come from a particular background will behave in a particular way. This is also called *prejudice* because you are prejudging a person. While stereotyping is unfair, learning about cultural practices may help you communicate with your client and understand some of your client's responses. For instance, people from some cultures, like the Italians, express themselves verbally when they are in pain. But a client who has an Irish or German background may find it difficult to tell you when he is in pain. Some clients may be very open and willing to tell you everything about themselves, but others, like some American Indians, will think you are asking very personal questions when you ask about their diet or minor health problems, even though you are a health care provider.

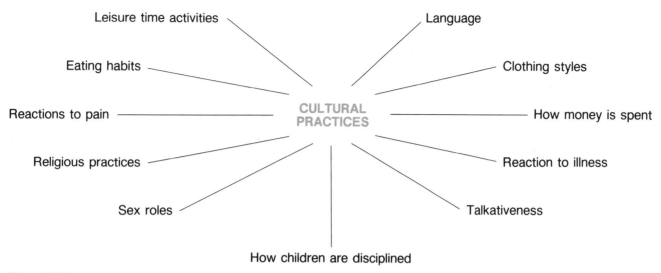

Figure 3-2
Cultural practices include beliefs about health and illness.

You will be a more effective HM/HHA if you try to understand the client's culture and method of doing things. At times, actions by clients may be misinterpreted because of cultural misunderstanding. Cultural beliefs are so much a part of our lives that many people cannot describe their own cultural practices. Sometimes it is hard to remember that everyone does not live the way you do. Answer the questions about health practices in the Cultural Health Quiz. Think about how your answers might differ from those of a person with a different cultural background.

Spiritual Needs

A minister, rabbi, or other religious leader may be able to offer a client emotional and spiritual support that no one else can provide (Figure 3-3). Spiritual and religious support can help the client and family deal with major life events such as birth, death, illness, and disability. Religion often plays an important part in a client's recovery. Even if your religious views differ from your client's, respect the client's choice and help him meet his spiritual needs.

If you are not familiar with your client's religion, find out if the client's religion has any practices that you need to know about, such as diet restrictions or days of fasting. For example, during the month-long celebration of Ramadan, many Moslems will not eat, drink, or smoke during daylight hours and will only eat and drink moderately after dark. This kind of information

---

Cultural Health Quiz

Circle all the answers that apply to you and fill in any answers that are not included in the choices. There is no correct answer.
1. I keep my good health:
   a. by eating well, exercising, and by getting enough rest and sleep.
   b. by getting health checkups regularly.
   c. by praying and attending church regularly.
   d. by being good and working hard.
   e. _____
2. I consider myself ill when:
   a. I have a headache.
   b. I have a headache, a runny nose, and no fever.
   c. I have a high fever and am too weak to get out of bed.
   d. _____
3. The reason I become ill is because:
   a. I have not worked hard or I have not been good.
   b. I have not taken care of myself.
   c. I picked up a germ from someone.
   d. _____
4. When I am ill and want treatment, I:
   a. call or visit a medical doctor, nurse practitioner, or health clinic.
   b. visit a healer.
   c. go to church and pray.
   d. perform ceremonies or rituals.
   e. use folk medicine.
   f. go for a massage or acupuncture treatment.
   g. _____

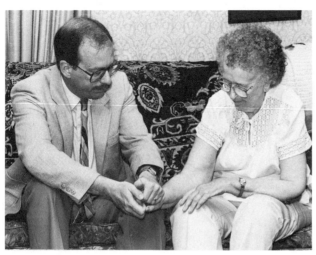

Figure 3-3
A pastoral call can be an important part of a client's recovery. Allow the client privacy at such times.

can be important when planning health care. Major Western religions are summarized here.

Guidelines for Working With People From Other Cultures

1. Recognize your own prejudices. No doubt, you have some ideas about how certain cultural groups behave. If you begin working for a client whom you think will be lazy or excitable because of his culture, you are being unfair to the client. Everyone has prejudices. When you are aware of yours, you can alert yourself to give the other person a fair chance.
2. Learn about and take an interest in the culture of your client. Accept the family's practices and customs without making judgments. Minorities have often been ridiculed for their beliefs, so they may not want to discuss their customs with you until you have gained their trust.
3. Clients may speak another language and sometimes a family member or friend may translate. If so, speak more slowly. Use short sentences and phrases. Do not use slang or medical terms because they may be harder to understand and translate.
4. Share what you learn about your client's customs with the home care team. You may know more about a client's customs because you spend more time in the client's home than other members of the home health care

Major Western Religions

Jewish Religion

A Jewish religious leader is called a rabbi and the place of worship is known as a synagogue or temple. Some clients may eat kosher foods. Kosher foods are those that are considered clean by Jewish law. Some foods, such as pork and shellfish, are not eaten. Other foods may be eaten if they are cleaned and prepared according to Jewish law. The day of worship is called the Sabbath. It begins at sunset on Friday and ends at sunset on Saturday. Before supper on Friday evening, the woman of the household will light candles in a ceremony to recognize the beginning of the Sabbath. The men may cover their heads with a small round cap called a yarmulke. During Yom Kippur, the day of atonement, no food is eaten for a full day from sunset to sunset.

Catholic Religion

The head of the Catholic church is the pope. Cardinals, bishops, priests, and nuns follow in religious authority. A local priest is often called "Father." Sins are confessed to a priest at least once a year and followers go to Mass, the worship service, on Sundays and holy days. Religious objects such as crosses, medallions, statues, and rosaries should be handled with respect. During the Easter season, a priest may visit so the client can receive the Holy Eucharist. It is customary for the client not to eat any food or fluids for an hour before receiving the sacrament.

Protestant Religions

The protestant faith includes many denominations. The minister, pastor, or clergyman is the head of the local church. Most have the sacraments of Baptism and Communion, and worship on Sunday. Seventh-Day-Adventists have their day of worship on Saturday.

team. This information can help the team provide better care.

Review Questions

True or False

1. ____ You may not always feel comfortable about the way your client lives his life.
2. ____ The nuclear family is the only real family.
3. ____ All people have the same basic human needs.

4. ____ Adults can always meet all their own needs.

5. ____ When a client's daughter talks with you, you do not need to listen because she is not the client.

6. ____ Do not take sides or interfere in a family disagreement.

7. ____ When you work for a family you will learn things about the family that you cannot share with your family and friends.

8. ____ Some cultures are better than others.

Fill in the Blanks

9. When you have formed certain expectations about how you think a person will behave before you have met him, this is known as _____ or _____.

10. The religious practices, the accepted reactions to pain or illness, food preferences, language, and the way a family lives are called _____.

Matching

Match the basic human need on the right with the activity you may do to help the client meet his basic human needs.

11. ____ preparing a nutritious meal

12. ____ changing a lightbulb or wiping up spilled water

13. ____ helping the client with a bath

14. ____ playing cards with a client

15. ____ spending some time listening to the client's stories about his life

16. ____ washing dishes after a meal

A. provide socialization

B. provide cleanliness

C. provide good nutrition

D. provide safety

Questions for Discussion

17. Think about the religious or cultural practices that your family follows. Can you describe them?

18. List five basic physical and emotional human needs. How would you react if you could not meet those needs?

19. What kind of adjustment will you have to make when caring for a client who has family values or religious practices different from your own?

Chapter 4
Caring for Children

Objectives

At the conclusion of this chapter, the homemaker/home health aide will:

1. Understand the basic characteristics of babies, toddlers, preschoolers, school-age children, and adolescents.

2. Explain major safety precautions for children at different ages.

3. Understand how the stress of illness in the family affects children and their parents.

4. Know the kinds of concerns or observations about children that should be reported to your supervisor right away.

5. Be able to describe appropriate play activities for children of all different ages.

Introduction to Caring for Children

The HM/HHA may care for children when the children are ill or disabled, or when a parent is ill, disabled, or not able to care for the children (Figure 4-1). You will also spend time with children who are visiting the client while you are working. This chapter will provide you with guidelines to use when working with children. Every child is an individual, so you will need the advice of your supervisor and home care team for details about particular situations.

Normal Growth and Development of Children

The Infant (Birth to 12 Months)

Infancy is a time of rapid growth and change. The baby depends on adults to meet all of his basic human needs. Although the baby may spend most of his day sleeping, one of the most important things he learns is trust. He learns trust when his needs for food, warmth, and love are met consistently by a caring person.

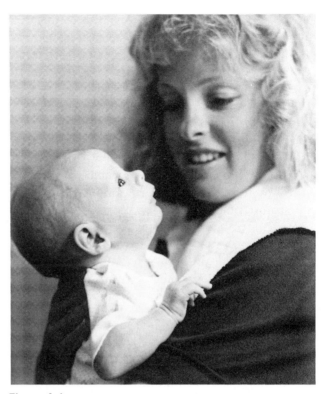

Figure 4-1
As a homemaker/home health aide, you may be assigned to care for a young baby if a parent is ill or unable to care for the child.

Characteristics of Infants

Sight and Reflexes
The newborn can see, but can only focus on objects 6 to 10 inches away from him for the first month. As he gets older, his eyes will focus better. When a young baby is frightened by a loud noise or feels he is not being held securely, he will tense his body and stretch out his arms. This position is called the *startle reflex*.

Food and Nutrition
Generally breast milk or infant formula provides all the nutrients needed during the first few months. Later the baby will start on cereals and solid foods. The feeding schedule should be followed according to the physician's directions. The first tooth usually appears between 4 to 7 months, and the baby will have about six teeth by the end of the first year.

Elimination
Babies urinate frequently each day. They should be washed and changed as soon as they are wet to prevent skin rashes. The baby may have several

bowel movements per day. Any sign of diarrhea should be reported right away because babies can become dehydrated very quickly. If a baby has had a dry diaper for more than 6 hours, this should also be reported to your supervisor.

Physical Milestones

During the first year the baby grows and changes rapidly. When first born, the baby is very limp, because he has very little physical control over his body. By the end of the first month, he may be able to hold his head up for short periods. While holding the baby, you must support his head. After 3 or 4 months, many babies are strong enough to hold up their own heads, but they still may need occasional head support. At about 6 months, the baby can sit without support for short periods of time. By 12 months, the baby can sit, crawl, climb stairs, and stand. Walking soon follows.

Social and Emotional Tasks

The baby gains a sense of trust when his cries are met consistently and when his physical needs and his need for love and affection are satisfied. The baby may smile at his parents at two or three months, and from then on continues to show a great interest in being with people. Young babies need to be held and cuddled so they can develop a sense of security. Between 8 and 18 months, many babies cry when their mothers leave the room or when the mother lets another person hold the child, even for a moment. This is a normal part of the baby's development.

Play

A baby learns about the world through his senses. Expose him to different sounds, textures, colors, and shapes. Introduce one object at a time instead of providing an overwhelming number of choices. Let the baby see what it feels like to gently roll from his side, to his back, and then to his tummy. Feeling a cool breeze or a light splash of water at bath time are new experiences for the baby. Talking and reading to the baby help him learn about language. Babies love games like "peek-a-boo," "pat-a-cake," and "so big," especially after they are about 6 months old.

Discipline

In only a few months, babies are able to get around fairly easily. Limits must be set for the child's protection. Because babies and young children are easily distracted, redirecting the baby's interest is one of the easiest forms of discipline. When the baby is going after a dangerous object, distract him with a safe toy and then move him away from the dangerous object. Most infants begin to understand the word "no" near the end of their first year.

The Toddler (1 to 3 Years)

The toddler wavers between wanting the comfort and security of adults and wanting to be independent. He can now get around by himself to explore his environment, but because he cannot think ahead of possible dangers he needs close supervision. He may be delighted to climb up a tall ladder, but scream with fright when he cannot get down. Toddlers are easiest to manage when a set routine for meals, naps, and playtime is maintained. They have little patience and want things done "now."

Characteristics of Toddlers

Toilet Training

Toddlers learn toilet training at different times depending on when they are physically and emotionally ready. Most are not completely reliable until after the age of 3 years. Bowel training is learned more quickly if started after 18 to 24 months. Learning to stay dry takes longer. Follow the toilet training plan that the doctor has recommended to the parents. During illness or times of stress or changes, it is normal for the child to temporarily lose some of his toilet training skills.

Everyday Care

The toddler can help with more of his everyday care. He can help with washing, brushing his teeth, dressing, and eating, and wants to do as much as he can by himself. The toddler likes to make a game out of everything he does, and is easier to handle if you play along while still getting the job done.

Playing and Learning

Play allows the toddler to learn about his world. He learns to imitate others, to practice new skills, and to vent his feelings. It is natural for a toddler to become attached to a favorite toy or object. The toddler learns about language when he is read to and talked to. Toddlers need to be shown how to do things, because they are just beginning to understand what words mean. They will use actions more than words to express themselves.

Discipline

Toddlers need rules, but too many rules will confuse them. Give choices between two things to encourage independence and decision making skills. Be sure that both choices are agreeable to you. For example, ask "Would you like green beans or peas as a vegetable tonight?" rather than "What vegetable would you like for dinner tonight?"

Reward the toddler's good behavior. Toddlers like to please adults and want attention. If they cannot get attention through good behavior, they may do something negative to get attention. Infants, toddlers, and preschoolers have very short memories and may not remember they have been told not to do something. The toddler has learned the word "no" and uses it frequently to assert his independence. Try redirecting the toddler's interest when he is doing something he should not do.

Safety Needs of Toddlers

Toddlers need close supervision, especially if visiting a house that is not childproof. See the Accident Prevention Checklist for details.

The Preschooler (4 to 5 Years)

The preschool period is characterized by the child's new ability and willingness to cooperate. Preschoolers use more words and fewer actions than toddlers to express themselves.

Characteristics of Preschoolers

Family Relationships

While infants and toddlers can focus only on their own needs, the preschooler is beginning to discover that other people have needs too. The preschooler likes to do simple jobs that make him feel he is helping people in the family. He also becomes aware of others outside the family and can be taught to speak to a police officer, mail carrier, or sales clerk if lost.

Playing and Learning

The preschooler can entertain himself for long periods of time alone. It is not unusual to invent a "pretend" friend because his imagination is very active at this age. The preschooler also loves to make up stories and have books read to him. Another common game is to imitate others and practice playing "mommy" and "daddy."

The child needs time to play alone without competition or criticism for mistakes. He also needs time to play with friends. He enjoys using physical skills when he plays in the water or with tricycles, scooters, teeter-totters, swings, skates, and balls.

Safety Needs of Preschoolers

The preschooler still needs fairly close supervision. For example, a child this age is not able to figure out how fast a car is coming down the street and he may not remember to stay on the sidewalk. Generally, the preschooler can be trusted to follow the safety habits that he knows when he plays alone. When playing with older children, he may take dangerous dares to prove himself. See the Accident Prevention Checklist for further details.

The School-Age Child (6 to 12 Years)

The school-age child has a desire to work, compete, cooperate, and achieve. As the school-age child begins to explore the world outside of his family, he learns how he fits in with other people.

Characteristics of School-Age Children

Gaining Independence

Many school-age children see themselves as independent, and do not realize that they depend on others to provide food, shelter, and other basic human needs. Assigning simple jobs that the child can easily do helps build a sense of accomplishment and a good self-image. Responsibilities can increase as the child grows.

The school-age child is greatly influenced by friends, although adults and family members are still an important part of his world. The child still looks to parents and other adults for direction and guidance.

Learning

The child at this age will learn things quickly if given the proper instruction and opportunity. Language continues to develop. The child will also use the slang, secret codes, and possibly swear words that are accepted by his friends, but often

Accident Prevention Checklist for Children

Car Accidents

Car accidents are the leading cause of accidental death for children over 1 year.

Children should always be secured in a properly fitting infant seat, child seat, or safety belt and placed in the back seat of the car. Children can wear adult seat belts with shoulder straps after they weigh 50 pounds.

Young children should be taught to look for cars before they cross the street. Older children should continue to watch for cars and learn to use hand signals when riding a bicycle.

Burns and Fire

Do not leave young children alone in a house for even 5 minutes.

Always check the temperature of the bath water for babies and young children with sensitive skin.

Matches should be kept well out of reach of young hands.

Hot coffee cups, burning cigarettes, and hanging tablecloths should be kept out of reach of infants and toddlers.

Turn saucepan handles away from the edge of the stove.

Keep electrical cords in good repair.

Drownings

Never leave a young child alone in the bath or wading pool for a second. Even swimmers can drown.

Keep bathroom doors closed and the toilet lid down when not in use.

Young children who cannot swim should always wear a life jacket and be supervised when near a swimming pool or body of water.

Falls and Other Injuries

Cribs and playpens should be sturdy, assembled correctly, and have bars that are close so the baby's head will not get caught.

Never leave a baby alone on a bed, couch, or chair. Babies can learn to roll over quite suddenly. If you need to leave the infant for just a minute, put the baby in a crib, playpen, or on the floor.

High chairs should be sturdy and have straps to keep the baby from climbing out. Even so, he should not be left alone in the chair. A high chair should not be used until the baby can sit without slipping.

Use gates at the top and bottom of all stairways until the young child can go up and down stairs with ease and stability.

Windows within reach of the young child should be securely locked.

Cover unused wall sockets with safety plugs or adhesive tape, so the baby or toddler is not tempted to stick a pin or a sharp object in the socket.

Sharp objects such as scissors or pencils should be taken away if a child runs with them or treats them carelessly.

Anything that is hanging, such as cords and tablecloths, can be of great interest and danger to a roaming baby or toddler. Close supervision is necessary to prevent such accidents.

Choking or Suffocating

Choking is the leading cause of accidental death in children under 1 year.

Small objects such as beads, buttons, and nuts should be kept out of reach of the baby and toddler when playing. These objects can easily get caught in the windpipe and cause choking.

To avoid getting food caught in a young child's throat, small round foods (such as hotdogs and grapes) should be cut into quarters.

A baby should never lie directly on a plastic mattress cover because of the risk of suffocation. A plastic cover should have a cloth mattress cover and a sheet over the plastic. For the same reason, the baby should not use a pillow. Plastic bags are never toys.

The safest sleeping position is on the abdomen with no pillow. The baby should have his own bed with a firm mattress for proper back support.

Poisoning

Toddlers and preschoolers are the most common victims of poisoning. Usually it occurs when materials that could be poisonous are stored improperly.

Kitchen and bathroom cupboards should have safety latches and locks installed to prevent babies and young children from opening doors where dangerous objects or poisons are kept.

Closets and cupboards with cleaning products and other toxic substances must be kept locked.

Put all medicines out of reach directly after use. Extra medicine left over after an illness should be flushed down the toilet by the parents. Use child-proof lids on medicine containers.

Never put a potentially toxic product into another container. A child may try a taste of the cleaning fluid in a soda pop bottle because he associates the bottle with a treat.

Among the most common substances that have caused accidental poisonings are aspirin and other drugs, insect and rat poisons, cleaning products, lead paint, turpentine, petroleum products, furniture polish, and indoor plants. Keep all of these things well out of reach of babies and young children.

not by parents and other adults. Children need to try new things and experience failure as well as success.

Play and Activities

When the child enters school, more time is spent on school than on play. Still, play and outside activities allow the child to make friends and continue his physical and emotional growth. School-age children learn that they must follow the rules of the group to be accepted by their friends.

Safety Needs of School-Age Children

As the child feels more independent, wants to explore the community, and wants to impress his friends, the risk of accidents can be a major concern. Towards the end of this period, the child has the primary responsibility for his own safety instead of depending on parents and other adults as he did in earlier years. The child should learn to follow the rules of the community and to take responsibility for his own actions. For example, he needs to be encouraged to read the instructions before operating a new piece of equipment and to use the proper hand signals when riding a bicycle in the street. He also should be taught to respect machinery and nature when doing chores and exploring the area where he lives. Usually the child will practice the safety habits of the adults he sees daily.

The Teenager (13 to 18 Years)

The teen years are sometimes characterized by moodiness. The young adult struggles between dependence and independence, undergoes rapid physical changes, and foresees leaving home in the near future. Adults who keep communication lines open, give guidance when needed, and maintain a sense of humor are best able to support a teenager.

Characteristics of Teenagers

Gaining Independence

Teens can contribute more to family discussions on budget matters, chores, activities, and nutrition, and have more responsible jobs in the family (Figure 4-2). Some families temper privileges with responsibility. As the teenager strives to be independent, he still needs and wants the support and guidance of caring family members.

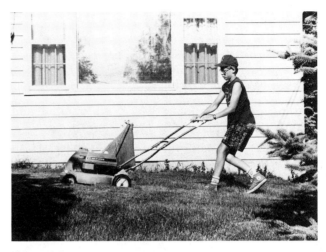

Figure 4-2
This young teenager is cutting the grass for his grandfather. Contributing to the family helps build a teenager's sense of self-esteem and responsibility.

Activities and Friends

During these years, the teenager develops an awareness of the world and some of its social problems. He may become active in causes or community programs.

Having a few close friends to confide in is very important during the teenage years. School and activities seem to consume all of the teenager's time. Adolescents are very conscious of their body image and will spend a great deal of time dressing and grooming. Dating starts as couples pair up during group activities and then separate from the group. In later adolescence, romantic relationships can become more important than other relationships.

Sex Education

Puberty usually begins between the ages of 10 and 15 years. This is when the body becomes capable of reproduction. The physical changes in the body during this period always seem to cause anxiety for the young teen. It is up to the parents, not the HM/HHA, to teach a child about sex education. If an adolescent in a home where you are working asks you questions about sex, discuss the situation with your supervisor.

Safety Needs of Teenagers

Teenagers are at an age of exploring and experimenting. An alarming number of teens use alcohol and other drugs regularly. If you suspect that a teen in a home where you are working is abusing alcohol or other drugs, discuss the situation with your supervisor.

Working With Children and Families

Working With Parents

Parents are the primary caregivers of their children. Don't be afraid to ask a parent for advice or help when caring for a child. Parents need to have a say in how their children are cared for when they cannot care for their children by themselves. Work with your supervisor on ways to keep parents who are ill or disabled involved in the care and discipline of their children.

When a child needs medical attention, his parents may feel guilty, even if they could not have prevented the illness, injury, or disability. Some parents may feel threatened that the HM/HHA is doing a better job of caring for the child than they could do. Give them support and encouragement so that they will participate in the care of the child and realize that no one can take the place of a parent (Figure 4-3). An important part of the HM/HHA's job is to help families work together.

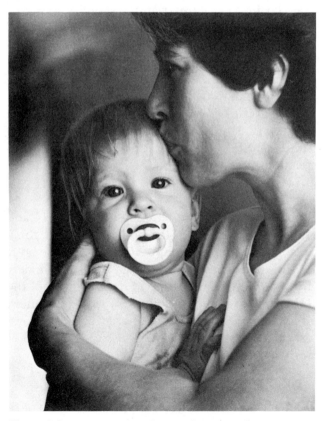

Figure 4-3
The bond between parent and child is important to both the parent and the child. Always encourage parents to take part in caring for their children.

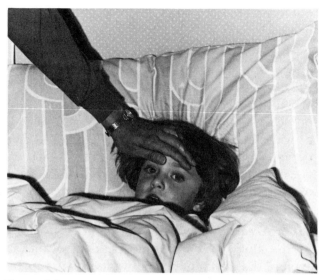

Figure 4-4
In this picture, the homemaker/home health aide is caring for a little girl who has recently had surgery.

Children and Illness

The HM/HHA is often called into a home to care for children when the family is going through a stressful period. The child who has an ill parent will experience many changes such as a new caregiver, less attention, and a change in routine. If an ill parent is home, the child may have to restrict play activities and keep quiet while in the house. The child will worry about the health of the ill parent and may be concerned about financial troubles as well.

The child who is seriously ill at home will have many strains on his life too (Figure 4-4). In addition to medical treatments that may be uncomfortable, the child must also deal with the fact that he cannot spend as much time with his friends. Because he will also be expected to keep up with his schoolwork at home, a visiting teacher may assist with lessons. A little time out for games or playtime can help take the child's mind off his worries. See Table 4-1 for activities that are appropriate for a child's age.

Understandably, many parents find it difficult to tell a child that he has a serious illness. Often children who are terminally ill know it without being told. If the child asks you questions about his illness, do not give the child any more details than his parents have already given him. Tell your supervisor about the child's concerns so the supervisor can help the parents deal with the child's

Table 4-1
Play and Activities

Birth to 1 Year	Colorful mobiles, soft cuddly toys, rattles, and stacking toys. Should be unbreakable and too large to swallow. Babies love company and even young ones like to be read to.
1 to 3 Years	Blocks, hammer sets, sandboxes, wading pools, dress-up clothes, balls, push and pull toys, and simple books
3 to 6 Years	Toy villages, farms, stores, and houses, puppets, dress-up clothes, trains, tractors, dolls, stories, simple games, crayons, and tricycles
6 to 12 Years	Board games, construction toys, puzzles, kites, sports equipment for team play, bicycles, sleds, musical instruments, and books. The younger ones still like clay, crayons, paints, and easier games, while the older ones enjoy craft kits and models.
13 to 18 Years	The teenager likes games and activities that adults enjoy. They may be interested in books, music, sports, adult card games, and school clubs.

questions. Table 4-2 lists signs of illness that you should report to your supervisor quickly.

All children who are receiving home care or whose parents or close relatives are receiving home care will feel a threat to their security. The way they react will depend on their age and stage of development. It is a good idea to let your supervisor know about any behavior changes so they can be dealt with before they become a problem. Here are some examples of behavior changes you should discuss with your supervisor:

- Children may test their normal routines and rebel against expected behaviors.
- A child who is normally cooperative may become temperamental, moody, or aggressive.
- A child who is outgoing may become unusually quiet, withdrawn, or shy.
- Others may regress and behave as a younger child would. For example, a child who has not wet the bed in years may begin wetting the bed again. Or a child may become afraid of the dark.
- A child who has confidence and is willing to try new things may become overdependent and conform to rules in ways that he never has before.

Nutrition

One of the most important factors in determining health is a well-balanced diet, especially when the child is growing and developing. Normal development of the brain and all the body system depends upon adequate nutrition. Nutritious foods should be served for all meals and snacks (Figure 4-5).

Table 4-2
Signs of Illness in Children that Need to Be Reported Immediately

Breathing Problems

Use first aid to clear the airway if you are qualified. If possible, have someone else call the rescue squad. When the immediate situation is in control, call your supervisor.

Fever

A young child's temperature can shoot up quickly and a high fever can cause convulsions. Report any fever.

Poisoning

Call the Poison Control Agency in your area if you suspect poisoning. The toll-free phone number is usually listed on the front page of the phone book. They will tell you what to do, notify an emergency service if it is needed, and stay on the phone with you until the situation is in control. When the situation is in control, call your supervisor.

Injuries or Accidents

Report any accident such as a cut that bleeds or a serious fall where a muscle might be strained or a bone broken.

Diarrhea

When a baby has loose stools, he can lose a lot of fluid quickly and become very ill. Tell your supervisor about the color, frequency, and whether there is pus or blood in the stools. Also report other signs of illness such as fever.

Vomiting

Call the supervisor if the child throws up. Babies often spit up after eating a meal so this does not need to be reported unless it is excessive. If you are unsure, report the incident.

Indications of Pain

A baby or young child may pull at a body part or cry or fuss when he feels pain or discomfort. Report these signs.

The Baby or Child Just Looks Ill

Even if the child does not have a fever, has not vomited, and does not have diarrhea, but seems listless and pale, report this to the supervisor. This is especially true if the baby is under 6 months old.

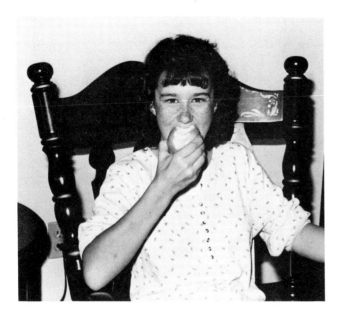

Figure 4-5
Nutritious snacks are especially important for growing children and teenagers, and for clients who are ill.

During times of stress, the child's appetite may come and go. The parents may be too busy to think about a balanced diet. If this happens, discuss the situation with your supervisor, so that the child can get the food he needs to grow. This and other concerns are listed under Situations to Report to Your Supervisor When Working With Children at the end of this chapter. For more information on nutrition, see Chapter 15.

Discipline

Discipline is not punishment, but guidance that teaches children reasonable ways of behaving. These rules for behavior also allow the child to feel secure and protected, and keep the child from having to make decisions he is not capable of making. It is *never* appropriate for the HM/HHA to punish a child using physical force such as a spanking. If you feel a child is not being disciplined properly, discuss the situation with your supervisor.

Discipline should be consistent and follow the rules of the household. If you do not agree with the rules of the household, discuss your concerns with your supervisor. Normal routines such as mealtime and bedtime should not be changed without the parent's approval.

Child Abuse

Child abuse is a serious problem in our country. Abuse can take many forms. It can be physical, such as beating a child, or verbal, such as making inappropriate threats. Or it can take the form of neglect, such as not feeding a child properly. If you suspect that there is any kind of abuse taking place within the household, promptly report your concerns to your supervisor. *Never* question the parents. The professionals at the home care agency are specially trained to deal with abuse and neglect situations. Do not discuss family situations with anyone other than your supervisor.

Situations to Report to Your Supervisor When Working With Children

Phone your supervisor if:
There is a shortage of food or clothing.
A parent becomes ill or is taken to the hospital.
A parent is not going to work or loses a job.
A parent or child is misusing medications, drugs, or alcohol.
A child is ill or not attending school.
You suspect child abuse or neglect.
There has been a serious argument in the family.
An accident occurs.

Review Questions

True or False

1. ____ Children have different human needs than older people.

2. ____ You can help the parents' relationship with their child by including the parents in the care of child whenever possible.

3. ____ It is all right to change a child's eating or sleep schedule without the parents' knowledge or consent.

4. ____ A teenager wants guidance, understanding, and support.

5. ____ The HM/HHA should always find out what an ill child knows about his illness before giving care to that child.

6. ____ Children seem to cope better when they

follow a regular schedule for meals, naps, and bedtime.

7. ____ All toddlers learn to be toilet trained at the same age.

8. ____ Discipline is guidance that teaches children reasonable ways of behaving for their protection.

9. ____ It is important to know how a young child develops so you will know what the child is capable of and whether he is developing normally.

Questions for Discussion

10. How would you discourage a toddler from playing with a piece of equipment that he should not touch, such as stereo equipment or your HM/HHA bag?

11. What would you do if the child of your client always wore dirty clothes and just never seemed clean?

12. What would you do if you think a child in the house is abusing drugs?

13. You are caring for a client who has a 3-year-old girl named Sally. Sally has been cranky for the last hour and you have a lot of cleaning to do before you leave in one hour. You know that Sally loves to play in the bathtub. Do you put her in the tub while you finish your work in the kitchen? Why or why not? What else could you do to entertain a toddler while you are finishing your work?

Chapter 5
Caring for Older Adults

Objectives

At the conclusion of this chapter, the homemaker/home health aide will:

1. Be aware of his or her own feelings about aging.

2. Understand and be able to describe the normal physical, social, emotional, and intellectual changes that take place with aging.

3. Be able to explain the role of the HM/HHA when caring for older clients.

Aging

We begin to age the moment we are born, but it may not be until we are well out of our teens that we begin to think about what growing older means. This chapter will cover some of the myths and facts about the aging process. After learning about normal changes that occur with aging, you will learn to recognize changes that are not normal and need to be reported. *Geriatrics* is the study of medical problems that are associated with aging. *Gerontology* is the study of aging. Few illnesses or diseases affect only the elderly, but many are associated with aging. Answer the Aging Quiz before you read this chapter to find out if your beliefs about aging are myths or facts.

Facts About Normal Aging

How Old Is Old?

In the health care profession, an adult is considered "young-old" when he is between 55 and 70 years old. The "old-old" are those clients over 85 years of age. After age 55, a client may face retirement and a change in social status; the death of a spouse, family members, or close friends; moving to a new home, moving in with children, or having children move away; and possibly a change in health or the health of a spouse. The chances of ill health and disability are much greater after a person is over 85 years old.

A Few Statistics on Older Adults

- In 1984, there were 28 million people over 65 living in the United States. That is nearly 12% of the entire population, or 1 in 8 people. By the year 2030, the percent of people over 65 is expected to grow to 21%.
- Men over 65 are twice as likely to be married as women over 65.
- In 1980, only 5% of those over 65 lived in institutions where they could receive care

---

The Aging Quiz

1. T or F   About 12% of the American population is over 65 years of age.
2. T or F   Older people are set in their ways and never change.
3. T or F   Most older people live with their families.
4. T or F   Over one third of all people over 65 live in nursing homes or retirement centers.
5. T or F   With advanced age, it is normal for a client to have spells of dizziness.
6. T or F   It is normal if your older client has a slight loss of memory.
7. T or F   It is normal for a client to lose some of his ability to think clearly if he is over 70 years old.
8. T or F   Generally, a 75-year-old person will have slower reactions than a 25-year-old person.
9. T or F   Older adults cannot learn new things.
10. T or F   When asked, most older people reported that they were often bored and lonely.
11. T or F   Some people do get shorter with aging.
12. T or F   Older people are just like children. They love to be babied.
13. T or F   All older people are alike.

(mostly nursing homes). Of the people who live outside nursing homes, over 80% of the men and nearly 60% of the women live with a spouse or relatives.

• In 1984, poverty level income in the United States was $6,282 per year for the household of an older couple and $4,979 for an older person living alone. In 1984, 12% of those over 65 were below poverty level compared to 15% of persons under 65.
• Most older adults have one or more chronic health problems. The four most common health problems for people over 65 in 1982 were (1) arthritis (50%), (2) high blood pressure (39%), (3) hearing loss (30%), and (4) heart condition (26%).
• Nearly 20% of those living at home needed help with personal care (bathing, dressing, using the toilet, getting in or out of bed or a chair, and walking) or home management (fixing meals, eating, shopping, daily chores, and using the telephone).

What Happens When People Age

Physical Changes

Hair and Nails

The loss of color or "graying" of the hair is one of the first signs of aging in many people. Some people begin to get gray hair when they are 16 years old, but others keep their natural color for several more decades. Hair on the head gets thinner with aging, while hair in the ears and nose and facial hair may become thicker and coarser. This maybe especially distressful for women. Fingernails and toenails become thicker, more brittle, and more difficult to cut. (This is why the HM/ HHA is not permitted to cut nails on an older client.)

Skin

The skin wrinkles with aging, especially if exposed to the sun and wind. The skin also becomes thinner and loses some of its ability to insulate and maintain the body temperature effectively (Figure 5-1). An older client may need an extra sweater or the heat turned up in the winter and a fan or air conditioning in hot weather. The thin skin of an

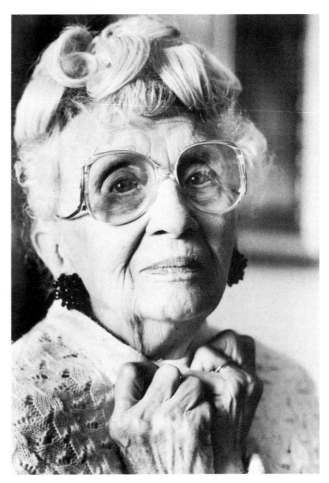

Figure 5-1
An older client may need a sweater for warmth even if the room does not seem cool to you.

older adult will burn more easily in hot bath water or with the use of a heating pad. A heating pad should never be set on a high temperature, and the bath water should be checked before allowing an older adult to get in the tub. The older client who is inactive or bedridden is more likely to get bedsores, partly because of thinner skin. Oil glands in the skin do not work as effectively so the skin may be drier and need more lotion than before. Older skin also seems to be more prone to skin problems such as rashes.

Muscles and Bones

An older client will not be as strong as when younger because the muscles lose some of their mass with aging. The older client with less muscle mass may prefer a more gentle backrub than the deep massage that a younger client enjoys. Clients who remain active will maintain more strength than those who are inactive. An older client should talk to his doctor before he starts a new exercise program.

One of the most well-documented physical changes that occurs with aging is that it takes more time for an older person to react physically than a younger person. This is known as *reaction time*. Because of the slower reaction time, many older people are discouraged from driving.

Older bones tend to be more frail and are more easily broken. Unfortunately, broken bones in an older adult also take more time to heal. Inactivity causes joints to become stiff, sore, and hard to move. A person who has been sitting in one position for 2 hours may find it difficult to get up and walk away quickly. Another common change is that the disks between the bones of the spinal column (backbone) may shrink and cause a person to become shorter.

Heart and Lungs

The circulatory and respiratory systems may not work as efficiently as they once did. This may affect the older client in several ways:

1. He may not be able to fight infection as easily and may get colds more easily.
2. He may not be able to maintain his body temperature as efficiently, so he may need a sweater or fan sooner than before.
3. He may tire more easily, so he may not be able to do as much without resting.

Digestion and Elimination

Normal aging causes few problems directly related to the digestive system. But poor eating habits may occur when the client is confronted with problems of getting older. For example, the client may find it harder or less pleasurable to eat when he has to deal with missing teeth or ill-fitting dentures, less saliva, an impaired sense of taste and smell, financial problems, loneliness, or confusion.

Constipation is another common complaint of older adults, but the bowel changes very little with aging. Constipation usually occurs because the client is not drinking enough fluids, is not eating enough fiber, or is not getting enough exercise. Figure 5-2 shows foods that contain fiber. Drinking plenty of fluids also helps keep the kidneys and urinary system working properly. Most clients should drink eight glasses of water each day.

Another common problem with older adults is

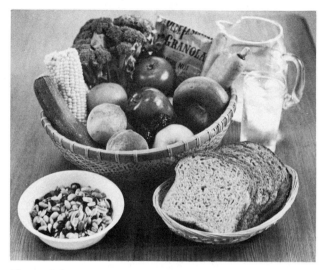

Figure 5-2
These foods all contain fiber, which aids digestion.

poor nutrition. A client who is ill may not feel well enough to prepare sound meals. A client who lives alone may not want to bother preparing meals for one person. Eating well-balanced meals is one of the best ways of preventing illness and maintaining good health. For more on nutrition see Chapter 15.

Sex and Intimacy

Growing old does not mean a client cannot be sexually active. Many couples are sexually active well into their nineties. Between the ages of 45 to 50 years, women experience menopause and stop ovulating. This means they can no longer get pregnant. Men are capable of becoming fathers throughout their lives. Both men and women have a need for intimacy and closeness even if they are not sexually active.

Sensory Losses

With aging, the senses (hearing, seeing, taste, smell, and touch) may become less efficient. This is known as *sensory loss*. Sensory losses are often so gradual they may not be noticed by the client. This can be difficult for the family and friends who may notice that the client is not hearing or seeing the way he used to. Some clients find it difficult to admit they are aging and losing their sight or hearing. A daughter may become concerned when her aging father fumbles for his glasses. Or an older parent may give up reading instead of admitting she should get new glasses and use the large-print books available in public libraries.

Guidelines for Working With Clients Who Have a Sensory Loss

	What Happens With the Sensory Loss	Suggestions for Working With Clients Who Have a Sensory Loss
Hearing	Many older people have a significant hearing loss. Not being able to hear well makes it difficult to be included in activities and conversations. Clients who are hard of hearing may feel isolated.	When talking, turn off the radio and television to eliminate background noises. If the client has a hearing aid, make sure it is clean, the batteries are working, and it is turned on. If the volume is set too high, the sound may become distorted just as it does when the volume is too loud on a radio. Speak at a normal volume and use a low tone. Shouting is unnecessary and inconsiderate. Lower-pitched sounds are easier to hear than high-pitched tones. Position yourself 3 to 6 feet from the client and face him so he can see your lips. Do not speak directly into the client's ear because he will not be able to read your facial expressions. Make sure the lighting is good and that you do not cover your mouth when talking. Avoid eating or chewing gum when speaking. Rephrase your statement if the client does not understand you. Clients who lipread cannot read every word that is said. Rephrase the message with new words. When a client has difficulty hearing, use short sentences, simple words, and gestures. Make an effort to include clients in conversations. If the client cannot hear at all, use a pen and notepad or a communication board.
Balance	Changes in the inner ear may cause problems with balance. The likelihood of serious falls increases.	If the client has a cane or walker, encourage him to use it. Rugs should be tacked down. Stairs and hallways should have plenty of light. Have your client use handrails on stairs. Encourage the client to sit on the edge of the bed for a minute before he gets up. Then he should rise slowly.
Vision	Vision dims with aging. Brighter lights are needed for reading and for simply getting around. Clients' eyes may not react to changes in light as quickly as they used to. It may take longer to adjust when going from a dark room to bright sunlight or from a light room to a dark room. Depth perception may be less accurate. A client may see a curb, but may not be able to tell how far to step down.	Report signs of impaired vision to your supervisor. Keep the client's glasses clean and within easy reach. Always return objects to the proper place after use or after cleaning. Use large letters and bright colors to label and color-code objects for easy identification. For example, label the numbers on the phone with large numbers.

(continued)

Guidelines for Working With Clients Who Have a Sensory Loss *(continued)*

	What Happens With the Sensory Loss	Suggestions for Working With Clients Who Have a Sensory Loss
Vision	Focusing may take longer. It may take longer for a client who has been reading to focus and recognize someone who has just walked in the room.	Give some warning (perhaps a cough) when you approach a client who cannot see to avoid startling him. Also, tell him when you are leaving the room.
		Replace dim lights with brighter bulbs if needed.
		Your home health agency may be able to help the client get large-print materials from the public library or a community agency.
		In a group, speak to your client by name or touch his forearm lightly so he knows that you are talking to him.
		Suggest that your client use sunglasses outdoors.
Touch	The ability to feel temperature changes may not be as great as when younger. It may take more intense hot or cold sensations before a client realizes a possible danger.	Caution clients to check the temperature of their bath, shower, or dish water. When alone, a tub thermometer can be used to see that the bath water is 90°F to 100°F.
		The water heater may need to be turned down so that water from the faucets is not too hot.
		Check foods that hold heat, such as french fries or baked potatoes, before the client eats them.
		Examine the feet daily for sores or signs of pressure.
Smell	The client may not be able to smell odors as well as when younger. He may not be able to smell his own body odor and may neglect to bathe frequently. Or he may not be able to smell food burning, a gas leak, or even a fire.	Encourage the client to wash daily, even if he does not need a full bath every day.
		Smoke detectors should be installed and checked monthly to make sure they are working properly.
Taste	The loss of taste buds on the tongue makes it harder to detect food flavors. This can make eating less pleasurable.	Encourage a balanced diet with attention to the food's appearance.
		Herbs and lemon can be used to enhance food flavor, especially for clients who cannot use salt.

Sensory losses can also be safety hazards. Consider the danger to the client who cannot detect the smell of gas or cannot tell that the bath water is too hot. These losses can also make it difficult for a client to participate in activities around him. Family members may think an older relative is confused or losing interest in things when he doesn't react the way he used to. For example, a man may not laugh at a joke that he cannot hear. Or a woman may stop commenting on news stories when she can no longer see well enough to read the newspaper. Sometimes people with a sensory loss are wrongly labeled "confused" or "senile." As a result, the client may be treated differently and left out of family activities. The more the client is isolated, the more out of touch he may become. That is why any change in behavior should be reported to your supervisor. Unless the client is examined by a doctor, he may have to continue to live with a problem that is treatable. Not all problems can be treated, but it is always worth reporting changes to your supervisor. See the Guidelines for Working With Clients Who Have a Sensory Loss.

Social, Emotional, and Intellectual Changes

Older adults experience many changes in their lives. Most older adults are able to cope with the stresses of daily life remarkably well. As a person adjusts to all the changes that go with aging, he continues to grow and develop. Old age is a time of reviewing the events in life from a more mature perspective. Now is the time to come to terms with the successes and failures of the past.

Retirement

Work provides people with a sense of identity, a social group, an opportunity to achieve, and the opportunity to earn an income. A sudden illness or disability can force a client to retire. If outside interests are not developed before retirement, a client can suddenly feel lost. Others see retirement as a chance to do all the things they never had time for (Figure 5-3).

Attitudes and Personality

A positive attitude can sometimes do more to improve health than anything else. People should follow the advice of doctors, but the mind is also important as a healer. When a client is in good health, his personality usually remains the same as it has always been. A man who is a grouch at age 80 was probably a grouch at age 30. If either you or a family member notices a change in personality in a client, it should be reported to your supervisor. A personality change is not a normal sign of aging.

Depression

One of the most common reactions to a sense of loss, whether it be the loss of health or the loss of a spouse, is depression. A depressed client may have trouble sleeping or may lose his appetite. Usually the low feeling is short lived, but it does need to be taken seriously and reported to your supervisor. If the client ever expresses a suicidal thought, it must be taken seriously and reported to your supervisor immediately. The incidence of suicide increases with aging and usually can be prevented with proper counseling.

It is commonly believed that most older people feel lonely and sad most of the time. This is not true. It may seem that way to you because when you work in the home health care field, most of

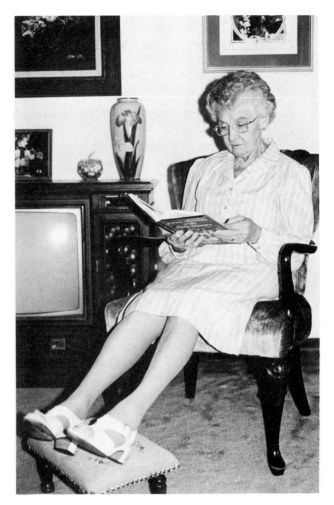

Figure 5-3
This client is taking the time to do things she never had time to do until she retired.

your clients are people who are ill, disabled, and under stress. During times of stress, a client may express more negative feelings in order to cope with his situation. Home health care is usually a temporary service that allows clients to adjust to new routines. Once a client has dealt with the initial crisis of the illness or disability, he can go back to a more normal life even if he still needs the assistance of the home health care agency. When asked, most older people report that they are happy with their lives.

The Myth of Senility

Senility is an inappropriate and outdated term used to describe mental impairment or an inability to think clearly. Normal aging does not cause any changes in mental abilities. Confusion or mental impairment is caused by other problems (disease or medications), which can usually be treated. Alz-

---

Caring for the Client Who Is Confused

1. Call the client by name. Use Mr., Ms., Mrs., Dr., or an appropriate title.
2. Use gentle reminders to let the client know the date and time. For example, "It is Wednesday, August 24th already." Or, "Mrs. Hart, it's 8:30 and time for breakfast."
3. Keep a calendar and clock with large numbers in view. Some clients mark the calendar each morning at breakfast.

---

heimer's disease (see Chapter 10) is one of the few diseases associated with confusion that cannot be treated. Signs of confusion are often not reported, because family and friends assume it is a normal part of aging. See Caring for the Client Who Is Confused.

Learning

It is a myth that older adults are set in their ways and cannot learn new things. An older client may need more time to learn than a younger person, but that is not always true. The person who keeps his mind active is more likely to keep his mental abilities strong. Some older clients will learn much faster than some younger clients. Always consider the individual person. Most home health clients are under stress, and that may also make learning more difficult. If you are working with a client who seems to be having trouble catching on to the material you are trying to teach, review the Guidelines for Teaching the Older Adult and the general section on teaching in Chapter 2. The HM/HHA will only reinforce material that has already been presented by the doctor, nurse, or another home health care professional.

Memory

It is well documented that older people can remember things in their distant past better than things that happened recently. A slight loss of memory is normal, but a greater loss might be cause for concern. Loss of memory is distressful and embarrassing for the older client. It can also cause safety problems. A client who forgets that a casserole is in the oven or that the iron has been left on can cause a serious accident. If the client is losing his sense of smell, the accident can become much worse. Memory tricks such as setting a timer

---

Guidelines for Teaching the Older Adult

1. The environment should be suitable for learning and without distractions.
   - Is the room clean and are the radio the TV off?
   - Is the client comfortable?
   - Is the client wearing his glasses and hearing aid?
   - Is the lighting adequate?
2. Explain why the material you are teaching is necessary or helpful. People at any age learn only if they want to learn. If the client is not interested, you may want to try another time. Meanwhile, ask your supervisor for suggestions for that particular client.
3. Keep your teaching sessions short. They only need to be a few minutes. Too much material can be overwhelming, frustrating, and confusing. Your supervisor will help you plan what is an appropriate amount to teach.
4. Allow the client plenty of time to ask questions. Do not try to rush the learning process. Tell the client you will get back to him if you cannot answer a question. Write the question down to help you remember to find out the answer.
5. At the end of the teaching session, have the client repeat information that has been presented to see if he has understood the material correctly.

   HM/HHA: "Mr. Smith, tell me which snack foods you cannot eat on your low salt diet."

   Mr. Smith: "I'm not supposed to eat potato chips, salted peanuts, or pretzels anymore, but I don't have to give up apples."

   HM/HHA: "That's right. Now, what else could you prepare for a snack?"

6. Give the client positive feedback or praise when the client gets the correct answer. If an answer is incorrect, correct the misunderstood information tactfully and immediately.
7. Give the client enough time to think about his answers. It may take longer for an older client to store and retrieve new information because his storehouse has grown quite large over the years.

---

or putting a frying pan on top of the TV can help remind the client about the meal. Eyeglasses and house keys should be kept in the same place so they are not lost easily.

Older people like to talk about their past. An important task of later adulthood is reviewing life events. It is not unusual for a HM/HHA to not know what to talk about with a new client the first time you meet or when providing personal care such as a bed bath. Ask questions about where the client lived, or what school was like for her, or any other general question about the client's life. Listen carefully and find out what interests your client. This will help you get to know your client and understand some of his feelings and past experiences.

The Role of the Homemaker/ Home Health Aide

Your job when working for an older client is to provide safe, effective care according to the care plan that has been ordered by the doctor and home health agency. Two other responsibilities are showing respect for your client's dignity and protecting your client from harm.

Respecting Your Client's Sense of Self-Worth and Dignity

Treat the client as you would like to be treated if you were in his position. Show respect for your client. More often than not, when you show kindness to a client, he will return that kindness to you.

Use formal titles when addressing your client. Do not call a client by his first name or a pet name such as "dear" or "honey." It may be considered disrespectful. Use Mr., Miss, or Mrs., unless the client tells you to use his first name. Most older adults that you care for will be unemployed and facing many life changes. Using a formal title is a way of recognizing the client's status in the world and respecting his dignity.

Never talk about a client in front of him. Never assume a client cannot hear or understand what you are saying just because he is hard of hearing or disabled. Sometimes a family member may start to do this. If so, include the client in the conversation ("Well, how do you feel, Mr. Smith?") or change the subject and continue the conversation at another time away from the client. Talking over a client's head can only make the client feel alone and insignificant.

Do not talk to an adult like a child. They are not children and do not appreciate being treated as such. Comments like "Eat all your breakfast because it is good for you" in a sing-song tone can only make a client feel resentful or encourage a poor self-image. Incontinence is one of the worst indignities a client can experience. This situation can only be made worse if the client is told he is "naughty" or made to feel he is "bad." Wetting the bed is not done on purpose and is handled best by making sure the client gets cleaned up quickly for his own comfort.

Encourage independence. Medical experts advise clients to participate in their normal daily activities as much as possible. Of course you will help the client follow the activity plan written by the home health care professionals. Occasionally a well-meaning but overprotective HM/HHA tries to do too much for the client. It may be difficult to watch someone who has had a stroke struggle with daily routines that were once done without thought. For example, it may be easier for you to button a shirt than to take the time to allow the client to do it himself. Doing too much encourages overdependence, and does not allow the client the chance to be self-reliant. Let your client know you believe he can do things without your assistance.

There may be times when a very ill client may need to have assistance with all aspects of his personal care. The HM/HHA who displays genuine caring and allows the client to give directions and make choices is still allowing the client some control over his situation. This can make all the difference in the world to the client who cannot care for himself. The ultimate goal of home health care is to help clients help themselves so they can live as normally and independently as possible (Figure 5-4).

Encourage your client to take an interest in his appearance. People who stay in pajamas all day are more likely to feel ill than those who get dressed and are well groomed. Men should be encouraged to shave and women to get their hair done if that is their normal routine when they are able to get around. Dentures, glasses, and hearing aids should all be kept clean and in good working order.

Recognize the need for social contact. Older clients need social contact as much as people of any age. Leaving the television on all day is not the answer. In some cases, you might be assigned to

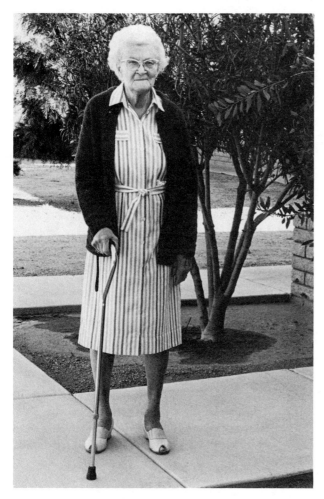

Figure 5-4
This 94-year-old woman rises early, gets dressed, eats breakfast, and takes a short walk as part of her daily routine.

play cards or checkers with a client who lives alone. Visits from family and friends or the company of a pet can make a day. Older people often enjoy talking about their past or historical events that occurred in their lifetime. They may like to listen to music from a show they saw or talk about a family photo. Socialization while you work can be interesting for both you and your client. If your client receives few visitors, the contact you establish will be an even more important part of his recovery. Most people can endure a great deal of suffering and pain if they know that someone cares about them.

Privacy. Everyone needs and has the right to privacy. There are three kinds of privacy that you need to respect when working for a home health client.

1. The client needs privacy during personal care procedures, such as when you assist with a bath or dressing. An older adult, like anyone else, may feel modest and embarrassed at needing assistance with bathing and other practices that have always been done independently and privately. Respect the need for privacy by closing doors and making sure the client is covered even if no one else is in the house.

2. The client has a right to expect that any personal information (about state of health, family relationships, money matters, and so on) will not be discussed with anyone who is not directly involved in the client's care.

3. The client has a need for time alone with his own thoughts. Some use quiet time for prayer or religious study, some use it to read books or listen to music. If a client is living in a family situation where he does not seem to get time to himself, let your supervisor know. While working for a client you can show respect for private time in many ways:
   - Knock before you enter a room even if the door is open
   - Ask before you turn on the television or radio.
   - Ask the client if he needs some time alone if it seems appropriate.
   - Do your work quietly and respect a client's occasional wish not to talk.

Protecting the Older Adult

Safety at Home

Because an older client's senses are not as sharp as before, there is a greater need for safety precautions. Often people do not feel they should spend money on themselves to fix up their homes. Even if they want to make changes, many may not be able to afford them. In some cases, the home health agency may be able to work with community agencies to get the funding. For more on safety, see Chapter 12.

- Lighting needs to be adequate for stairways and hallways.
- Floors should be kept clear of clutter and loose electrical cords.
- Carpets and throw rugs should be securely fastened to the floor.
- Banisters and handrails for stairways must be sturdy.

Protecting Your Client Against Fraud

Unfortunately, older adults are often targets for con artists. Here are some suggestions to help prevent fraud.

- Encourage your client to have service (including home health care staff) and repair persons show identification before entering the house.
- If someone comes to the door and wants to use the phone, your client should make the call for that person without letting the man or woman enter the house.
- Many "miracle cure" products are aimed at older adults. Sometimes they are harmless, but sometimes they can interfere with medication the client is taking. Let your supervisor know if your client is using these types of products. Your supervisor can decide how to handle the situation.

Protecting Your Client Against Abuse

Sadly, many older adults are abused in their homes. Abuse can be in the form of physical harm (hitting or slapping) or physical neglect (not enough food or a very dirty house). It can also take the form of threats or teasing. People who are the abusers need as much help as those who are being abused. Suspected abuse is a delicate situation that must be reported to your supervisor. Never confront a client or family member directly. Leave that to a trained professional.

Review Questions

True or False

1. ____ Older adults have slower reactions than younger people.

2. ____ It is normal for an older adult to be confused after the age of 75.

3. ____ Abuse of the elderly is not a problem that exists today.

4. ____ Only a small percentage of older people live in nursing homes or other institutions. Most live in their own homes.

5. ____ The skin becomes more delicate with aging and needs more care.

6. ____ The HM/HHA may file, but not cut, a client's fingernails and toenails.

Exercise

7. How does it feel to have a sensory loss?
   a. Cover your glasses or a pair of sunglasses with plastic wrap and then try to read a newspaper. Now try reading a book with large print.
   b. Put cotton in your ears and try to have a conversation with someone. This will help you understand how difficult it is to hear conversation when you are hard of hearing.
   c. Try to write a letter with the hand that you do not usually write with. This will help you understand how difficult it is for a client who has had a stroke to write with his other hand.

Questions for Discussion

8. How can you help orient a client who is confused?

9. Have you ever seen a health professional talk to an older client as though he was a child? Do you think that you will want to be addressed in that manner when you are older?

Chapter 6

Working With the Client Who Is Ill or Disabled

Objectives

At the conclusion of this chapter, the homemaker/home health aide will:

1. Be able to explain the difference between an illness and a disability.

2. Be able to describe some of the changes that may occur in a client's life if he becomes seriously ill or disabled.

3. Describe some of the ways the client or his family may react to an illness or disability and the way people in our society react to people with disabilities.

4. Understand when professional members of the home health care team need to be called to help a client deal with the emotional side of an illness or disability.

The Difference Between an Illness and a Disability

What Is an Illness?

Health is not only the absence of physical and mental illness, but it also includes a personal sense of well-being. A client is *ill* when he is sick or has a disease. An illness can be mental or physical. Because the body works as a unit, a client's feelings or sense of well-being may be affected when he is physically ill. When a client has a mental illness, he may have physical symptoms too.

Illness can be acute or chronic. An *acute illness* occurs suddenly and only lasts a short period of time. A *chronic illness* is a long-term illness that may last as long as the person's life. Diabetes and heart disease are both chronic illnesses. Appendicitis and the common cold are acute illnesses.

What Is a Disability?

A *disability* refers to a permanent physical or mental limitation. It may be caused by an illness or an accident, or it may occur at birth for known or unknown reasons. Disabilities include blindness, deafness, an inability to use an arm or leg, paralysis, mental retardation, speech disorders, and other conditions. Over 35 million people in the United States have some type of disability.

How It Feels to Have an Illness or Disability

A sudden illness or disability will be a shock to the client and his family. The stress of living with an illness or disability can cause other physical or mental health problems such as ulcers, digestive problems, or headaches. The stability of the family may also be threatened. The client who is ill or disabled may not be able to return to work for a long time, and may even lose his job. Even if the disability looks minor to you, the uncertainties of the future may cause great stress for the client and the family (Figure 6-1).

Often the client who has just become disabled will need to learn new skills in order to work and to take care of himself. Household chores that the client has always done may have to be handled by someone else.

The client who has had a disability for years may still feel the loss. A client who has been blind since birth may still feel sad that he cannot see a beautiful autumn tree even though he has never experienced vision. The child who has been in a wheelchair for most of her life may grieve at the loss of her legs when she is old enough to see other children running and playing sports. Some clients cope well with these feelings and others do not.

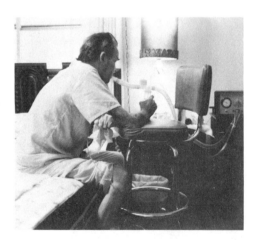

Figure 6-1
This client is using a hand-held nebulizer for a breathing treatment. Many home health clients use medical equipment that a homemaker/home health aide is not permitted to adjust. If you suspect that some of the equipment is not working properly, phone your home health agency right away. Do not try to adjust the equipment yourself. (Walsh J, Persons CB, Wieck L: Manual of Home Health Care Nursing, p 523. Philadelphia, JB Lippincott, 1987)

Living With a Disability

Most people with disabilities realize that the general public finds it difficult to deal with people who are disabled. A client who has lived with his disability for years may still feel angry or frustrated when people focus their attention on his physical limitations instead of talking with him as they would with anyone else.

The client who has lived with a disability for years will often have a system for bathing and dressing, and will be able to tell the HM/HHA exactly how to help him with his personal care (Figure 6-2). As long as the client's system is safe and approved by your supervisor, the client will take the lead in his plan of care. The client who is newly disabled or newly ill will need more help from the home health agency in learning the best way to do his daily care with his particular physical limitation.

Prejudices and Stereotypes

The language you use as a HM/HHA can help promote understanding between you and your client. Not so many years ago people with disabilities were known as "handicapped." Handicapped people were seen as second-class citizens. The term "disabled person" is not liked by many because it is a negative description of a person who happens to have a disability. When you use the term "client with a disability" instead of "disabled client," it stresses the person first and his limitation second. This lets the client know that you realize there is more to him than his disability. The terms "physically challenged" or "mentally challenged" also give positive descriptions of a person with a disability.

Compare the way these two homemaker/home health aides describe their clients. Which HM/HHA seems to understand that a physical limitation is a small part of who that person is?

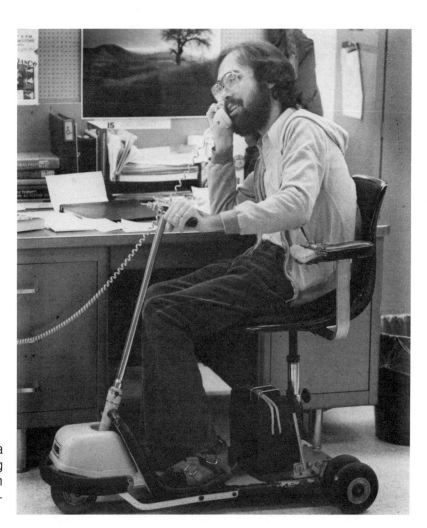

Figure 6-2
A motorized wheelchair helps the client with a disability lead an independent life. (Lindberg JB, Hunter ML, Kruszewski AZ: Introduction to Person-Centered Nursing, p 29. Philadelphia, JB Lippincott, 1983)

HM/HHA 1: Did you see the blind woman across the street?

HM/HHA 2: Did you see the woman who is blind across the street?

HM/HHA 1: I have to go take care of the spinal cord on Elm Street.

HM/HHA 2: I'm going to take care of the man with spinal cord injury on Elm Street.

Reactions to Disability and Illness

Coping Mechanism	What the HM/HHA Should Do
Denial	
A difficult diagnosis or disability can be hard to accept and the client may deny that he has a problem. A client who is denying his illness may not take his medications or follow the treatment plan. Or, a client may go doctor shopping trying to find one who will tell him what he wants to hear.	When the client and family use denial, they are trying to protect themselves. You need to deal with these situations carefully and not by yourself. Let the supervisor know what you have observed. You and the supervisor can work together to figure out how best to assist the family.
Depression	
Depression is the most common reaction to an illness or disability. People usually experience depression when they have to deal with a loss. Signs of depression include: • a feeling of hopelessness • a poor appetite • the inability to sleep • sleeping more than usual • a lack of interest in people, hobbies, and interests he used to have	Keep in mind that no one can be talked out of depression. One of the most helpful things you can do is listen to your client carefully. Encourage the client to take part in his care, but don't push if the client is not ready. A regular daily schedule may help the client regain a sense of control. Try not to appear too cheerful and happy when you are providing care. If you do, this may remind the client of what he can no longer do, or it may cause the client to think you do not care about the seriousness of his condition. Give the client support by letting him know his feelings are normal.
Overdependence	
People often regress a little when they are ill. It is normal to want someone to take care of us during a difficult time. Some clients become overdependent because they get more attention when they need assistance than when they are well and able to care for themselves.	Encourage your client to do as much for himself as the care plan will allow.
Difficult Behavior	
During a long illness, a client may begin to feel he is losing control of his life. Needing help with even the most basic activities of daily living such as brushing the teeth can be frustrating. It is not unusual to see a client who was once described as a good, kind neighbor become impatient, difficult, and uncooperative. A client may be abusive to you or to his family. Always let your supervisor know if a client's behavior is aggressive or difficult. Usually the problem can be solved with your supervisor's assistance.	Complaints or uncooperative behavior are usually a result of the pain or discomfort a client is experiencing and not his true feelings toward you as the HM/HHA. The best response is to stay calm and cheerful and continue to do your job. Always let the supervisor know about changes in the client's condition or any unusual behavior even if the situation resolves itself. If the incident occurs again, there is a record and you and the supervisor will have already discussed how to handle such problems. In the extremely rare situation that looks dangerous, leave the house and phone the supervisor immediately.

In these examples, the first statement is impersonal and the focus is on the importance of the illness or injury rather than the client as a person. A client with a disability has the same basic human needs as any other person, including the need for acceptance, love, and recognition.

Reactions to a Serious Illness or Disability

Reactions to an illness or disability will vary depending on the seriousness of the health problem and the personality and coping abilities of the family and client. *Coping mechanisms* are behaviors people use automatically to help them deal with difficult situations. Coping mechanisms are normal and are used by everyone for short periods of time. They can be harmful if they are used too much and the person never faces his real problem. Some common coping behaviors are described in Reactions to Disability and Illness.

Situation Exercise

Read the situations below and decide which coping mechanisms are being used by the client. Did the HM/HHA respond appropriately? How else could the situation have been handled?

Situation 1

Mr. Oscar was hospitalized for major surgery. After the surgery, he wanted the hospital nurses to give him a daily bed bath even after he was well enough to do most of it himself. He made such a fuss that it was easier for the nurses to give the bed bath than to try to get him to take care of himself. When Mr. Oscar went home, his wife continued to give the bed baths. Mrs. Oscar hired a local home health agency to help care for Mr. Oscar while he recovered.

The home health agency supervisor assigned Jim, a HM/HHA, to help Mr. Oscar with his morning care. Jim was told to help Mr. Oscar with his bath, but only with the areas of his body he couldn't reach. Mr. Oscar complained at first, but Jim was firm about how much he would help with the bath. Soon Mr. Oscar was able to do the entire bath himself. It would have been easy for Jim to give the entire bath, but if he did Mr. Oscar may never have tried to care for himself.

Situation 2

Mrs. Brown recently had her right leg amputated and was home from the hospital. Her family said she made good progress in the hospital and were surprised she had kept her good spirits after losing her leg. Several friends visited Mrs. Brown in the hospital and the visits always cheered her up. When she had been home awhile Sue Jones, a HM/HHA from the local home health agency, was assigned to help with her daily bath and breakfast. Sue noticed that Mrs. Brown hardly talked and never seemed to eat much of her meal. Sue told her supervisor right away and learned from the family that Mrs. Brown had always been outgoing and talkative before the surgery. What could Sue and her supervisor do to help Mrs. Brown?

Family Reactions

Families of a relative who is severely disabled may have to spend a lot of extra time and energy caring for the relative at home. They also need to deal with their own feelings about the disability. Parents may feel guilt even when they were not responsible for a child's disability. Even the most caring families will feel anger, frustration, and disappointment at some times. Some families may want their relative to stay at home, and then find they resent the extra time and effort needed to care for the relative who is very ill or very seriously disabled.

Review Questions

True or False

1. ___ A chronic illness is a sudden, short-term illness.

2. ___ A chronic illness is an illness that lasts a long time.

3. ___ Many clients with disabilities will be able to tell you exactly how you can help them with personal care.

4. ___ The HM/HHA must be sensitive about the terms used when talking about people with disabilities.

5. ____ Do not let your client do anything for himself if you can do the job faster and better.

Questions for Discussion

6. List four reactions that a client may have when he has an illness or disability. What are some ways that you could respond to those reactions?

7. What are some of the changes that would happen in your life if you had a physical disability and needed assistance with personal care and other activities of daily living?

Chapter 7

Promoting Mental Health and Understanding Mental Illness

Objectives

At the conclusion of this chapter, the homemaker/home health aide will:

1. Understand the basic characteristics of good mental health.

2. Be able to describe some of the myths about mental illness.

3. Be able to explain why coping mechanisms can be helpful and give some examples of coping mechanisms used in healthy and unhealthy ways.

4. Be able to discuss ways the HM/HHA can promote mental health and the role of the HM/HHA in a home situation where there is mental illness.

The Promotion of Good Mental Health

Most of the time the HM/HHA works with clients who have good mental health. During times of stress such as a severe illness, the client's mental health may be threatened (Figure 7-1). The HM/HHA needs to understand the characteristics of good mental health so she can recognize behaviors that need to be reported to the supervisor.

Characteristics of Good Mental Health

A person who has good mental health:

- Accepts himself, knowing his abilities and limitations.
- Accepts others without trying to change them.
- Can adjust to changes, frustrations, and disappointments in life.
- Treats others the way he would like to be treated.
- Takes responsibility for his decisions and actions.
- Guides his actions by long-term plans and not by short-term rewards.
- Can give and receive love and affection graciously.
- Can ask for help from family, friends, or others.

An *emotion* is a feeling. Your *mood* is the way you feel most of the time. Some people seem to be

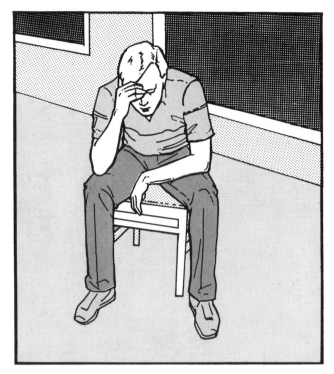

Figure 7-1
You will provide care during times of crisis for your client and his family. During such times, it is often normal for your client to display feelings of sadness or loss.

happy most of the time and others always seem to look at the dark side of life. Your mood can affect the way you feel and the way your clients will feel about you. A cheerful HM/HHA can make a client feel much better about himself. When you are feeling just a little down, try to think of something that makes you feel good. You might be surprised to see how quickly you can make yourself feel better. It is normal for your moods to vary, but a mentally healthy person can control his own moods so they can work for him.

Everyone has good days and bad days. A person with good mental health is not always happy. Instead, he has to work hard to get through difficult times. But, overall, a well-adjusted person can cope with life's highs and lows.

Understanding Mental Illness

Mental illness occurs when a person loses touch with reality and cannot cope with the stresses of daily life. The client may not respond or interact appropriately with other people. Mental illness is unfortunate, but it is not any more unfortunate than a physical illness. The majority of people who have a mental illness can be helped. Advances in medications and treatment programs have been tremendous. Still, many people think that a person who has had a mental illness is dangerous and will not get better, is unable to work, and is unable to contribute to society. This is not true, but it is difficult for many families to talk about the mental illness of a family member without feeling embarrassment and shame. Let the family know that you understand that mental illness is unfortunate, but that there is hope for improvement or recovery.

Coping Mechanisms

When the pressures of life become too much, people use coping mechanisms to reduce the tension. Everyone uses coping mechanisms. A client with a mental illness uses them more than healthy indi-

Table 7-1
Coping Mechanisms

Coping Mechanism	Explanation	Example
Denial	Refusal to believe a situation is true	"I can't possibly be seriously ill. I'm going to another doctor." A second opinion is often advisable, but a client who keeps changing doctors may not be dealing with reality.
Depression	Extreme sadness with feelings of hopelessness and discouragement. Not to be confused with the occasional blue feeling we all experience from time to time.	"I'm such a burden to my family. I just don't feel like eating today."
Repression	Temporarily "forgetting" to do something that the client may not have wanted to do in the first place	A client who hates to take his medication may say, "Oh no, I forgot to take my pills again yesterday."
Regression	Acting less mature in order to get others to take care of him. Normal if used for short periods during times of stress or illness, but can become a problem if the client will not cope with his life situation.	A client who can feed himself says, "Please feed me today."
Projection	Blaming others unjustly. The client projects blame onto someone else when the client is responsible.	"I know I would have gotten better sooner if my sister had come to visit me twice a day instead of only once a day."
Rationalization	Explaining an action as though it were acceptable even though it wasn't	"I took twice as many pills today because I forgot to take my medicine yesterday."
Hostility	Signs of anger or hostility. It is very rare for a client to become violent, but if you ever sense that happening, leave the house immediately. Your first concern should be your own safety.	"Get out of here! I don't need a bath today."

viduals. This client may have trouble understanding reality. Some of the common coping mechanisms are described in Table 7-1.

The Role of the Homemaker/ Home Health Aide

- Report unusual behavior to your supervisor right away. If a client ever makes comments or jokes about hurting himself or someone else, let your supervisor know immediately.
- Show caring and understanding for the client and the family. Your behaviors should serve as a role model for promoting healthy behavior.
- You must want and expect to see the client make progress. Progress is usually slow, but a positive attitude by all health care providers makes a difference. The HM/HHA who sees a client with a mental illness as a "lost cause" will not help the client recover. Instead, focus on the client's strengths.
- Keep the environment calm and maintain a regular routine.
- Allow the client to do things for himself in accordance with the care plan. The goal of treatment is to allow the client to become more independent.
- Observe the client and let the health care professionals know how the client is doing and whether he is taking his medication and following his treatment plan.
- Build a trusting relationship with the client and family. The client may feel more comfortable talking with the HM/HHA than with the doctor, nurse, or social worker.
- Be honest with your client. Do not lie or try to trick your client. If a client says "I'll tell you something if you promise not to tell my doctor," stop him and let him know that you cannot make that kind of promise.
- Help the confused client know what is real. If a client thinks she sees a white bunny sitting in the corner of her room, never

agree with her. Gently let the client know that you do not see a white bunny in her room, but do not force the issue. The supervisor should be called if a client is seeing things or hearing things that are not real.
- Counseling and diagnosing are jobs for professional members of the home health care team. They are not the job of the HM/HHA. Do not give advice to a family or client when you are not qualified to do so.

Review Questions

True or False

1. ____ A person who has good mental health is always happy.

2. ____ It is normal for all people to feel a little blue once in a while.

3. ____ Everyone needs some encouragement, understanding, and support during times of trouble.

4. ____ Anyone who has a mental illness can never work or live a normal life.

5. ____ Most mental illnesses can be treated.

6. ____ A person who is well adjusted has a good self-image and is flexible, but he may still have trouble dealing with some difficult situations.

7. ____ Coping mechanisms are used by everyone.

Questions for Discussion

8. Have you ever used a coping mechanism?

9. How would you react to an ill client who denies that he is ill?

10. Are you generally a happy person? When you feel a little down, what do you do to pick yourself up?

Chapter 8
Caring for the Client Who Is Dying

Objectives

At the conclusion of this chapter, the homemaker/home health aide will:

1. Be able to define *hospice*.

2. Have explored some of his own feelings about death and caring for a dying client.

3. Understand the five stages of the dying process as described by Dr. Elisabeth Kübler-Ross.

4. Be able to describe the HM/HHA's role and responsibilities to the client, to the family, and to the home care team.

5. Understand the emotional and physical needs of the dying client.

6. Know what to do if a client dies while you are in the home, who to notify, how to assist the family, and how to follow the policies of the home health agency.

Hospice and Home Care

Everyone has thought about death at one time or another, when a close relative, a friend, or even a pet has died. Death is the final part of the life cycle. Everyone must die. Despite this fact, most people still find it difficult to talk about death or to work with people who are dying. In our society, we tend to think it could happen to someone else, but not to us.

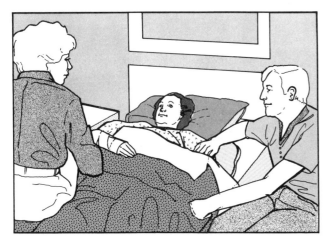

Figure 8-1
Support from family and friends is an important element of care.

The majority of people die in hospitals, but more and more people are choosing to die in their own homes surrounded by loved ones. One of the reasons for this shift is the hospice movement that began in a London hospital in the 1960s. A separate section of this hospital was opened to care for those who were unlikely to recover from an illness or injury, the *terminally ill*. The purpose of the program was not to cure patients, but to keep them comfortable and to include their families in the care. Now, *hospice* programs are operating in hospitals, clinics, and homes. Instead of simply treating the physical needs of the client, the hospice program considers the physical, emotional, and spiritual needs of the client and his family (Figure 8-1). We now realize how important it is to work through our feelings about death and dying.

Getting to Know Your Feelings About Death and Dying

1. Try to recall your first experience with death. How old were you? Can you describe how you felt the first time a relative, a friend, or even a pet died?

   _____
   _____
   _____

2. What do you think happens when you die?

   _____
   _____
   _____

3. Do you have any fears about dying?

   _____
   _____
   _____

4. Would you want to be told if you were ill and probably had only a few months to live? How would you want to spend the time you had left?

   _____
   _____
   _____

5. How would you feel if you needed help with bathing, dressing, and other activities of daily living?

   _____
   _____
   _____
   _____

This is important for you because one of your roles as a HM/HHA might be to care for clients who are choosing to die at home.

Understanding Your Feelings About Death

It is not possible to care for a dying client effectively unless you have explored your own feelings about death. To clarify your own thoughts about death and caring for the dying client, answer the questions under Getting to Know Your Feelings About Death and Dying. First answer the questions alone, and then discuss your answers with family members or a close friend. You may be surprised at what you learn.

The Five Stages of the Dying Process

Dr. Elisabeth Kübler-Ross is a well-known physician who has studied dying patients and their reaction to the dying process. She found that people go through five stages when they are dying:

1. Denial
2. Anger
3. Bargaining
4. Depression
5. Acceptance

These reactions to the dying process are normal and allow the person to deal with his feelings. Often family members of a client who is dying will go through the five stages too. A person may spend only a few minutes in a single stage, or several months. Sometimes a person will go back to a previous stage after he has been through it (Figure 8-2). You will not always recognize the stage a client is in, but at times it may help explain your client's behavior.

Denial

Denial ("No, not me.") is a natural reaction when a person first learns of his illness. A client may not hear all the medical facts or may go to several different doctors trying to find one who will find the others wrong. Denial often helps the client cope with the seriousness of his situation.

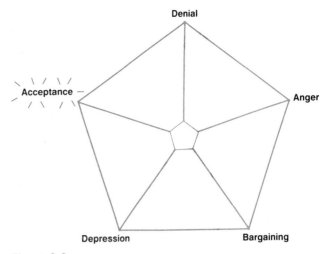

Figure 8-2
This diagram shows the five psychological stages of the dying process. Most terminally ill clients will skip from one stage to another instead of passing through the five stages in order.

Anger

The second stage is characterized by feelings of anger and resentment ("Why me?"). This stage may be especially difficult for the HM/HHA and the family, because the client may be critical of everything and everyone he comes in contact with. The client may express anger towards those who are healthy, cheerful, and able to live their lives normally. The client can move on to the next stage after he has been allowed to express his anger. If you understand why the client is showing anger, it can help you to act as a sounding board so he can release his feelings.

Bargaining

After working through his anger, the client may now want to bargain for more time. ("Yes me, but . . .".). For example, a person may promise to be a better husband or make promises to God to pray or go to church more often. This is also the time when people tend to organize their insurance policies, files, and wills in preparation for death. Sometimes a person may wish to see a relative who lives out of town, or to go to a favorite restaurant once more. If the client wants to bargain with you by changing the personal care routine that your supervisor has assigned, let him know that you cannot change the care plan without notifying your supervisor.

Depression

Depression ("Ah, me.") sets in as the client considers the loss of everything and everyone he has ever loved. He may also be sad because of things he will miss in the future. For example, he may never see an expected grandchild or his 50th wedding anniversary. This is a time of quiet reflection for the client. A warm touch can show your caring and understanding at this time.

Acceptance

Acceptance ("Yes, me.") is the final stage of preparing for death. It occurs when all the unfinished business is done. The client no longer sees death as defeat, but has accepted it as the last part of the life cycle. The client still sees a glimmer of hope, but he is ready to let go. People who have reached acceptance may want to spend most of their time alone or with just one or two members of the family.

The Role of the Homemaker/ Home Health Aide

Personal Care and Light Housekeeping

The HM/HHA will always be instructed how to care for individual clients by the supervisor. You will be told what to observe and what to report to the supervisor. The type of care you provide may be changed frequently by the supervisor according to the client's condition. Always allow and encourage the client to participate in his care as much as he is able to. This helps the client to maintain independence and a good self-image.

Respect, Encouragement, and Support of the Client and Family

Many HM/HHAs are afraid to care for a person who is terminally ill for fear that he will ask questions about his condition. Most people want to know about the seriousness of their illness, but it is up to the physician and family to discuss these matters with the client. Usually the physician and nurse discuss the client's condition in a family conference, so the family can support one another

and the client when they first hear the news. In the unusual situation where the family does not want the client to know the seriousness of his illness, the client may realize it anyway after observing the behavior of family and health care staff. If the family does not wish the client to know about his condition, you must respect their wishes. It is never appropriate for you to give details of the client's medical condition to the client, to the client's family, or to the client's friends. Only the physician or nurse may do this.

The HM/HHA provides physical care for the dying client, but providing emotional support for the client and family is just as important. If there has been a recent death in your own family, you should work through your own grief before caring for a client who is dying. The client and family members will need support, and you may not be able to provide it effectively if your grief has not been resolved.

If you ever are reluctant to care for a dying client for any reason, your supervisor will appreciate your honesty if you tell him directly. Not everyone can or should care for the terminally ill.

Emotional Needs of the Dying Client

Hope

When interviewed by Dr. Kübler-Ross, terminally ill patients all said that they wanted to know the seriousness of their illness, but they also wanted some degree of hope. Even if it seems the client will not live long, always give the client realistic hope. False hope is not helpful or comforting. The family and the client may have different ideas of hope. While the family may hope for an improbable cure, the client may simply hope to live another 3 months and have the strength to walk his daughter down the aisle at her wedding, or to see the spring flowers bloom. Hope is a powerful force. It can improve the quality of life and sometimes extend life itself.

The Need to Have Someone Listen

In our society, people are often afraid to talk about dying. If your client wants to talk with you about his illness or worries, you will be doing him a great service by listening carefully to his thoughts. A client may feel more comfortable talking about his feelings while you are giving him a bath or preparing his lunch than during a formal counseling session with a doctor. Let your client take the lead. If a client asks you questions you cannot answer, simply say you do not know the answer, but will try to find out for him. Usually the client does not want advice or answers from you, but simply someone who will listen.

Listen with understanding to family members who wish to express their grief and experiences. Let your supervisor know what the family and client are discussing, because she is trained to assist them in dealing with their difficult situation.

The Need to Live a Normal Life

A client who has a terminal illness has the same basic human needs as other people. He will probably want to do as much for himself as he can in order to make his life as normal as possible.

Children's Needs

Children who have a terminally ill parent or close relative should be told the seriousness of the situation in words they can understand. The HM/HHA should not be the person to disclose this information to the child. The parents, close relatives, or nurse should do this. The child will need reassurance that he will be cared for if a parent dies. A child is never too young to understand death.

The dying child should also be told about his situation, but not by the HM/HHA. Always try to find out what the child has been told so that you can answer questions honestly with consideration for the family's wishes. Terminally ill children also need to lead normal lives, which includes laughing and crying, playing with friends, and fighting with their brothers and sisters.

Spiritual Needs

The spiritual needs of the client must be recognized and supported. The client may want to talk to a clergyman even if he does not attend a church regularly. Your supervisor will be able to assist the client with this need.

Physical Needs of the Dying Client

Mouth Care

It is normal for the client to lose his appetite or to have trouble swallowing. The client should be kept on his side while lying down if he is having trouble swallowing saliva so he will not choke on secretions that may collect in his mouth. Help the client brush his teeth several times each day and let him have the opportunity to rinse his mouth out with a pleasant-tasting mouthwash or plain water as often as he wishes. Keep the client's lips lubricated with petroleum jelly or lip gloss.

Face and Eye Care

Encourage the client to wipe his face with a warm washcloth before and after meals and after naps for refreshment. You may need to help wipe the secretions from his eyes using plain water and a clean washcloth.

Positioning

Improper positioning causes fatigue and muscle soreness. See Chapter 16 for proper positioning. If the client is restless, he may need more frequent repositioning and perhaps side rails. If he has trouble breathing, use pillows to help him sit up comfortably, or try raising the head of the bed if a hospital bed is used.

Hearing

As death approaches, a person may lapse between consciousness and unconsciousness. Hearing is the very last sense to leave, so always assume your client can hear and understand every word you say even if it does not appear so. Tell your client the date and time and something about the weather. As always, explain what you are doing as you assist with bathing, dressing, or anything else. Normal conversation may be a comfort and will help your client feel less isolated.

Pain

Pain is one reason many people fear death. Usually, there is greater physical pain earlier in the illness, before an effective pain reliever for that person is found, than just before death. Not surprisingly, it has been proven that people who have sound emotional support often need fewer pain medications than those without support. Still, pain can be very difficult for the client and family. Methods of pain relief such as positioning and backrubs that do not involve medications will be discussed with you by your supervisor for individual clients.

The Actual Time of Death

The client who is actually dying may or may not be unconscious. His feet and hands may begin to feel cool as his circulation loses its effectiveness. Breathing may become irregular, and there may be a gurgling sound as fluids get caught in the windpipe. When the heart stops, the face and skin lose color as the blood stops circulating.

Usually a family is prepared for a death that occurs at home. They have often made the funeral arrangements and know the steps to take at the moment of death. A physician needs to be notified to pronounce the person dead. If you are there when a client dies, make a note of the time the client died and phone the home health agency. Then follow the instructions given to you by your agency and the doctor.

The Need to Grieve After Death

Even for the most prepared person or family, the death of a loved one can be a great shock. The HM/HHA can help most by offering to make some of the initial phone calls to the home health agency and the funeral home, and by listening as the family expresses feelings of sadness and disbelief. People express grief in different ways. Try to show caring and acceptance to people who seem to have trouble expressing their feelings.

After working closely with a dying client and his family, the HM/HHA and other home health staff who have worked closely with the client will also need emotional support. It helps to talk about your relationship to the client. The home care team will often have a staff meeting after the death of a client where you can discuss your feelings. You and others who have worked with the client may wish to attend the client's funeral.

Review Questions

True or False

1. ____ The five stages of dying are normal reactions and help the person deal with his feelings about dying.

2. ____ Most people who are dying want to know there is some hope, no matter how small.

3. ____ The HM/HHA should find out what the client knows about his illness before going to the client's home.

4. ____ Listening to a client's family is not necessary, because HM/HHAs are hired only to care for the client.

5. ____ A client who is terminally ill is unlikely to recover.

Questions for Discussion

6. Why is it necessary for you to have come to terms with your own philosophy of death before caring for a client who is dying?

7. Have you ever been around a close relative or friend who was dying? Did you notice that person going through any of the five stages of dying? What happened?

Part Three

The Human Body and Health Problems

Chapter 9
How the Body Works

Objectives

At the conclusion of this chapter, the homemaker/home health aide will:

1. Be able to explain the difference between a cell, a tissue, an organ, and an organ system.

2. Be able to explain what the skin does and discuss the kinds of observations the HM/HHA may need to make about a client's skin.

3. Be able to explain the purpose of the skeletal system and the kinds of observations the HM/HHA may need to make about the skeletal system.

4. Be able to explain the purpose of the muscular system and explain how knowledge about this system will help you give better care to a client.

5. Understand how the circulatory system works and discuss seven health problems that affect the circulatory system.

6. Understand how the respiratory system works and understand why a client with a respiratory problem may tire easily.

7. Be able to explain how the digestive system works and know the kinds of observations the HM/HHA should report to the supervisor.

8. Be able to explain the purpose of the nervous system and its importance.

9. Understand how the urinary system works and discuss the kinds of observations the HM/HHA should report to the supervisor.

10. Know how the male and female reproductive systems work.

11. Understand the endocrine system's role in the human body.

12. Appreciate how all the organ systems work together.

13. Explain how knowledge of the organ systems will help the HM/HHA provide better care to clients.

What Are Living Things Made Of?

The human body is made up of cells, tissues, organs, and organ systems. The *cell* is the smallest living unit in the body. Similar cells work together to form *tissues*. Several tissues form an *organ*, and various organs work together to form an *organ system* (see box). For example, the cells that line the stomach form a tissue called epithelial tissue. The stomach, which is an organ, is made of several kinds of tissues. The digestive system consists of several organs, including the mouth, the esophagus, the stomach, and the intestines. There are ten organ systems that work together to create a person.

> Cell→Tissue→Organ→Organ →Person
> systems

Cells

The cell is the basic unit of life. All living things are made of cells. Some human cells are so small that 5000 cells are the size of a single grain of sand. An egg is an example of a large cell. Even though a single cell is small, each cell has the needs of any living thing.

Characteristics of Cells

Every individual cell

- Has a specific job to do in the human body.
- Needs oxygen, water, and nourishment to live and produce energy.
- Removes its own wastes.
- Has the ability to grow and reproduce. Most have the ability to repair themselves.
- Will die.

Tissues

When similar cells group together, they form *tissues*. There are four basic kinds of tissues found in the human body.

1. Connective tissue: Examples are cartilage, tendons, ligaments, blood, lymph, and fat.
2. Epithelial tissue: Examples are skin, glands, and blood vessels. Epithelial tissue lines most body surfaces such as the respiratory, digestive, and urinary tracts.
3. Nerve tissue: Examples are brain, spinal cord, and nerves.
4. Muscle tissue: There are groups of muscles throughout the body.

Organ Systems

Skin

The skin has three primary jobs.

1. It covers the body and protects the internal organs from infection and disease.
2. It helps maintain body temperature by sweating when it is hot or shivering when it is cold.
3. It provides information about the world around us by its ability to feel sensations such as temperatures, textures, and pressure.

The skin is made up of three layers: the epidermis, the dermis, and the subcutaneous layer (Figure 9-1).

The epidermis is the thin outer layer that we can see. The epidermis is made of cells that die and flake off easily when we wash. It holds *pigment*, which gives our skin its natural color.

The dermis and the subcutaneous layer are the two deeper layers of the skin. They house the sweat and oil glands, the hair follicles, blood vessels, and fatty tissue.

Oil glands keep the skin and hair lubricated. Older people often have drier skin because the oil glands lose some efficiency with the aging process. Hair keeps the body warm, and protects it. Eyelashes and eyebrows keep dirt from entering the eyes, and the hairs in the nose and ears keep particles and germs out.

How the Skin Helps Control Body Temperature

The skin helps maintain body temperature in three ways.

1. Sweat glands release a salt water solution (sweat) through the pores. The sweat cools the body as it evaporates.
2. The blood vessels in the skin help regulate the temperature. When the body is hot, the blood vessels get larger (dilate). This makes them closer to the surface of the skin, so the body's heat can be released through the skin. When the body is cool, the blood vessels get smaller (constrict), so heat cannot be released through the skin easily.
3. The skin also controls body temperature through the hair follicle muscles. When cold, the hair follicle muscles contract to hold in body heat. This is commonly known as *goose bumps* or *goose flesh*. Babies and older adults are not able to generate and retain heat as

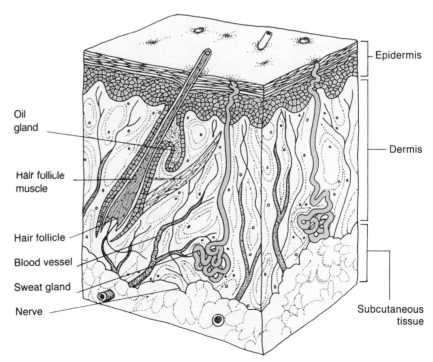

Figure 9-1

A cross section of the skin. (Wolff L, Weitzel MH, Zornow RA et al: Fundamentals of Nursing, 7th ed, p 379. Philadelphia, JB Lippincott, 1983) well as healthy adults, so they need to be protected from cold temperatures.

Observations to Make About the Skin

Observations about the skin that should be reported include the following.

- Changes in skin color such as yellowing of the whites of the eyes in clients with dark sink, or a yellow tint to the skin of a white client
- Rashes or bruises
- A blister, especially on the feet
- An ulcer or open sore
- Changes in texture
- Temperature changes
- A red, tender area that might be the start of a pressure sore

Common Skin Problems

A common skin problem is the *decubitus ulcer*, which is also known as a *pressure sore* or *bedsore*. Bedsores occur when blood cannot reach an area of skin due to prolonged pressure. An ulcer can develop quickly and take a long time to heal. Once a pressure sore develops, a client's rehabilitation process may be slowed down until the sore has healed. Decubitus ulcers are most likely to develop over the *bony prominences,* places where the bone is close to the skin's surface. To prevent decubitus ulcers, good nutrition and good skin care techniques must be followed carefully. See Chapter 20 for more complete information on pressure sores.

Skin Care Products

Many clients use lotion for dry skin. Lotions that simply lubricate the skin can be refreshing, but be wary of products that claim to replace protein or prevent wrinkles. Because our culture is so oriented towards youth, older people are especially vulnerable to such advertising claims. Let your supervisor know if your client is spending a lot of money on skin products or expecting miracles. A talk with an informed health professional, such as a doctor or nurse, may help the client decide whether he wants to continue buying these skin care products.

Skeletal System

There are 206 bones in the human skeletal system (Figure 9-2). The skeletal system has three purposes.

1. It supports the muscles
2. It gives the body a protective frame.
3. It stores calcium and produces red blood cells.

Bones change throughout a person's life. A child's bones are more flexible than an adult's bones. As people age, bones become harder and less flexible, and do not heal as easily. The bones of some older adults are quite brittle and easily broken.

A *joint* is where two bones meet. Bones are held together by fibrous strands of connective tissue called *ligaments*. The ends of bones are made of *cartilage,* a soft flexible tissue that cushions the joint.

There are several kinds of joints, which allow a person to move body parts in a number of ways. It helps to think about the way joints move when you are assisting a client with dressing or bathing. Refer to Chapter 16 for information on how to assist a client with repositioning.

Observations to Make About the Skeletal System

Tell you supervisor if a client's joint becomes

- Red and swollen or
- Painful.

Notice the condition of your client's joints and how easily he moves. Some clients do not like to talk about their own pain, but you may notice that they move more slowly, or grimace when they move. An older client may need more time to move than a younger client. Let the client move at his own pace. When helping a client change positions in bed, be sure to support the joints when moving a limb.

Common Bone Problems

You may see two basic bone problems. First, there are chronic long-term problems, like arthritis. With arthritis, the joints swell and become quite painful. For more information about arthritis, see Chapter 10.

Second, there are short-term problems, like broken bones and muscle or ligament strains, that

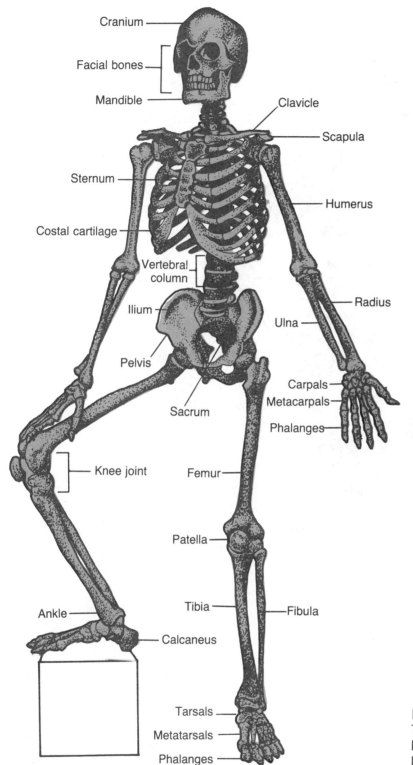

Figure 9-2
The skeletal system. (Rosdahl CB: Textbook of Basic Nursing, 4th ed, p 99. Philadelphia, JB Lippincott, 1985)

happen when a client has an accident such as a fall. These problems can be especially serious in older clients whose bones are more brittle and take longer to heal. Prevention is the best way to deal with this type of bone problem. When stairways are well lighted and rugs are secured to the floors, falls are less likely to occur. If a client does fall and you think he may have broken a bone, call for professional help and do not move the client. A bone fracture can become much worse if the client is not moved properly, especially if it involves the back.

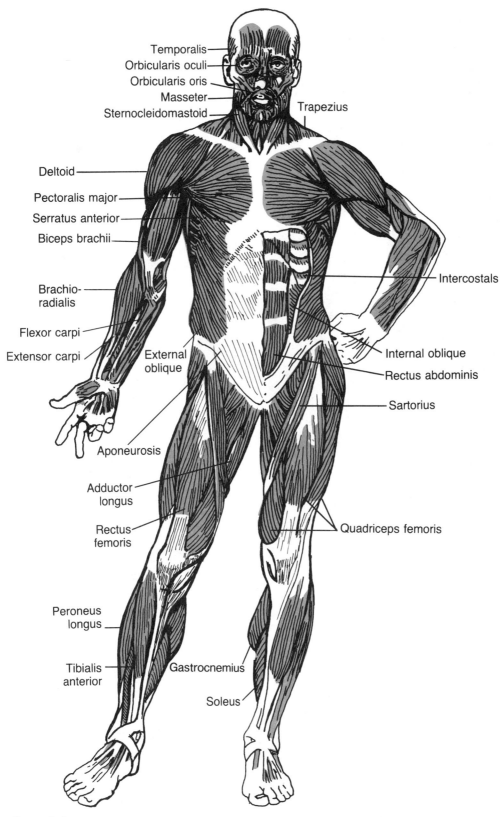

Temporalis
Orbicularis oculi
Orbicularis oris
Masseter
Sternocleidomastoid
Trapezius

Deltoid
Pectoralis major
Serratus anterior
Biceps brachii

Brachio-
radialis

Flexor carpi
Extensor carpi

External
oblique

Aponeurosis

Adductor
longus

Rectus
femoris

Peroneus
longus

Tibialis
anterior
Gastrocnemius

Soleus

Intercostals

Internal oblique
Rectus abdominis

Sartorius

Quadriceps femoris

Figure 9-3
The muscular system (front view). (Rosdahl CB: Textbook of Basic Nursing, 4th ed, p
107. Philadelphia, JB Lippincott, 1985)

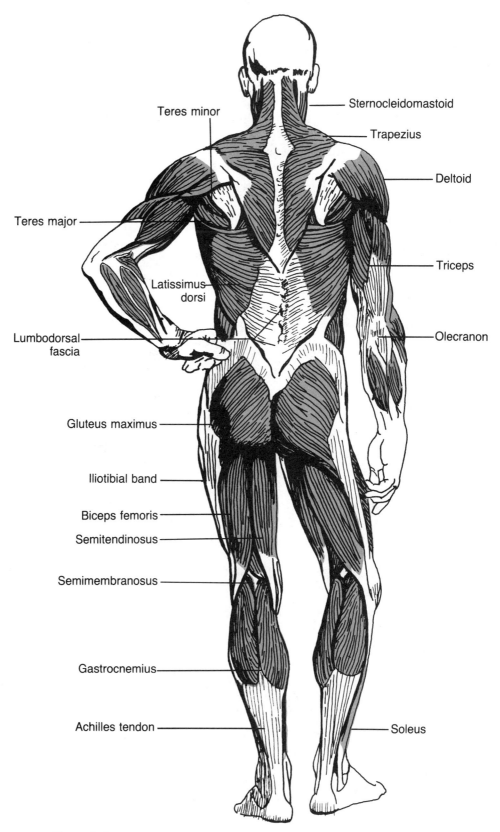

Teres minor

Sternocleidomastoid

Trapezius

Deltoid

Teres major

Triceps

Latissimus dorsi

Lumbodorsal fascia

Olecranon

Gluteus maximus

Iliotibial band

Biceps femoris

Semitendinosus

Semimembranosus

Gastrocnemius

Achilles tendon

Soleus

Figure 9-4
The muscular system (back view). (Rosdahl CB: Textbook of Basic Nursing, 4th ed, p 108. Philadelphia, JB Lippincott, 1985)

Muscular System

The human body has over 600 muscles (Figures 9-3 and 9-4). The muscles allow the body (1) to move and (2) to generate heat to keep warm during activity.

Muscles are attached to bones by fibrous tissues called *tendons* (Figure 9-5). Muscles move by contracting and extending. A muscle is considered in good *tone* when it is partially contracted and ready for action. This is the normal state of the muscle.

There are two kinds of muscles, voluntary and involuntary. *Voluntary muscles* are the ones that you consciously control. For example, when you turn the pages of this book you are using voluntary muscles.

Involuntary muscles act without your conscious control. Examples include the pumping of your heart, the contractions of your stomach, and the expanding and contracting of your blood vessels. These movements occur without your thinking about them.

As a HM/HHA, you may come across the following terms to describe muscle and bone movements.

- *Flexion:* Decreasing the angle between two bones. Flexion is used when you bring your hand to your shoulder (Figure 9-6).
- *Extension:* Increasing the angle between two bones. Extension is used when you straighten your arm (see Figure 9-6).
- *Abduction:* Moving away from the midline of the body (Figure 9-7).
- *Adduction:* Moving towards the midline of the body (see Figure 9-7).

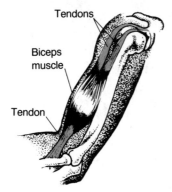

Figure 9-5
Muscles are attached to bones by tendons. (After Rosdahl CB: Textbook of Basic Nursing, 4th ed, p 83. Philadelphia, JB Lippincott, 1985)

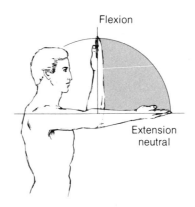

Figure 9-6
This sketch demonstrates flexion and extension of the arm. (Lindberg JB, Hunter ML, Kruszewski AZ: Introduction to Person-Centered Nursing, p 49. Philadelphia, JB Lippincott, 1983)

Observations to Make About the Muscular System

Report complaints of swelling, redness, or pain. Preventing accidents prevents strained muscles and tendons. If you are helping a client to reposition himself in a bed or a chair, be sure to give adequate support by holding the joints carefully.

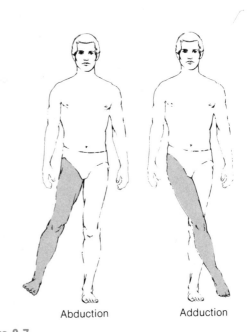

Figure 9-7
This sketch demonstrates abduction and adduction of the leg. (Lindberg JB, Hunter ML, Kruszewski AZ: Introduction to Person-Centered Nursing, p 50. Philadelphia, JB Lippincott, 1983)

Common Muscle Problems

Sprains, strains, atrophy, and contractures are common muscle problems that you will see. Careful safety precautions to prevent accidents will reduce sprains and strains. Range of motion (ROM) exercises prevent contractures and atrophy and keep the muscles in good tone and function. See Chapter 16 for more information on range of motion exercises. Two terms you may hear when talking about a client's muscle problems are explained below.

Atrophy. When muscles are not used, they shrink and become weak. This condition is called atrophy. Is can occur in a short time. Clients need to use their muscles as much as the doctor will allow to keep atrophy from occurring.

Contracture. When muscles are not used, they shorten and can get stuck in a fixed contracted position. This is called contracture. A contracture can result in permanent damage and loss of function. Following the doctor's activity and exercise orders will prevent contractures.

Circulatory System

The circulatory system does the following jobs.

1. It carries blood to all the cells in the body.
2. It provides all the cells in the body with oxygen and nutrients.
3. It helps fight infection.
4. It helps maintain body temperature.
5. It helps control fluid balance.

The circulatory system consists of the heart, the blood vessels (arteries, veins, and capillaries), the blood, and the lymph nodes and vessels.

The *heart* is about the size of a fist and pumps nearly 3500 gallons of blood every day. *Arteries* carry "clean" blood rich in oxygen and nutrients to individual cells. *Veins* carry "dirty" blood back to the heart. The blood in the veins is "dirty" because it is carrying the waste from cells, called *carbon dioxide.* The "dirty" blood is pumped to the lungs, where carbon dioxide is released through exhaling and oxygen is picked up through inhaling. After the blood is "cleaned" in the lungs, it goes back to the heart and begins the journey through the body again (Figure 9-8).

The *lymph vessels* and *nodes* are responsible for

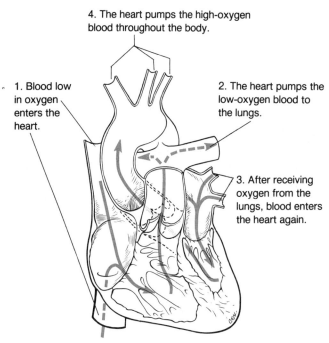

4. The heart pumps the high-oxygen blood throughout the body.

1. Blood low in oxygen enters the heart.

2. The heart pumps the low-oxygen blood to the lungs.

3. After receiving oxygen from the lungs, blood enters the heart again.

Figure 9-8
A cross section of the heart. Blood low in oxygen enters the heart and is pumped to the lungs. In the lungs, blood gives off cell wastes (carbon dioxide) and picks up oxygen. Then the blood is pumped to the other side of the heart, which pumps blood throughout the body. (Porth CM: Pathophysiology: Concepts of Altered Health States, 2nd ed, p 256. Philadelphia, JB Lippincott, 1986)

filtering and removing excess fluids in the tissues. The *spleen* also filters impurities out of the blood.

Observations to Make About the Circulatory System

- Measuring the *vital signs* (temperature, pulse, respiration, and blood pressure) helps the home health team learn about the condition of the client's circulatory system.
- Report any changes in the skin color. A client may become pale or flushed for many reasons that may indicate a medical problem.
- Report any complaints of swollen lymph nodes. Lymph nodes are found under the arms, in the neck, and in the groin.

Common Circulatory Problems

A problem in the circulatory system can affect every part of the body, because this system provides all the body cells with oxygen and nutrients. There are a number of disorders that can occur in the circulatory system. Some of these will be discussed in more detail in Chapter 10.

Anemia. Anemia occurs when there are too few red blood cells in the blood. The job of the red blood cells is to carry oxygen and iron to the body's cells. People who are anemic tend to be pale and to tire easily.

Atherosclerosis. Atherosclerosis happens when fatty deposits collect in an artery and cause it to become more narrow. When the arteries are more narrow, the heart must pump harder to get the blood to the cells. There is also the danger that a blood clot could form in the narrowed vessel (Figure 9-9).

Angina. Angina is a temporary tightening or painful sensation in the chest or left arm. The pain occurs when the heart muscle cannot get enough blood to function properly.

Heart Attack. A heart attack is also known as a *coronary* or a *myocardial infarction*. It occurs when the blood supply to the heart is completely blocked. Because blood can no longer get to the heart, the heart tissue dies. If only a small part of the heart muscle dies, the heart can repair itself under strict medical care. If too much of the heart muscle dies, the heart will not work and the person will die.

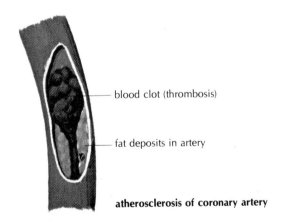

blood clot (thrombosis)

fat deposits in artery

atherosclerosis of coronary artery

Figure 9-9
Atherosclerosis occurs when fat deposits collect in an artery. This condition makes the artery more narrow and makes it necessary for the heart to work harder when pumping blood. It also may increase the chance for a blood clot (thrombosis). (Memmler RL, Wood DL: The Human Body in Health and Disease, 6th ed, p 210. Philadelphia, JB Lippincott, 1987)

Edema/Swelling. Edema is a term used to describe swelling caused by an excess of fluid in the tissues. You may see a client with swollen ankles. The best way to reduce the swelling is to have the client put his feet up on a stool with his legs uncrossed. Edema should be reported to your supervisor, because it is a sign that the client's fluid balance is not stable.

Hemorrhage. A hemorrhage is a sudden loss of blood. It can be either internal or external. People can bleed to death within 1 minute if the wound is extremely severe. The basic first aid measure to stop a bleeding wound is to cover it with a clean cloth and apply firm pressure. For more on first aid for bleeding, see Chapter 22.

Varicose Veins. Varicose veins occur when the valves in the veins are damaged and the veins swell. They are found most often on the legs. Hemorrhoids or piles are varicose veins in the rectum.

Respiratory System

You are familiar with the main job of the respiratory system—*breathing*. The purpose of breathing is to provide the cells with oxygen and to remove carbon dioxide wastes from cells.

The respiratory system has several parts (Figure 9-10):

- The *nose* and *mouth* take in and release air.
- The *trachea* or windpipe leads to the upper chest and becomes the bronchi.
- The *bronchi* take air into the lungs.
- The *lungs* are where the exchange of oxygen and carbon dioxide takes place.
- The *diaphragm* is a thin, flat muscle that lifts the lungs and helps the breathing process.

A person inhales oxygen into the lungs when breathing. This oxygen is picked up by the blood and delivered to the cells of the body. The blood carries carbon dioxide, a cell waste products, back to the lungs. Carbon dioxide leaves the body when a person exhales (breathes out).

Observations to Make About the Respiratory System

Observations about the respiratory system that should be reported include the following:

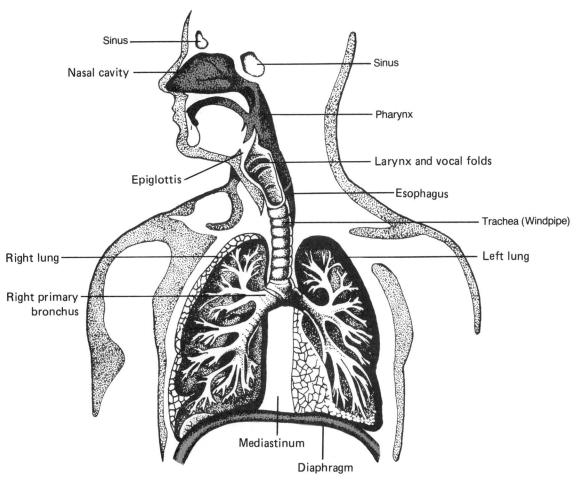

Figure 9-10
The respiratory system. (Rosdahl CB: Textbook of Basic Nursing, 4th ed, p 138. Philadelphia, JB Lippincott, 1985)

- Unusual breathing patterns or changes in breathing such as pauses, noisy sounds, or breathing difficulty;
- Excessive or persistent coughing;
- Hoarseness;
- Nasal congestion; and
- Changes in the color of sputum (mucus coughed up from the lungs).

Common Respiratory Problems and Care Guidelines

Because the lungs are responsible for providing oxygen to and removing carbon dioxide from all the cells in the body, lung disorders can be very serious. A client with respiratory problems may tire easily and need more time to do a task. Allow him time to work at his own pace. A client may need to do breathing exercises that have been prescribed by the physician in order to increase his lung efficiency. See Chapter 20 for more information on breathing exercises.

Smoking and air pollution interfere with the lungs' ability to work effectively, so smoke and air pollution should be avoided by any client with health problems. If a client is having trouble breathing, have him sit up straight because this is the easiest position for clearing the air passages.

Chronic Obstructive Pulmonary Disease.
There is a range of serious lung disorders called chronic obstructive pulmonary disease (COPD). In each disease, the lungs are not able to keep a good flow of air either going into or leaving the lungs. Asthma, bronchitis, and emphysema are the three most common diseases included in COPD. See the Quick Reference Chart in Chapter 10 for details.

Digestive System

The digestive system has two purposes.

1. It breaks food down so that nutrients can be absorbed into the blood and nourish cells throughout the body.
2. It moves the waste products of digestion through the intestines and out of the body.

Digestion begins when food is put into the mouth (Figure 9-11). Food begins to break down when it is mixed with saliva and chewed. Swallowing pushes the chewed food down the *esophagus*, which is the tube that leads to the stomach. When you swallow food, a cartilage structure called the *epiglottis* covers the trachea (windpipe) so that the food does not get into the lungs. In the *stomach*,

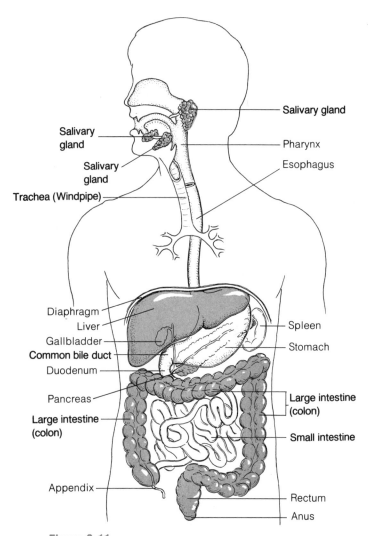

Figure 9-11
The digestive system. (Lindberg JB, Hunter ML, Kruszewski AZ: Introduction to Person-Centered Nursing, p 382. Philadelphia, JB Lippincott, 1983)

the food is churned and mixed with digestive juices for 3 to 5 hours until it passes into the small intestine. The stomach of an adult can hold about a half gallon of food and liquid at a time. In the *small intestine*, the food encounters the last set of digestive juices from the *pancreas*, the small intestine, and the *gallbladder*. The food is absorbed by fingerlike projections called *villi* within the small intestine. The villi have very small blood vessels called capillaries, which permit food to enter the bloodstream. Because not every bit of the food that we eat can enter the blood, the waste products of digestion are pushed into the *large intestine* in a liquid form. In the large intestine, a large part of the liquid is absorbed. The waste products that are left, known as feces, are passed out of the body through the *rectum* and *anus*.

The pancreas, liver, and appendix are three other parts of the digestive system. The *pancreas* produces digestive juices used in the small intestine during digestion. It also produces insulin, which is used to convert sugar into energy for cells.

The *liver* produces bile. Bile is stored in the gallbladder and released into the small intestine during digestion to break down fats. The liver also filters drugs and alcohol out of the blood and stores sugar, minerals, vitamins, protein, and fats.

The *appendix* is a small pouch-like structure where the small and large intestines meet. Appendicitis occurs when particles get caught in the appendix and become infected. Surgery is usually required to remove the appendix when it is infected.

Observations to Make About the Digestive System

Report any of the following to your supervisor.

- Nausea or vomiting
- Indigestion or heartburn
- Diarrhea or changes in the color, frequency, or texture of stools
- Sores, redness, or pain in the mouth or throat
- Problems with teeth or dentures

It is important for the HM/HHA to realize that even though asking a client questions about bowel habits may be embarrassing for you at first, changes in the digestive system can indicate serious health problems such as colon cancer. Colon cancer is one of the easiest types of cancer to treat successfully if detected early.

Common Digestive Problems

You may see any of the following common digestive problems:

- Anorexia: The loss of appetite or a lack of interest in eating food
- Diarrhea: Loose, watery, or unformed stools
- Nausea: An unpleasant feeling in the abdomen. Vomiting may or may not follow.
- Vomiting: The sudden expulsion of food from the stomach. *Emesis* is another word for vomiting.

Nervous System

The nervous system consists of the brain, the nerves, the spinal cord, and the sense organs.

The purpose of the nervous system is to keep the body informed. The sense organs and nerves pick up messages and send the messages to the brain. The brain decides how to respond.

The *brain* (Figure 9-12) is the controlling center where messages are received and decisions are made. Certain parts of the brain control specific jobs for the body. If the blood supply to one

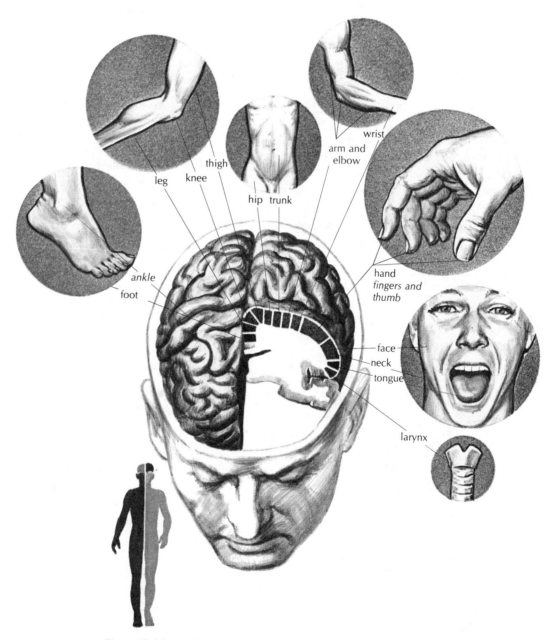

Figure 9-12
Each area of the brain has a specific job. (Memmler RL, Wood DL: The Human Body in Health and Disease, 6th ed, p 112. Philadelphia, JB Lippincott, 1987)

part of the brain is cut off or reduced, the cells in that part of the brain will not be able to work. This is what happens when a client has had a stroke. For more information on strokes, see Chapter 10.

The *nerves* are message pathways that branch off the spinal cord. The nerves allow messages to travel all over the body, sending information to and from the brain. For example, if you touch a hot iron, a message travels from the tip of your finger along the nerve pathways, up the spinal cord, and into the brain (Figure 9-13). The brain reacts by sending messages to the appropriate body parts so that you can pull your hand away from the heat. All of this happens very quickly. The time that it takes for the messages to travel to the brain and back is called *reaction time*. Reaction time is faster in young people than in older people. This means that an older adult cannot step on a car brake or pull his hand away from a hot iron as quickly as a younger adult can.

The soft *spinal cord* is located within the spinal column, which is also known as the *backbone*. The backbone protects the spinal cord, which is the main pathway for nerve messages to get to and from the brain. If the spinal cord is damaged, some body parts cannot send or receive informa-

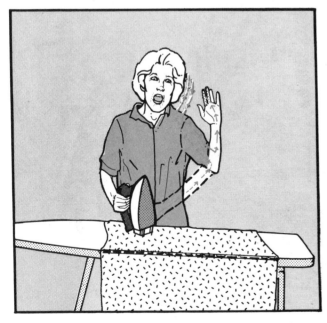

Figure 9-13
When this homemaker/home health aide touched the hot iron, an impulse traveled to her brain and back to her hand in a quick moment telling her to pull her hand away from the iron right away. This series of reactions happens very quickly and is part of the nervous system.

tion to or from the brain. A client who has had a spinal cord injury or a broken back may not be able to move his arms or legs, depending upon where the injury occurred on the spinal cord.

The Senses

Through the senses, we get information from inside and outside of the body. The eyes see objects. The ears hear sounds. The inner ear and muscles help us know the body's position and balance. The skin feels textures, pressures, and temperature (Figure 9-14). The tongue senses taste. The senses of hunger and thirst occur in several parts of the body.

Observations to Make About the Nervous System

Report the following problems to your supervisor.

- Problems with touch, sight, hearing, smell, or taste should be reported. Hearing and visual problems are often treatable. A sensory problem may be a sign of a more serious health problem. Sensory problems should always be reported to your supervisor.
- Report any seizures or convulsions to your supervisor. Epilepsy is another disorder of the nervous system. For emergency care of the client who has had a seizure, see Chapter 22.

Urinary System

The urinary system has two main jobs.

1. It removes waste products from the blood.
2. It maintains the water balance in the body.

The structures in the urinary system include two kidneys, two ureters, the bladder, and the urethra. Figure 9-15 shows the urinary system.

The *kidneys* are about 4 inches long, and are shaped like lima beans. They are located just above the waist and under the rib cage and back muscles. The kidneys filter the blood and produce urine.

The *ureters* carry the liquid waste products from the kidneys to the bladder.

The *bladder* is a holding tank for the urine. It is a thick muscular sac that has several layers. The bladder is quite small when empty. As the bladder fills with urine, the walls become thinner, just as a balloon does when it is filled with air.

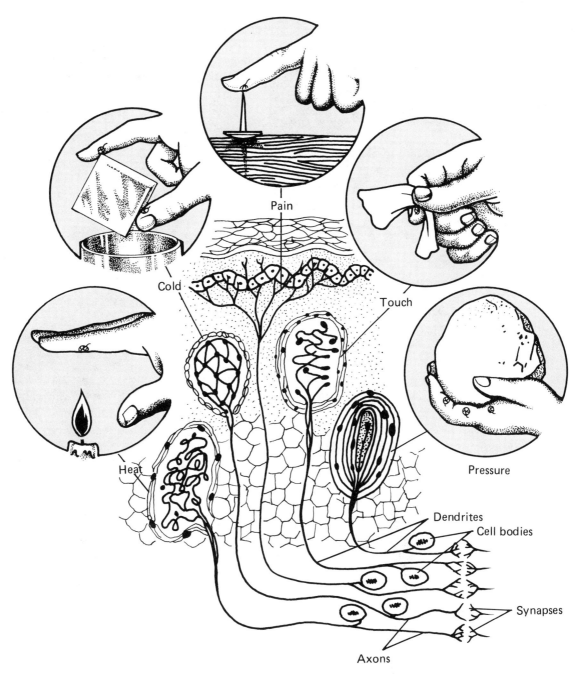

Pain

Cold

Touch

Heat

Pressure

Dendrites

Cell bodies

Synapses

Axons

Figure 9-14
This sketch shows examples of receptors in the skin that pick up sensations. The receptors are part of the nervous system. Their job is to carry messages to and from the brain. (Rosdahl CB: Textbook of Basic Nursing, 4th ed, p 116. Philadelphia, JB Lippincott, 1985)

The *urethra* is a tube that leads from the bladder and out of the body. During *urination*, urine is released from the bladder and travels down the urethra. The urethra is about 8 inches long in men, and 1½ inches long in women. Because women have a short urethra, it is easier for germs to get into the urinary system and cause infections.

During digestion, food is absorbed into the blood and carried to individual cells. Cells wastes are picked up by the blood and taken to the kidneys where the blood is filtered. These wastes leave the body as urine. Body wastes are also removed from the body as feces, as sweat, and during exhalation.

Observations to Make About the Urinary System

- You may be asked to keep records on how much fluid the client takes into his body and how much he voids (urinates). For more information on measuring intake and output, see Chapter 20.
- Note changes in the color of urine. Normally urine is light yellow and clear, but the color may change if the client is on medications. Urine should never have blood or sediments.
- The urine may need to be strained if a kidney stone is suspected.

Common Urinary Problems

Incontinence occurs when a client cannot control his bladder or bowels. Note whether the person releases large quantities of urine periodically, or dribbles small amounts throughout the day. Follow the bladder control program that your supervisor recommends. For more information on incontinence, see Chapter 18.

A more serious problem occurs if a person is unable to urinate for about 8 hours. If a client has not voided for a long period of time, the bladder becomes firm and distended, and can be felt above the pubic bone. Sometimes a client may dribble small amounts of urine, but retain most of it in the bladder. Running water may help the client void, but a problem with voiding should always be reported. If the client cannot void, a nurse may need to come to the house to catheterize the client. The HM/HHA is not licensed to catheterize a client. (See Chapter 18 for more information.)

Reproductive System

The purpose of the reproductive system is to create life. The male and female reproductive systems are different, so they will be discussed separately.

Male Reproductive System

A man's reproductive organs are inside and outside of his body (Figure 9-16). The *scrotum* is the sac located behind the penis. The scrotum contains the *testes*. The testes are the male sex glands, which produce sperm. *Sperm* is the male sex cell.

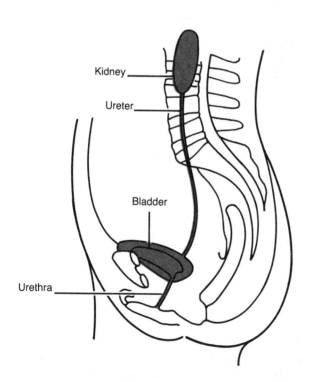
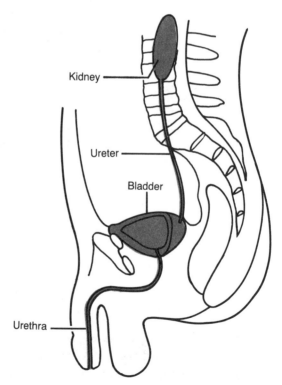

Figure 9-15

The female and male urinary tracts. (Wolff L, Weitzel MH, Zornow RA et al: Fundamentals of Nursing, 7th ed, p 550. Philadelphia, JB Lippincott, 1983)

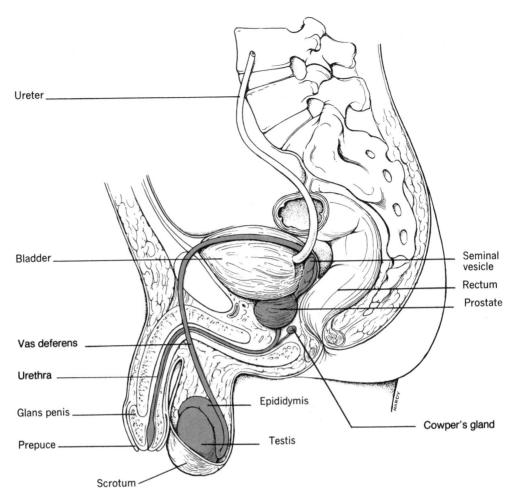

Ureter

Bladder

Vas deferens

Urethra

Glans penis

Prepuce

Scrotum

Seminal
vesicle

Rectum

Prostate

Epididymis

Cowper's gland

Testis

HARDY

Figure 9-16
The male reproductive system. (Rosdahl CB: Textbook of Basic Nursing, 4th ed, p 157.
Philadelphia, JB Lippincott, 1985)

When the testes produce sperm, it is stored in the *epididymis*, which is also located in the scrotum. The testes also produce hormones responsible for male sex characteristics such as facial hair, broad shoulders, and a deep voice.

During intercourse, millions of sperm cells travel in a fluid called *semen* through the *vas deferens* to the *urethra*. The urethra, located in the penis, is also used to empty urine from the bladder. (During intercourse, the opening from the bladder to the urethra closes tightly and urine cannot get into the semen.) The *prostate gland, seminal vesicles,* and the *Cowper's gland* produce fluid and nutrients for the sperm to swim in as it travels out of the body. At the same time, the *penis* erectile tissue fills with blood, becomes firm, gets larger, and releases the semen into the woman's vagina in a process known as *ejaculation*. The sperm then swim up into the woman's uterus and

fallopian tubes to unite with a female egg, if one is available.

The prostate gland is located below the bladder and it encircles the urethra. As men age, the prostate gland often enlarges and squeezes the urethra, making urination painful. Surgery is often needed. Many men fear this surgery will end their sex lives. This is not true. If a client expresses these fears, have him talk with his physician or nurse.

Female Reproductive System

The female reproductive organs are all internal (Figure 9-17). The two *ovaries* produce sex cells. The female sex cell is called the *egg* or *ovum*. The ovaries also produce the female sex hormones, which are responsible for female characteristics such as breasts and the ability to bear children.

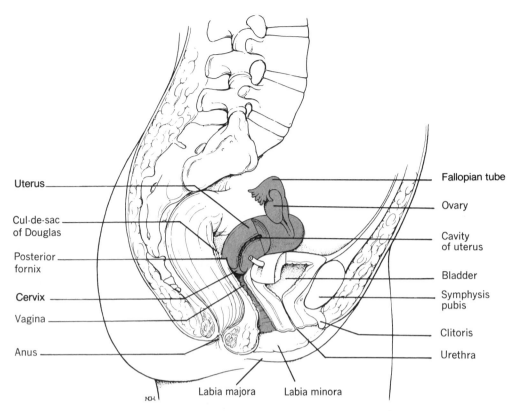

Labels on the figure:
Uterus
Cul-de-sac of Douglas
Posterior fornix
Cervix
Vagina
Anus
Labia majora
Labia minora
Fallopian tube
Ovary
Cavity of uterus
Bladder
Symphysis pubis
Clitoris
Urethra

Figure 9-17
The female reproductive system. (Rosdahl CB: Textbook of Basic Nursing, 4th ed, p 158. Philadelphia, JB Lippincott, 1985)

Although a man produces millions of sperm at a time, a women can produce only a single ovum each month. The *fallopian tubes* are the site of fertilization, and allow the egg to travel from the ovary to the uterus. The *uterus* is a muscular organ that is the size of a woman's fist. The uterus carries and protects the fertilized egg (fetus). The *cervix* is the opening of the uterus where sperm are deposited by the male during intercourse. The *vagina* is the stretchable opening that allows for the birth of an infant, and it is also the organ of sexual intercourse.

The Menstrual Cycle

The menstrual cycle is a process that women of childbearing age (from puberty to menopause, or approximately from ages 13 to 50 years) undergo each month to prepare for pregnancy. For most women, this cycle repeats itself every 28 days, although the cycle does vary among individuals. On day 1, the menstrual period begins when the bloody lining of the uterus is discharged. The lining continues to be released, and the woman bleeds for 2 to 6 days. As soon as the menstrual period has ceased, the lining of the uterus begins to rebuild in preparation for pregnancy.

Ovulation and Pregnancy

Even though the ovaries house many eggs, only one will be released midway through the menstrual cycle. The release of the egg is called *ovulation*. During ovulation, the egg begins the short journey through the *fallopian tubes*. If it unites with a single sperm, the egg becomes fertilized, implants itself in the lining of the uterus, and grows into a *fetus*, an unborn baby. The menstrual periods stop during the 9 months of pregnancy. If the egg does not meet a sperm, the egg disintegrates and passes out of the body. Normally only one egg is released from one ovary each month. If two eggs are released and fertilized, then *fraternal twins* will be produced. Fraternal twins share the same womb, but do not look alike. *Identical twins* are produced when a single egg is fertilized and divides into two identical pieces, which grow into two identical people.

Menopause

Between the ages of 45 to 55 years, a woman goes through *menopause*. Some people call this the "change of life." It is a normal part of development, when the ovaries no longer produce eggs and the menstrual periods become less regular and less frequent until they stop altogether. Naturally, the woman can no longer become pregnant. Sometimes women will experience dizziness, hot flashes, or other physical changes while their bodies are adjusting to this change. If your client asks you questions about these symptoms, talk with your supervisor, because they can often be treated with medication.

Endocrine System

The endocrine system is an unusual system because the various organs do not work together in the way that organs in other systems do. This system consists of separate glands, which produce and release substances that send messages to parts of the body (Figure 9-18).

Glands in the Endocrine System

Pituitary Gland. The pituitary gland is a small gland located under the brain. It has several functions. The pituitary gland influences growth; the thyroid gland; sperm production in men; ovula-

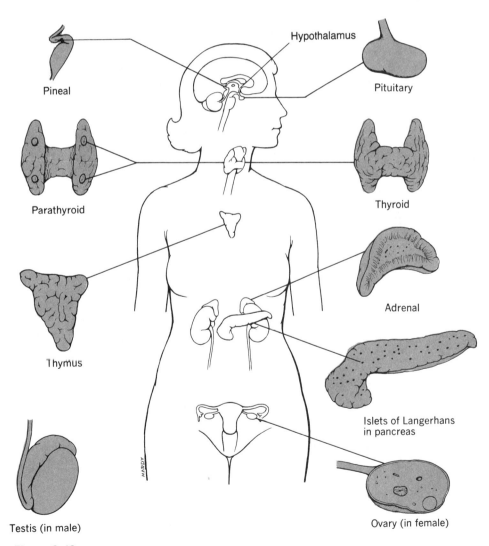

Figure 9-18
The glands of the endocrine system. (Rosdahl CB: Textbook of Basic Nursing, 4th ed, p 163. Philadelphia, JB Lippincott, 1985)

Summary of the Organ Systems

Organ	Purpose	Observations to Make
Skin	Covers the body; prevents infection; maintains temperature; regulates fluids; removes waste	Rashes, warts, sores or blisters, bunions, yellowing of skin, temperature, dry or oily
Skeletal	Gives the body a protective frame; supports muscles	Red or swollen joints; pain with movement
Muscular	Allows movement; generates heat for the body	Soreness or stiffness; strains or sprains; redness or swelling
Circulatory	Provides nutrients and oxygen to all the cells in the body; removes cell wastes; helps fight infection; controls temperature; controls fluid balance	Shortness of breath; tires easily; changes in vital signs; changes in skin color (pale or flushed); swollen lymph glands; edema
Respiratory	Takes oxygen into the body through inhalation; removes wastes through exhalation	Shortness of breath; excessive coughing; changes in the color or amount of mucus; hoarseness; nasal congestion
Digestive	Breaks food down so it can be used by cells for energy; removes waste	Nausea; indigestion; vomiting; diarrhea; changes in stools (blood, mucus, or consistency); changes in appetite; weight changes
Nervous	Picks up information; controls thought, movement, and other activities of the body	Difficulty hearing or seeing; loss of touch, smell, balance, or taste; confusion; loss of ability to move or control body
Urinary	Filters wastes from blood and produces urine; removes urine from the body; controls water balance; maintains temperature	Changes in color or contents of urine (blood or pus); inability to void; incontinence; change in frequency of urination
Reproductive	Reproduce the species	Refer questions about sexuality or the reproductive system to your supervisor
Endocrine	Each gland produces hormones that control different body functions.	

tion, uterine functions, and milk production after pregnancy in women; water and salt balance; and the body's reactions to stress.

Thyroid Gland.   The thyroid gland is located in the throat. It controls energy and metabolism, growth, mental functioning, and the amount of calcium in the blood. People who have too much thyroid hormone released into their systems will be jittery and nervous. Those whose thyroid is not producing enough will appear slow and lethargic.

Parathyroid Gland.   The parathyroid gland is located right behind the thyroid gland. It works with the thyroid to control the level of calcium in the blood and the bones.

Adrenal Glands.   The adrenal glands are located on the tops of the kidneys. They influence sexual characteristics, water and salt balance, the amount of minerals in the blood, and the stress responses. An inner part of the gland releases adrenaline, which gives the body extra energy when needed during times of stress.

Sex Glands.   The ovaries and testes produce the hormones that determine sexual characteristics, as discussed earlier in the section on the reproduction system. The ovaries and testes also produce the sex cells, the ovum, and sperm.

Pancreas.   The islets of Langerhans in the pancreas produce two hormones that control the blood sugar. The hormone *insulin* decreases the amount of sugar or glucose in the blood by helping the sugar enter the cells where it can be used for energy. Another hormone called *glucagon* stimulates the liver to release glucose into the blood so that the blood sugar is raised. Diabetes is one of the most common endocrine problems. It is discussed in Chapter 10.

Review Questions

True or False

1. ____ A decubitus ulcer (bedsore) can slow down the recovery of the client.

2. ____ When helping a client move, the major joints (hips, knees, elbows) should not be supported.

3. ____ When muscles are not used, they shrink and become weak very quickly.

4. ____ You notice that your client, Mrs. Peeples, has swollen ankles. You should have her put her feet up on a footstool and tell her not to cross her legs.

5. ____ A client with a respiratory illness may find it easier to sleep sitting up than lying down because it is easier to breathe.

Matching

Match the organ system on the right with its function.

6. ____ Produces new life.
7. ____ Each gland in this system produces hormones that control different body functions.
8. ____ Covers the body and prevents infections.
9. ____ Provides a frame for the body and supports muscles.
10. ____ Brings oxygen into the body through inhalation and removes carbon dioxide (a cell waste) through exhalation.
11. ____ Allows movement and generates heat for the body.
12. ____ Carries nutrients and oxygen to all the cells in the body and carries waste products away from the cells.
13. ____ Cleans and filters the blood and produces urine. Removes urine from the body.
14. ____ Breaks food down so it can be used by the body for energy, growth, and development. This system also removes wastes.
15. ____ Picks up information and processes it so the body will know what to do. Responsible for thinking, movement, and other body activities.

A. Skeletal
B. Reproductive
C. Muscular
D. Endocrine
E. Circulatory
F. Digestive
G. Respiratory
H. Skin
I. Nervous
J. Urinary

Chapter 10

Common Health Problems

Objectives

At the conclusion of this chapter, the homemaker/ home health aide will:

1. Understand what happens to the client who has Alzheimer's disease and will be able to explain the kinds of things the HM/HHA may be expected to do when caring for the client.

2. Understand what diabetes is and what the HM/HHA may be asked to do for the client with diabetes.

3. Know what may happen to the client who has had a stroke and describe the kind of care the HM/HHA may be asked to provide.

4. Know how to use the Quick Reference Chart for Common Health Problems at the end of the chapter.

In your job as a homemaker/home health aide, you will care for clients who have many different kinds of health problems. Some clients will have only one health problem and others will have many. This chapter will explain Alzheimer's disease, diabetes, and stroke in detail. It also provides a more general quick reference chart for other health problems that you are likely to encounter while working as a HM/HHA.

Alzheimer's Disease

Alzheimer's disease is a gradual loss of mental abilities. A client with this disease will have a loss of memory, an inability to think clearly, and a decline of physical abilities. Alzheimer's is not a normal part of aging and is not caused by a personality flaw, but by physical changes in the brain. It may comfort families to know there is a physical cause for this disease. There is no cure for Alzheimer's. Only a physician can determine if a person has Alzheimer's.

Generally, Alzheimer's disease begins after age 65, but it can happen at any age. It affects 5% of those over 65, and over 2 million Americans have it. The client with Alzheimer's may live only a few years or up to 20 years, but the disease always causes mental deterioration and the inability to care for oneself.

Portrait of a Client With Alzheimer's Disease

Early in the disease, a person with Alzheimer's may forget things. He may forget not just the name of a person he's just met, but where he is and why he's there. Then, the client's behavior, personality, and ability to make judgments will change. The client may realize he is not all right. He may confuse the hot and cold faucets in the shower or put on a winter coat in the summer. Or he may forget personal information such as where he went to school. Physical movements will slow down and become less coordinated.

Later, he will not remember his own phone number or address. Even when the client has been badly affected by the disease, he may keep skills that were important to him. For example, a musician may not be able to tell you his address, but he might be able to play some of his favorite pieces on the piano. Eventually, the client may not know his spouse's name and will need help with everything he does (dressing, meals, making decisions, and so on.) In the end the client cannot talk, walk, or function.

Loss of Memory and Problems With Thinking

An early sign of Alzheimer's disease is forgetfulness, but not the kind that people experience daily. A person who has Alzheimer's may forget the names of friends, parts of recent conversations, or how to do simple tasks.

Language and Speech

The client may not understand you. When you say, "It is 1:30 in the afternoon," he may hear your words, but not understand their meaning. You may have trouble understanding him. Your client may make up phrases or speak in unclear and incomplete sentences. Ask the client what his words and phrases mean. ("Does noise ringer mean doorbell?") Use the phrases he uses when talking with him. Use simple words and short sentences. Give the client time to respond to your questions or comments. Communicate nonverbally with a smile or a touch on the arm. Look directly at him when talking, and point to objects or gesture with your hands to help him understand.

Physical Changes

The family may tell you the client's handwriting has changed or that his walk has changed. You may also notice that the client has a blank look. His movements may be slow and uncoordinated. Over time, he will be unable to do his own personal care and will not be able to live alone. Your supervisor or an occupational therapist may have ideas about how to help the client adapt or learn a new skill. But with declining mental ability, the client will have trouble learning new skills.

The Role of the Homemaker/Home Health Aide

Develop a Warm, Trusting Relationship With the Client

- Try to stay calm and relaxed when you are with a client who has Alzheimer's disease. Use a quiet voice and avoid sudden movements, especially when you first meet.
- Explain what you are about to do before you do anything. This will help make the client feel safe.
- Keep a consistent routine for the client. Schedule meals, activities, and rest periods at the same time each day.
- Use eye contact and a light touch on the arm when talking.
- Reassure the client when he is frightened. Tell him you care about him and want to keep him safe.
- Let him know that you do not mind repeating things and that you will keep explaining things when he forgets.
- When you leave the house, tell the client you enjoyed being with him and that you look forward to seeing him again.

Safety

Always be alert for potential safety problems for the client who is confused. He may wander out of the house in the night or forget that people cannot drink household poisons. He may forget to turn off the stove or other appliances. You may have safety suggestions that the family has not thought of, like sewing address labels in the clothes of a client who likes to wander. (For more on general safety, see Chapter 12.)

Maintain the Client's Skills With Meaningful Activities

One of the main goals of care is to help the client with Alzheimer's keep skills he already has. You may be assigned to a client to help remind him how to care for himself, not to do the work for him. Work with your supervisor and the family to find simple activities the client can do that will be meaningful to him. If he likes to garden, watering the flowers or planting seeds indoors may interest him. Watching television is not helpful because the client is not working to maintain his skills.

The client may realize he is not able to do much, and may appreciate doing something for someone else. You might have him make two cups of tea, one for each of you. To help a client get the tea, explain each step. Praise each step that he completes successfully.

HM/HHA   "First we need to go to the kitchen." (HM/HHA leads client to the kitchen.)

HM/HHA   "OK, now get a cup from the cupboard."

Client   "I forget what I was doing."

HM/HHA   "That's all right. You were going to make a cup of tea for each of us. We need two cups from that cupboard."

Client   "Oh, that's right. I'll get the cups."

HM/HHA   "Good. Now get two teabags from the box on the counter . . . "

Personal Care

The client may need help with personal care. Have the client get dressed every day. Wearing pajamas all day tends to make people feel they are not well. Put powder and lipstick on a woman who is used to wearing makeup, and help a man to shave. Compliment the client on his clothes. The client with Alzheimer's, like anyone else, may have trouble accepting help with activities that he has always done privately. For example, it may take longer to use the toilet if someone else is in the room. Allow time and show understanding for the client's situation.

Understanding Problems With Thinking, Judgment, and Decision Making

The client may forget that he cannot do all the things he used to do. Some activities, such as using a sharp knife, may be dangerous for him. Do not take the client's word when he tells you what he can and cannot do. Follow the care plan strictly as you would with any other client. For clients who have trouble making decisions, keep the choices simple. Ask the client, "Would you like to wear your blue shirt or your green shirt today?" instead of "What do you want to wear today?" Use large notes to remind the client to turn off the stove or what to say when he answers the telephone.

Dealing With Emotional Outbursts

A client with Alzheimer's can become extremely upset when he is overwhelmed. Too much noise, too many questions, and too much to do can all frustrate and confuse the client. A man who can't tie his shoes may scream and cry. The client does not have these outbursts on purpose. He may say offensive things to you or someone in the family and then forget he said them. ("You're not helping me" or "I hate you.") It will be hard not to take his comments personally and difficult to convince the family that he does not mean what he says. You may be able to avoid extreme reactions by getting to know the client well enough so that you know when he is getting tired or overstimulated.

To calm the client, take him away from the upsetting situation. Turn off the loud music or have the client leave a crowded room. Then, sit down with the client and hold his hand. Speak quietly and stay calm. When you become upset, that can only make the client even more upset. If you feel yourself getting upset, take a deep breath and remind yourself that a person with this disease has little control over his emotions. If a client ever becomes physically combative, keep your distance and do not try to interfere.

Food

The client must eat a well-balanced diet and drink plenty of fluids. There are no foods that will cure Alzheimer's, but poor nutrition might make the client more confused. The client may have trouble eating. He may forget how to cut his food or may not have the coordination to do so. A messy eater can use an apron as a bib. Some clients will forget that they have eaten 5 minutes after a meal. For those who like to nibble all day, leave carrots and crackers out. Others do not want to eat at all. Your supervisor will have suggestions for individual clients. (For more on nutrition, see Chapter 15.)

Home Management

A clean, uncluttered house is safer and easier for the client with Alzheimer's disease to live in. It will be easier for him to know where things are and it will help to avoid accidents.

Working With the Family

The HM/HHA is often assigned to give the family some time off. Alzheimer's is a frightening disease, and families usually need a lot of support and encouragement. Even families who are providing excellent care may feel they are not doing enough. Let the family express their feelings and frustrations. Toward the end of the illness the client will need so much care that the family may consider a nursing home. Your supervisor will have information that will help the family make an informed decision. Tell your supervisor when this issue or other serious issues arise.

Taking Care of Yourself

Working with a client with Alzheimer's can be rewarding when you have developed trust, have helped the client participate in meaningful activities, and are able to calm the client when needed. But it can also be very demanding. Although it is good for the client to have the same caregiver over a period of time, it is recommended that an individual HM/HHA work no more than 4 hours per day and 3 days per week with a client who has Alzheimer's disease.

Diabetes Mellitus

What Is Diabetes?

Diabetes mellitus is a serious disease that occurs when the body does not produce or does not use insulin normally. Insulin is a hormone produced in the pancreas that is needed to convert sugars and starches into energy for the cells to use. Without insulin, sugar stays in the blood, causing a condition known as *hyperglycemia* or *high blood sugar.*

Types of Diabetes

There are two basic types of diabetes, type I diabetes and type II diabetes.

Type I diabetes is also known as *insulin-dependent diabetes*. It was formerly called *juvenile onset diabetes* because it usually begins in childhood. Treatment includes insulin shots as well as careful meal planning and exercise programs. With type I diabetes, the pancreas is not producing any insulin, so the insulin must be replaced.

Type II diabetes is also known as *noninsulin-dependent diabetes*. It was formerly called *adult onset diabetes*. Type II diabetes is more common than type I diabetes. It occurs most often in people who are over 40 years old and overweight. With type II diabetes, the pancreas produces insulin, but not very efficiently. Most clients do not have to take insulin shots because they can control their diabetes through diet, exercise, and sometimes oral medications that stimulate the pancreas to produce more insulin.

How Diabetes Is Detected

Diabetes, like any other illness, can only be diagnosed by a doctor. If diabetes is suspected, a blood test will be done. In recent years there has been a greater push to inform the public about the signs and symptoms of diabetes. This has allowed more people to recognize the early signs of the disease and seek treatment from their doctors. The classic signs and symptoms of diabetes include:

- increased thirst,
- increased need to urinate,
- fatigue,
- unexplained weight loss,
- a sore that heals slowly, and
- sugar in the urine.

Urine Testing

Urine testing is a method of estimating the blood sugar level and the amount of ketones in the blood. Some clients have a special instrument that allows them to perform a home blood test with just a drop of blood. Urine testing is not as accurate as a blood test, but it is an inexpensive and simple procedure. While most diabetics will check only for glucose (sugar), occasionally they will check for ketones, too. *Ketones* are produced when fat is used by the body for energy. Usually most of the energy we use comes from carbohydrates.

Diabetic Emergencies	
Insulin Shock	Also called hypoglycemia or diabetic shock.
Cause	Two much insulin and not enough food
Reaction	Confused, pale, nervous, weak, hungry, dizzy, sweats, and may become unconscious. Anytime a client who takes insulin behaves unusually, assume it is due to an insulin reaction and give the client some sugar.
Treatment by HM/HHA	Give sugar, candy, or orange juice and follow with a cracker or piece of bread. Call for help.
Diabetic Ketoacidosis	Also called hyperglycemia or diabetic acidosis.
Cause	Too little insulin
Reaction	Loss of appetite, heavy labored breathing, fruity breath, abdominal pains, and flushed dry skin. Will go into a coma without treatment.
Treatment by HM/HHA	Call for help.

People who are dieting will have ketones in their urine, and that is normal. But when a type I or insulin-dependent diabetic has ketones in his urine, it could be a serious problem that may need medical attention.

The client who needs to test his urine will have his own test kit. Usually the client will test his own urine, but if you ever help, read the directions carefully. The kits usually contain a chemically treated plastic strip with a patch on the end that changes color when dipped into fresh urine. To read the strip, match the patch with the color strip on the bottle (Figure 10-1). The timing on these tests is very important. Be sure to read the directions carefully before you start and time the procedure with the sweep hand of your watch.

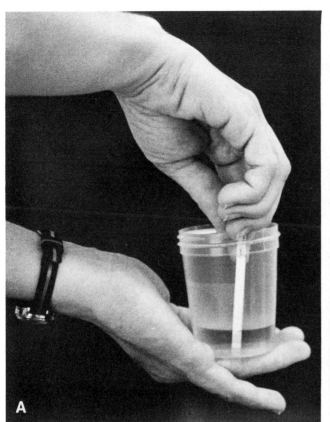

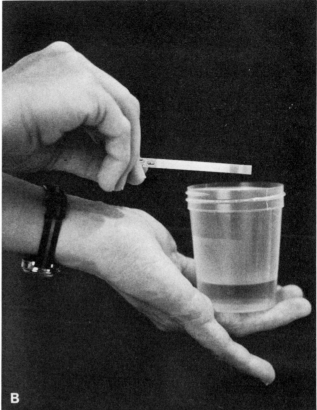

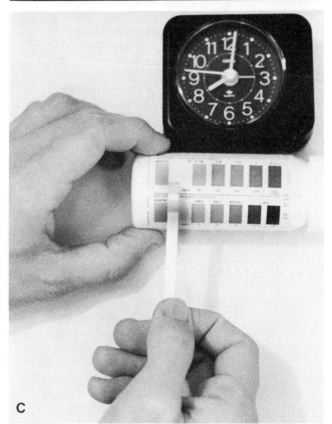

Figure 10-1
Testing urine for glucose and acetone. (*A*) Step One: Without touching the end of the dipstick, dip the plastic stick into the urine so that the patches at the end are covered. (*B*) Step Two: Remove the dipstick and tap it gently on the side of the container to remove excess urine. (*C*) Step Three: Compare the dipstick patch to the color chart. This procedure must be timed carefully to get an accurate result.

Complications of Diabetes

Complication	Description of Complication
Infection	Because of the disease process and poor circulation, diabetics are at high risk for infections. Sores and cuts should be treated promptly. The feet need daily attention to prevent infection.
Vascular complications	One of the more serious complications is that the circulatory system becomes less efficient and affects every organ in the body.
Neuropathy	Neuropathy is a disorder where nerves are damaged from the high levels of glucose in the blood over a long period of time. This causes pain, tingling, numbness, and loss of sensation, especially in the hands and feet. Safety precautions such as wearing shoes or slippers, and testing bathwater before getting in the tub will help prevent accidents.
Retinopathy	High blood sugar levels may cause serious eye problems and loss of vision. Good diabetic control in the early years may help slow the damage to the eyes.
Atherosclerosis	Atherosclerosis occurs when fatty deposits collect on the large vessel walls and block or cut off the flow of blood. Diabetics are more prone to atherosclerosis than a healthy person.

Treatment and Care of the Client With Diabetes

Medical experts can treat and control the symptoms of diabetes, but there is no cure. Diabetes is a lifelong illness. Treatment involves diet planning, exercise programs, and prescribed medications. Treatment is individual and must be supervised by a doctor. It is important to support the client and help him realize that keeping his diabetes in control now will make a difference in his health 20 years from now.

Diet

Diet is the cornerstone in the treatment of diabetes. Sometimes diabetes can be controlled by diet alone. Most people do not like diets, so imagine how difficult it can be for the client who must follow a strict diet that may include eating at certain times each day and weighing portions of foods for the rest of his life.

The doctor and dietitian or nurse will consider the client's age, sex, weight, activity level, meal patterns, food preferences, and state of health before planning a diet. The main goals of diet therapy are to provide adequate nutrition for health, to maintain or attain an ideal body weight, and to keep the blood sugar within normal limits.

Many clients follow a *diabetic exchange list* that has been recommended by the doctor. The exchange list divides nutritious foods into six categories (milk, breads, vegetables, fruits, meats, and fats) and then lists foods that can be substituted for one another. A client who knows he can have a fruit exchange for a snack can look at the fruit category to see the different fruits that are acceptable and the amount that is considered a single serving. On a typical exchange list, the client who would like to eat some kind of apple would see that he could have either 1 small apple, or ½ cup applesauce, or ⅓ cup apple juice. Find out about the diet that your client is following. Your client will have the complete diabetic exchange list from his doctor if he follows the exchange diet.

Foot Care

Due to circulatory problems, the diabetic needs to be particularly careful about his feet. The client with diabetes does not have a good sense of feeling and is prone to infections. He may not notice an infected sore on the bottom of his foot until he sees it. Follow the Guidelines for Foot Care.

Guidelines for Foot Care

1. Feet should be washed daily with a mild soap without soaking for very long. Rinse well and use a clean, dry, soft towel to dry the entire foot gently, making sure to get between the toes (Figure 10-2).
2. While washing the feet, inspect them carefully for small sores or blisters. The client may find it helpful to use a small mirror when checking his feet. Blisters may mean that the shoes are too tight. If there are sores, report this to your supervisor so they can be treated.
3. To prevent cracks in dry skin, a lanolin lotion or petroleum jelly should be applied. Dusting powder can be used if the feet are sweaty.
4. Your client should be encouraged to keep his feet warm and protected. He should wear well-fitting shoes or slippers with white cotton socks. Cotton absorbs moisture, keeps the feet warm, and is not irritating. Mended socks, garters, or anything else that will irritate the skin should be avoided. Clean socks should be worn every day.
5. Shoes with low heels and closed toes are safest. New shoes should be broken in slowly. On the first day, they should be worn only for a half hour. On the second day, wear them for 1 hour. On the third day, they can be worn for 2 hours. Double the time every day until the shoes are comfortable. This will help prevent blisters.
6. Do not cut the toenails of a client with diabetes. This should be done by a nurse or doctor. You may be assigned to file the nails. File them straight across to prevent an ingrown toenail.
7. Discourage the use of heating pads or electric blankets. A hot water bottle wrapped in a towel and loose bed socks will keep the feet warm at night.
8. Follow your care plan directions carefully. Encourage your client to seek medical advice for foot problems.

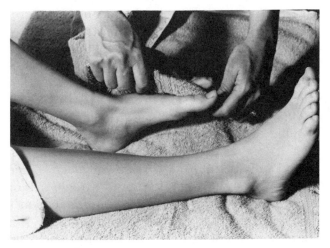

Figure 10-2
After washing the feet, dry between the toes carefully to prevent skin irritation.

Exercise Programs

The client should not begin an exercise program without consulting his doctor. The client may need to adjust his insulin or diet when beginning or changing exercise programs. Daily exercise is encouraged for most clients, but the amount and kind of exercise must be carefully monitored by the doctor.

Medication

When a client cannot produce enough insulin, it may need to be given by injection. Most clients give themselves their own shots or have a nurse or family member give it. The HM/HHA is not allowed to give an insulin shot, but it is helpful to know the amount and kind of insulin your client is taking in case there is a health emergency. Insulin should be stored away from heat and sunlight, in a cool dry place.

The second type of medication that is commonly used is called an *oral hypoglycemic agent*. It comes in the form of a pill. Many clients think they are taking insulin orally, but it is not insulin. This medication is used by people with type II diabetes because it stimulates the pancreas to produce more insulin. Because people with type I diabetes cannot produce insulin, oral agents cannot be used.

Social and Emotional Support

Having a lifelong disease naturally causes emotional stress. Keep in mind that even though a client may look fine, it is not normal for a person to have to watch his diet, check his urine, or give himself an injection each day. The diabetic client needs support. If it appears your client or a member of his family is unusually depressed, let your supervisor know so the home care team can offer appropriate assistance.

Stroke

What Is a Stroke?

A *stroke* may also be called a *cerebral vascular accident* (CVA). A stroke occurs when an area of the brain does not get the blood it needs because of a blocked or ruptured blood vessel. Blockage can occur from a blood clot or from fatty deposits that collect in the lining of the blood vessel. When blood and oxygen are cut off from a part of the brain, the brain cells in that area will be damaged. Each part of the brain has a different job. How the client is affected by the stroke depends upon where the damage to the brain occurred. A stroke can affect voluntary movement, sensations (temperature, touch, pressure), memory, emotions, and communication. Stroke victims may have one-sided weakness or paralysis. *Paralysis* is the inability to move.

The client will receive his initial care in the hospital where the rehabilitation program begins. It is nearly impossible to predict how much progress a stroke victim will make after he returns home. Never promise anything about the success of a rehabilitation program, because it will be extremely discouraging for the client and family if your promises for recovery are not met. Treatment programs will vary considerably between stroke clients based on their condition and individual needs.

A stroke is a frightening experience for both the client and the family. The care plan may have suggested tasks for the family so they can learn to do procedures correctly. Most families want to stay involved in the care, but a HM/HHA may be assigned to give the family some time off.

The Role of the Homemaker/Home Health Aide

Build Confidence and Self-Esteem

Encourage the client to follow the exercises and activities prescribed by the doctor. Progress may be slow, but succeeding at these activities will help the client regain physical strength, self-confidence, and independence. Your genuine understanding and support for the client can help keep his spirits up. Attitude plays a large part in recovery. An uncooperative client who is discouraged may need your encouragement and support even more than a severely disabled client who accepts his condition. To accent the positive, talk about the client's accomplishments and strengths, not his limitations.

Working With Communication Problems

A client may have slurred speech and trouble talking if the muscles in his mouth and face are affected by the stroke. Another common problem is aphasia. *Aphasia* is the loss of the ability to communicate. Aphasia is most often caused by a stroke.

The client with *expressive aphasia* can understand written and spoken words, but cannot express himself. He knows what he wants to say, but he cannot find the words or say the words he wants to use. Because the client cannot communicate well, it is common for people to assume he has lost the ability to think. This is not the case. Some clients are able to speak slowly and not very clearly. Encourage the client to talk because practicing does help. Do not correct mistakes he makes while talking, because that is likely to discourage the client. Those who cannot talk may be able to write or to communicate by pointing to letters and pictures.

Receptive aphasia occurs when the client has trouble understanding what you are saying. To him, it may seem as though everyone around him is suddenly speaking a foreign language. Some clients will be able to understand written words or short, simple phrases. Gestures and pictures may also be used. You do not need to talk louder, just more slowly. You may need to repeat yourself and allow enough time for the client to respond. Listening to excessive chatter can be frustrating and confusing for the client with this problem.

Clients who have difficulty speaking may have a speech therapist. The therapist and your supervisor will let you know other ways to help communication. Here are some suggestions to aid communication.

- Talk to the client, not above his head to someone else. Let the client know that you believe he can understand you, even if he has trouble speaking.
- Use touch, gestures, a communication board, or flip cards with words and pictures to communicate with your client.
- If client is able to write, provide a thick, easy-to-hold pen and some paper.
- Ask questions that have "yes" or "no" answers.
- Leave a call bell within reach. The client must be able to call for help if he is left alone, even for a minute. Place a bell on the client's lap or someplace within reach.
- Keep hearing aid, glasses, a clock, and a calendar within sight and within reach.
- For more on communication, see Chapter 2.

Understanding Loss of Movement and Sensation

One of the most common problems for a stroke victim is that one side of the body may become weakened or paralyzed (unable to move voluntarily). Sometimes just an arm or leg is affected. It may help the client to know that most people who become paralyzed or lose muscle control will regain some of it when they follow the prescribed exercises. Still, rehabilitation is a tremendous amount of work. A right-handed client who becomes paralyzed on his right side after a stroke will need to learn how to do everything with his left hand.

Many safety problems can occur if a client experiences the loss of feeling or sensation on one side of the body. Unless the client looks, he may not be able to tell you where his weak arm is. When in a wheelchair, he may not be able to tell if his foot has fallen off the footrest. Remind your client to check the position of his weak arm or leg periodically. Many stroke victims with a loss of feeling have been badly burned without knowing it by leaning on a hot stove or touching a hot iron.

Positioning

Good positioning is important because it prevents pain, stiffness, contractures, swelling, fatigue, and bedsores. The client who cannot reposition himself must be turned and repositioned every 2 hours. Check the skin for redness and signs of skin breakdown each time the client is turned. Follow the positioning guidelines on the care plan. For more on positioning, see Chapter 16. For more on skin care, see Chapter 18.

Be Aware of Problems With Swallowing

If the client has lost feeling or muscle control in one half of his mouth and throat, swallowing can be difficult. To avoid choking, have the client take a small bite of food and place it on the stronger side of his mouth. He should chew the food well and hold his breath while he swallows. This helps prevent food from going down the windpipe. The client may find it easier to swallow if he is told to concentrate on swallowing as he swallows. Liquids should be taken only in small sips. It may help to have the client tip his head toward the stronger side so the liquid will go down easier.

Prevent Fatigue

Even the smallest tasks seem to make the stroke victim tired. This can be frustrating and discouraging. Allow the client adequate rest periods. Let him know that getting tired is normal because of the changes his body is going through. Your reassurance will help the client and family feel better.

Follow Activity and Exercise Instructions

The client should not do any exercises that are not approved by his doctor. Range of motion (ROM) exercises may be ordered by the doctor to stimulate circulation and to keep the muscles in good tone. For more on ROM exercises, see Chapter 16.

Common Health Problems

The following chart will give you a basic understanding of the client's health problem and the role of the HM/HHA. It is only a general guide. It should never replace the instructions for an individual client that are given to you by your supervisor.

Quick Reference Chart for Common Health Problems

Acquired Immune Deficiency Syndrome (AIDS)

The job of the immune system is to fight disease. When a person becomes infected with the AIDS virus, the immune system weakens and cannot fight common germs that a healthy person could fight easily. AIDS is a fatal disease that is growing rapidly among all people, although it is most often associated with homosexuals and drug abusers who share needles.

Treatment

No cure. AIDS is a relatively new disease that is spreading rapidly. Medical experts are working hard to find a cure, but that may take several years. The goals of care for the HM/HHA are to prevent infections, provide comfort, and give emotional support.

HM/HHA Care

1. HM/HHAs will not get AIDS by caring for a client who has AIDS or who carries the AIDS virus. In most cases, AIDS is spread through sexual intercourse or exposure to the blood. The Centers for Disease Control recommend that health care workers use appropriate precautions such as gloves or masks whenever "contact with blood or other body fluids of any patient is anticipated."
2. Always use good handwashing techniques.

Alzheimer's Disease

See pages 87 to 89.

Arthritis

Inflammation (swelling) of the joints. There are hundreds of kinds of arthritis. Joints may be painful, warm, red, and stiff, and have limited movement. Fingers can become permanently disfigured.

Treatment

No cure. Medications, prescribed exercises, heat therapy, and bedrest may be ordered by the doctor to control the symptoms. The goal of care is to relieve pain and prevent deformity.

HM/HHA Care

1. Follow the care plan and keep the client comfortable.
2. If client is on bedrest, good skin care is needed to prevent bedsores. (See Chapter 20.)
3. Range of motion exercises may be prescribed. (See Chapter 16.)
4. Encourage a good diet to promote healing. (See Chapter 15.)
5. Provide emotional support.

Cancer

Cells that grow abnormally and form masses are called *tumors*. If the tumor is not cancerous, it is *benign*. When cancer is present, the tumor is *malignant*. Cancer warning signs include a sore that does not heal; a lump or thickening under the skin; a change in a wart or a mole; trouble with swallowing or indigestion; hoarseness or a cough that does not get better; a change in bowel or bladder habits. A person with any of these problems should see a doctor.

Treatment

Cancer can be treated using surgery, radiation, or chemotherapy. These treatments can be given alone or in combination.

HM/HHA Care

This disease is very trying both physically and emotionally. It takes a special person to provide home care for the cancer client. This disease can differ so much between clients you'll need to follow the care plan written for your particular client carefully. Good nutrition (Chapter 15) is always important and good listening

(continued)

Quick Reference Chart for Common Health Problems *(continued)*

	will be a valuable skill. (See Chapter 2.) When the client or family has questions you can't answer, talk to your supervisor to let him know of their concerns.
Cataracts	When the lens of the eye gradually clouds over making it difficult for the client to see, this is a cataract. Generally, cataracts strike people over the age of 65.
Treatment	There are several different types of surgery to treat cataracts.
HM/HHA Care	When the client has limited vision, the HM/HHA may be assigned to assist with meals, do light housekeeping, and help with bathing and other personal care activities. Safety will be a prime concern. (See Chapters 5 and 12.)
Colds or Viruses	The client may have a high fever, a runny nose, trouble breathing, aching muscles, and coughing spells.
Treatment	Bedrest, plenty of fluids, medications as prescribed (may include oxygen or a vaporizer)
HM/HHA Care	1. Take vital signs as directed. (See Chapter 17.) 2. Encourage fluids and a nutritious diet (Chapter 15). 3. Good handwashing and keeping the house clean will help prevent the spread of germs. (See Chapter 13.)
Chronic Obstructive Pulmonary Disease (COPD)	COPD is a term for several kinds of lung diseases (asthma, bronchitis, and emphysema). Your client may have pain, difficulty breathing, and coughing spells, and he will tire easily.
Treatment	Smokers will be encouraged to stop smoking. Oxygen treatments may be necessary

	to aid breathing. The client will need to avoid crowds and situations where he could get a respiratory infection.
HM/HHA Care	1. Support for the client who has given up smoking. Discourage family and friends from smoking near client to keep the air clean. 2. Follow instructions on the care plan regarding activity levels. These clients may tire very easily. Do not overdo activities. 3. Client may find it easier to breathe sitting up in a chair. 4. Use good handwashing. (See Chapter 13.) Client will be more susceptible to infections.
Deafness	Deafness means a total loss of hearing. Hard of hearing (HOH) is a limited loss of hearing. Deafness may occur gradually with aging or suddenly during an injury or illness.
Treatment	Usually a hearing aid is prescribed, although sometimes surgery may be used.
HM/HHA Care	1. Speak clearly, but do not shout. 2. Allow the client to see your lips so he may lipread. 3. Help with the care, cleaning, and operation of the hearing aid after you've been instructed about the model your client uses. 4. Learn to adjust the volume on a hearing aid. Turning the volume up all the way may make the sound distorted, so turning the volume down a little may help. 5. See Chapter 5 on aging for more information on sensory losses.
Diabetes Mellitus	See pages 89 to 94.

(continued)

Quick Reference Chart for Common Health Problems *(continued)*

Fractures/Broken Bones	A fracture is a broken bone. A fracture may occur after a fall or accident. Pain, bruises, and swelling may occur. Older clients are more likely to have fractures because of their brittle bones.
Treatment	Casts, metal pins, or joint replacements are all used to treat fractures depending on the location of the broken bone.
HM/HHA Care	1. Check cast for unusual signs (pain, blood stains, foul odor, or swelling in fingers and toes). 2. Note and report color (warm/pink or cold/bluish) and sensations (numbness, tingling) in the fingers or toes beyond the cast. 3. Follow positioning directions given by your supervisor or physical therapist. For swelling, elevate the limb and phone the supervisor. 4. Keep the cast clean and dry. For more on cast care, see Chapter 20.
Glaucoma	Glaucoma is caused by high fluid pressure within the eye. Glaucoma is painful, can develop slowly or quickly, and can cause partial or total blindness if not treated. It occurs more often in people over age 40.
Treatment	No cure, but symptoms can be controlled with medication.
HM/HHA Care	1. Assist with personal care as instructed. 2. Give support and assist in client's adjustment to changes in vision.
Recovering From a Heart Attack	When the blood supply is cut off from an area of the heart muscle, the heart tissue will die. This is called a heart attack or myocardial infarction.
Treatment	The client may need to stop smoking, lose weight, eat less salt and fat, and decrease stress. A client who is recovering from a heart attack will have an exercise program that increases gradually. The exercise plan is prescribed by the doctor.
HM/HHA Care	1. Follow the care plan. 2. Assist client with the activities prescribed by the doctor as instructed on the care plan. 3. Report to your supervisor if the client appears to be doing too much. This can damage the heart further. The doctor or nurse may need to explain the treatment plan to the client again. 4. Support the client. He's been through a frightening experience. It will be difficult for him to change habits (smoking, diet, activities) that he has lived with for years. 5. See Chapter 22 for emergency information.
Heart Diseases	There are many types of heart disease, including congestive heart failure, coronary emboli, and coronary artery occlusion. The client may have chest pain, difficulty breathing, and cold feet and hands because the blood is not circulating properly. In addition, clients will tire easily and may have pain when breathing.
Treatment	The doctor may prescribe medications, oxygen, bedrest, or activity limitations and a low-salt diet.
HM/HHA Care	1. Take vital signs as ordered (Chapter 17). Report changes to the supervisor. 2. Note and report any changes in client (swelling, color, level of pain, breathing patterns). Have *(continued)*

**Quick Reference Chart for Common
Health Problems** *(continued)*

the client sit up if he has
shortness of breath or if
breathing becomes
difficult.

3. Assist the client and
family with meal planning.
(see Chapter 15.)

High Blood Pressure/ Hypertension	Hypertension means that the blood pressure is too high after several readings. This puts stress on the arteries and heart. The American Heart Association says that blood pressure is too high if it is over 140/90 for those under age 40 or over 160/90 for those over age 40. Only a doctor can diagnose hypertension.
Treatment	A change in lifestyle including one or all of the following is recommended: lose weight, stop smoking, eat less salt and fatty foods, eat a well-balanced diet, exercise, and lower stress. Medication may be required, too.
HM/HHA Care	1. Help client adjust to lifestyle changes as instructed by supervisor. For example, you may help teach ways to cook enjoyable meals that are low in fat and salt. (See Chapter 15.) 2. It may be appropriate for you to help remind the client to take medication. 3. If you are asked to take the blood pressure, you will be instructed when to contact your supervisor.
Pain and Discomfort	Because of cultural background or personality, many clients will not tell you when they are in pain. You want to know so you can help the client. Signs of pain include tense facial expression (clenched jaw, frowning, and anxious look), uncooperativeness, or restlessness.
Treatment	The HM/HHA is not licensed to give medications, but there are often better ways to treat pain than using medication. Give a backrub, listen while the client talks, help the client get repositioned comfortably, have the client wash his face and brush his teeth.
HM/HHA Care	1. Ask direct questions such as "Are you uncomfortable?" "Does your leg hurt?" "Is something hurting you?" "Does it itch?" 2. Keep the client calm. Look at the client while you talk to him calmly and clearly. 3. Hold his hand or touch his arm to reassure him. 4. Ask him what has helped him in the past such as repositioning, a backrub, or a nap. Then reassure the client and say "Now this will make you feel more comfortable" as you give the backrub. 5. Let your supervisor know when the client complains of discomfort.
Parkinson's Disease	The client may have tremors (shaky hands), lean forward and shuffle his feet when walking, and have a blank, expressionless look on his face. There is a gradual loss of muscle control with this disease. The physical deterioration may be striking, but the client will maintain his ability to think and understand others.
Treatment	Medications as prescribed by a doctor.
HM/HHA Care	1. Safety is a primary concern. Stairs must be well lighted and floor rugs secured to prevent an accidental fall. Other safety measures can be found in Chapter 12. 2. Your supervisor may have you encourage the client

(continued)

<table>
<tr><td colspan="2">**Quick Reference Chart for Common Health Problems** *(continued)*</td></tr>
<tr><td></td><td>to do his own personal care to encourage his independence.
3. Treat the client with respect and understanding. Let the client know you realize Parkinson's disease does not affect his mental ability.</td></tr>
<tr><td>Stroke or Cerebral Vascular Accident (CVA)</td><td>See pages 94 to 95.</td></tr>
</table>

Review Questions

True or False

1. ____ A person in the early stages of Alzheimer's disease may realize that he cannot think or remember things as clearly as he once did.

2. ____ A regular schedule helps the client with Alzheimer's feel safe.

3. ____ When helping a client with diabetes bathe, the HM/HHA should always inspect the feet for sores, blisters, or possible infections.

4. ____ The first thing to do for a diabetic who becomes pale, confused, and hungry is have him eat some sugar or candy.

5. ____ Most stroke victims can understand what you are saying even if they cannot respond.

6. ____ A benign tumor is not cancerous.

Question for Discussion

7. Do you know anyone who has had any of the health problems described in this chapter? What happened and how did that person react to his health problem?

Part Four

Reporting Information

Chapter 11

Recording and Sharing Information

Objectives

At the conclusion of this chapter, the homemaker/home health aide will:

1. Know when it is appropriate to make a verbal report and understand the need to follow up with a written report.

2. Understand why each client who is receiving health care has a medical record and the need for keeping information in the chart confidential.

3. Be able to demonstrate how to write a clear, accurate progress note after visiting a client.

4. Know when it is appropriate to fill out an incident report form.

5. Understand the kinds of changes that need to be reported and know how to report both verbally and in written notes.

Verbal and Written Reports

The HM/HHA is an important link between the client and the home health care team. In most cases you will see the client more often than any other team member. This means your observations can be very important. The HM/HHA uses both verbal and written reports to let the home health agency know about a client's condition.

Verbal Reports

The *verbal* report is what you tell your supervisor about a client. It is used to report sudden changes in the client's condition. For example, if you call your supervisor to say that your client has a high fever, that is a verbal report. You would also need to write a progress note about the fever for the client's chart. Another less formal type of verbal report occurs when you discuss your feelings or opinions about a client's family situation with your supervisor.

Written Reports

Medical Records

All clients have a *medical record,* which is also called a *medical chart*. The medical record contains doctor's orders, lab reports, progress notes, and other information about the client's health. Every home health staff member makes a short progress note each time he visits the client. The chart is the way the home health care team keeps the lines of communication open between individual team members. The chart also allows the team to keep track of the client's progress over a period of time. The client always has the right to read his chart. If your client wants to read his chart, this must be arranged by the home health agency.

Confidentiality and Legal Aspects

The client's chart is a confidential document. Only home health care team members who are directly involved in the case are allowed to read the client's chart. It is ethically wrong to discuss a client's case with your family or friends, and it may be illegal. By doing so, you would be violating the client's right to privacy.

Remember, too, that the chart is a legal document that can be used as evidence in a court of law. If you forget to write a progress note, it may be difficult to prove that you made the visit and provided care. That is one reason it is necessary to make a written report even after you have called the agency with a verbal report.

How to Prepare Written Reports

Every home health agency will use different forms for recording information about the client's condition. Your agency may use a checklist with room at the end to write a few lines as in Figure 11-1. Or your agency may use a narrative progress note where you will write a short paragraph about the care you have provided, as shown in the charting example in this chapter.

Progress Notes

Guidelines for Writing Progress Notes

Progress notes are written every time you visit the client. This is to document the care you have provided and to record your observations about the client's condition. The following guidelines will help make your progress notes accurate.

1. *Write the progress notes immediately after the visit.* This helps you remember to include

Homemaker/Home Health Aide Progress Note

Client's name _____

Date _____

Time from: _____ to _____

Vital signs
- ☐ Temperature (O, R, A) _____
- ☐ Pulse _____
- ☐ Blood pressure _____
- ☐ Respirations _____
- ☐ Observations _____
  _____

Mental status
- ☐ Alert and oriented _____
- ☐ Confused (describe) _____
  _____
  _____

Mouth care
- ☐ Assisted with brushing teeth
- ☐ Assisted with flossing teeth
- ☐ Cleaned dentures
- ☐ Observations _____
  _____

Bath
- ☐ Bed bath ☐ Shower
- ☐ Tub bath ☐ Sponge bath
- ☐ Assisted in and out of tub/shower
- ☐ Bath/shower stool used
- ☐ Assisted with dressing
- ☐ Observations _____
  _____
  _____

Skin care
- ☐ Backrub ☐ Shave
- ☐ Repositioned client at (time) _____
- ☐ Observations about skin: cuts, bruises, sores, etc. _____
  _____
  _____

Foot/nail care
- ☐ Soaked feet
- ☐ Soaked hands
- ☐ Filed toenails
- ☐ Filed fingernails
- ☐ Observations _____
  _____

Hair care
- ☐ Shampoo
- ☐ Shampoo in bed
- ☐ Comb/brush
- ☐ Observations _____
  _____

Elimination/toilet care
- ☐ Toilet ☐ Bedside commode
- ☐ Bedpan ☐ Urinal
- ☐ Catheter ☐ Ostomy appliance
- ☐ Emptied catheter drainage bag
  time _____ amount of urine _____
- ☐ Color of urine _____
- ☐ Urine test _____
- ☐ Bowel movement
- ☐ Fluid output _____
- ☐ Observations _____
  _____

Activity/exercise
- ☐ Cane ☐ Crutches ☐ Walker
- ☐ Wheelchair ☐ Bedrest
- ☐ Walks with assistance
- ☐ Walks without assistance
- ☐ Transfers with assistance
- ☐ Range of motion exercises; describe ____
  _____
- ☐ Observations _____
  _____

Meals/nutrition
- ☐ Prepared breakfast
- ☐ Prepared lunch
- ☐ Prepared dinner/supper
- ☐ Assisted with eating
- ☐ Encouraged to eat
- ☐ Encouraged fluids
- ☐ Restricted fluids
- ☐ Fluid intake
- ☐ Meals on wheels
- ☐ Special diet _____
  _____
- ☐ Observations _____
  _____
  _____

Home management
- ☐ Laundry ☐ Number of loads _____
- ☐ Changed linens
- ☐ Cleaned bathroom
- ☐ Cleaned kitchen
- ☐ Tidied house
- ☐ Vacuumed
- ☐ Other (with nurse approval)
  _____
- ☐ Observations/condition of home ____
  _____
  _____
  _____

Miscellaneous
- ☐ Weighed _____ lbs.
- ☐ With shoes ☐ Without shoes
- ☐ Other procedures (with nurse approval); describe _____
  _____
  _____

Additional comments _____
_____

Changes/problems reported to home health supervisor ☐ Yes ☐ No Date/time reported _____

Sign here _____
   Homemaker/home health aide signature   Date/time

Figure 11-1

This is an example of a homemaker/home health aide progress note. Each day after caring for a client, you will need to fill out a short report describing the care you provided and the client's general condition. This is an example of the type of form you may be asked to fill out for your client. On this form you would put a check mark by the services that you provided and write additional notes whenever appropriate.

details that you can easily forget by the end of the day.

2. *Report facts, not guesses or personal opinions.* When quoting a client or family member, use quotation marks to mark their words. The

sentence "I slept well last night" is enclosed in quotation marks.

3. *Use your own words, not technical medical terms.* Your progress notes will be easier to understand when you use your own words.

4. *Do not erase.* When you make a mistake, simply drawn a single line through the mistake and rewrite the entry properly. Above the mistake, write "error" and your initials as shown in Figure 11-2.
5. *Keep handwriting neat and easy to read.*
6. *Sign and date every entry.* Also include the time and your full signature and title.

Subjective and Objective Reporting

There are two kinds of information that are acceptable for the written progress note: objective and subjective reports.

The *objective report* is based on information that you have gained by directly observing your client. If you report something you can see, hear, feel, touch, or smell, then you are making objective observations. With objective reports, if five people were observing a situation at the same time, all five reports would be very similar.

A *subjective report* contains information the client has told you. It may include information that you have not had the chance to observe directly or things you cannot observe, such as feelings. It would be a subjective report if you wrote that Mrs. Green said, "My leg hurts today." This information could be as important as any that you get by directly observing the client. Try to make it clear in your report what the client has told you and what you have observed directly.

It is not appropriate for the HM/HHA to give an opinion or make a guess about a client's condition in the medical chart. Describe behaviors ("He didn't smile and didn't talk") instead of making a guess about what the client was feeling or why he was not smiling.

How to Tell if You Have Written a Good Progress Note

Pretend that you are your supervisor or someone else on the home care team. You know nothing about the visit the HM/HHA made, and you want to find out what happened that day. Read the progress note and see if it explains what the HM/HHA did during the visit and how the client is progressing. If you think the report is clear, factual, and complete, then you've probably done a good job. The chart is meant to explain things clearly without an additional verbal explanation.

Situation Exercise

Imagine you are the HM/HHA and write a progress note on the form provided. Examples of good and poor charting can be found with the answers at the back of the book. Before you look at the answers, have your supervisor review your answers. Your charting will not be exactly like the sample answer in the book, but your supervisor will be able to tell you if your charting is done well.

Friendly Home Health Agency
HM/HHA Progress Note

Client's name_____

_____
_____
_____
_____
_____
_____
_____
_____
_____
_____
_____
_____
_____
_____

HM/HHA Signature _____
Date _____ Time _____

The sore on the upper right arm was red, tender, and the size of a ~~dime~~ quarter. *error S.H.*

Figure 11-2
How to correct a charting error.

Mrs. Brown is an 85-year-old client who is receiving home care from the Friendly Home Care Agency because she has arthritis and needs assistance with personal care. Sandy Holmes, the HM/HHA, has been helping Mrs. Brown with her morning care on Mondays, Wednesdays and Fridays between 8:30 and 10:30 AM for the past 7 months.

On Monday, April 3, Mrs. Brown was talkative and cheerful as usual. Sandy assisted Mrs. Brown with her bath. During the bath, Sandy noted that a red area was developing on Mrs. Brown's lower back. She washed the area very gently and after the bath applied some lotion around the reddened area. Mrs. Brown asked Sandy to cut her toenails. Sandy said she could not, but that she would tell her supervisor so she could assign a nurse to cut the toenails. Then Sandy prepared breakfast.

Incident Reports

Accidents happen to everyone. Report accidents that happen to you, to your client, or to anyone who is visiting the client. When an accident happens, fill out an incident report form promptly. A report keeps the agency informed and prepares the agency for cases in which the client phones with a complaint or damage claim. If you do not know whether to file an incident report form, ask your supervisor.

Situation Exercise

While bringing breakfast to the table, Sandy, the HM/HHA, broke a juice glass. Sandy apologized and Mrs. Brown said not to worry. Sandy made a note in the progress notes and also filled out an incident report form. Sandy realized that even though Mrs. Brown did not seem to be bothered by the broken juice glass, she was only protecting herself by reporting the accident in a formal incident report. Here is what she wrote in the progress notes.

> While preparing breakfast, a small juice glass was broken by HM/HHA. Mrs. Brown said, "Oh, that happens. It's no problem." Incident report filed with agency today. Mrs. Brown ate two fried eggs, toast, juice, and one cup of coffee. HM/HHA left at 10 AM. ————
> ———————— *Sandy Holmes HM/HHA*

Summary on How to Report a Client's Condition

Who to Report to	When you have a question or notice a change in the client's condition, call your supervisor. Your supervisor will call the doctor if it is necessary.
When to Report	Phone your supervisor during the visit if your client has a sudden change in his condition. Follow your home health agency's policy as to when your written progress notes need to be turned in.
How to Report	After calling your supervisor to report a change in the client's condition, make a written note in the progress notes. Report accidents and incidents verbally and on the incident report form.
How to Report Emergencies	In a life-threatening situation, call the emergency services before you notify your supervisor. Then phone your supervisor as soon as possible.

Observations to Make When Caring for a Client

The observations that you make about your client's health can be valuable to the home health care team. Your supervisor will give you specific instructions on what you are to observe with a particular client. As you gain experience as a HM/HHA, you will gain a better sense of the important things to report. The main thing to remember is to *report any changes in the client's condition*. Changes in the client's appearance and mood should be reported, as well as physical changes. Your supervisor can decide what action needs to be taken.

Review Questions

True or False

1. ____ Personal information about a client's health or home life should never be discussed with anyone who is not directly involved with that client.

2. ____ An objective report means reporting information that you have observed directly.

3. ____ The HM/HHA progress note allows other members of the home care team to know the kind of care you provided and what you observed about the client during the visit.

4. ____ You are breaking the confidentiality rule when you tell a friend, "I had such a good day. I made one of my clients a spinach salad today and she loved it."

5. ____ One of the best ways to chart accurately is to write your progress notes right after your visit.

6. ____ The client has the right to read his medical chart, which includes the HM/HHA progress notes.

Multiple Choice

7. Frank James has had recent gallbladder surgery and has been home only one day. He is taking a nap when a neighbor comes to the door and says to you, "I heard Frank was in the hospital. What happened?" Circle the appropriate answer.
   a. "Mr. James had gallbladder surgery last week and just got home yesterday. I know that he is supposed to get up and walk a couple of times today, but he won't do it. His wife is worried sick about him. I was just about to call my supervisor to see if she had any ideas."
   b. "Perhaps you should speak with Mrs. James. I'll tell her you are here."
   c. "Mr. James is not available right now. If you tell me your name, I'll tell him you stopped by."
   d. "You haven't heard about Frank's gallbladder surgery? I thought you said you lived next door? Come on in. I'll get you a glass of ice tea."
   e. b or c
   f. c or d

Questions for Discussion

8. Why is it necessary for the HM/HHA to keep accurate records after visiting a client?

Part Five

Practical Home Management Skills

Chapter 12

Safety for You and Your Client

Objectives

At the conclusion of this chapter, the homemaker/
home health aide will:

1. Know how to prepare for a safe home visit and
   know under what circumstances you should leave
   a client's home for your own safety.

2. Know how a fire starts and be able to explain
   what to do if a fire starts.

3. Be able to do a safety check of a client's house
   and know what to do if a situation looks unsafe.

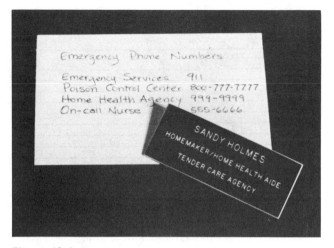

Figure 12-1
Always carry your list of emergency phone numbers and
wear your home health agency identification badge.

An important part of your job as a HM/HHA
is to think about safety, both for you and for your
client. Thinking about safety simply means thinking about how to prevent accidents and injuries. If
you ever see a safety hazard in a client's home that
you can't fix yourself, report it promptly to your
supervisor.

Safety and the Homemaker/ Home Health Aide

Remember to think about your own safety. Before
you make your first home visit for any client, review the following safety guidelines for the HM/
HHA. These suggestions are not meant to scare
you, but instead to make you aware of possible
dangers so that you can prevent them. Crime can
and does happen in all neighborhoods whether
they are suburbs, inner cities, or rural areas.
Wearing an agency uniform does not necessarily
prevent crimes. Before you make a first visit with a
new client, know:

how to prepare for the home visit,

where the client's home is and the mode of
transportation you will use,

precautions to take when you get to the client's
neighborhood, and

when to leave a client's house for your own safety.

Guidelines for a Safe Home Visit

How to Prepare for a Home Visit

Dress appropriately. If your agency does not have a
uniform, wear conservative clothes such as a white
top and a navy skirt or slacks. Wear comfortable
shoes with low heels.

*Carry identification and emergency phone num-
bers.* A name tag with your name, title, and the
home health agency's name will clearly identify
you (Figure 12-1). Also, take along the following
phone numbers:

- Your home health agency
- The emergency services, police, and fire
  departments
- The client's phone number

Money. Carry only enough money to pay for an
emergency phone call, transportation, and lunch.
Keep your money and identification cards in your
pocket. A purse can be a temptation both on the
streets and in someone's home.

HM/HHA bag. Your agency may have you
carry a bag with handwashing supplies, blood
pressure equipment, progress notes, and so on. In
the rare event that someone tries to steal your
bag, perhaps thinking you are a nurse carrying
drugs, don't be a hero. Just let them have it.

*Plan what you will say before you get to the client's
house.*

HM/HHA	(rings doorbell)
Client	(opens door partway) Hello.
HM/HHA	Hello. Are you Mrs. Walters? I am Sandy Holmes, a HM/HHA from the Tender Care Home Health Agency. (HM/HHA shows identification card.) I am here to help you with your bath and breakfast. I met you last Thursday when

my supervisor Mary Jones brought me over here.

Client   (opens door) Well, I didn't recognize you. Come in.

Know Where You're Going and How You'll Get There

Use a map. Before you leave for the client's home, know exactly where you are going and how to get there. When using a car:

- Make sure it has enough gas and that it runs well.
- Park close to the house and lock the doors of the car.
- Lock packages in the trunk of the car.
- When returning to your car, carry your keys in your hand so you don't have to search for them.

When using public transportation:

- Know which bus or train to take before you leave.
- Carry the correct change.

When you are walking:

- Cross the street to avoid groups of people who are loitering.
- Never accept a ride from someone you do not know.
- Walk on the sidewalk and avoid alleys.
- Walk with confidence. Look as though you know exactly where you are going even if this is a first visit.

Traveling in pairs. In some neighborhoods, the agency will have HM/HHAs travel in pairs. If this is the policy of the agency, follow it.

Precautions to Take When You Get to the Client's Neighborhood

Do not disturb the neighbors. Do not ring a neighbor's bell if the client does not answer his door. Do call and let the agency know the client did not answer his door as soon as you can.

Play it safe. If you ever feel it is not safe to enter a client's home or apartment, leave. Return to your home health agency and let your supervisor know why you did not visit the client.

Know When to Leave a Client's House for Your Own Safety

Situations to watch. When you enter a new client's house, look around and think about how you can leave quickly in case of a fire or an unpleasant situation. Leave the house calmly and quickly if:

- You are concerned about your safety.
- Someone in the house is drunk and uncooperative.
- There are weapons out in the open.
- A serious family argument is taking place.

Pets. If a pet is bothering you, ask the owner to put him in another room. If they will not do so, cut the visit short in a friendly manner. Talk with your supervisor for further advice.

Sexual advances. If a client or person in the client's home makes an inappropriate advance, leave the house calmly and quickly. In a rare situation, a client may misunderstand your kindness and make a sexual advance, thinking you have a personal interest in a relationship. End the visit quickly if you are uncomfortable. Discuss the situation with your supervisor.

Fire Safety

If one of these three elements is removed during a fire, the fire will go out.

1. Fuel—something that will burn
2. Oxygen—to feed the fire
3. Flame or sparks

What to Do if There Is a Fire

If there is a fire, leave by the closest escape route. Help your client and others in the house to leave, too, if you can do so without putting yourself at great risk. If it is dangerous to help others, leave the house immediately and call the fire department for help. They are experts at getting people out of burning buildings.

If you think the fire is behind a closed door that leads to your exit, feel the temperature of the door. If it is hot, do not open the door or the flames may fly into the room. Leave through another exit. If you must go through a smoke-filled hall, you and your client should put wet cloths over your noses and mouths, crawl along the floor, and move quickly. The air is fresher along the floor. Once you get outside, stay outside. You are not trained to rescue people from a burning building. Call the fire department from a neighbor's house. For what to say when calling the fire department, see the box.

When calling the fire department:

- Give the house address twice
- A quick description of the house or building
- Where the fire started
- Who is in the house (young children, disabled person)
- Your name
- Stay on the phone in case they have questions.

"I would like to report a fire at 3000 Elm Street. There is a fire at 3000 Elm Street. It is a brick house with white shutters. Some curtains caught fire in the family room in the basement. No one is left in the house. My name is Sandy Holmes."

Important note: You are not paid to be a fire-fighter, but there may be times when you can safely put a fire out before it gets out of hand. See How to Stop a Fire Quickly. Do not try to put out a fire if you do not think you can. Your responsibility is to get yourself (and your client, if possible) safely out of the house and call the fire department.

Home Safety Checklist

Think about each of your clients' homes as you review this list. If there is a potential safety problem in a client's home, bring it to the attention of your supervisor. A client who has several safety hazards in his home probably cannot correct them all at once. Your supervisor can work with the family and help them meet the most urgent safety needs first.

Fire Safety

____ Does everyone in the house know what to do in case of fire? (Locations of the fire extinguishers, exits, and alternate exits; keep low if there is smoke in the house; stay outside once you escape; and how to call the fire department.)

How to Stop a Fire Quickly

What's on Fire?	How to Stop It
Clothing	*Stop, drop, and roll.* Stop what you are doing and drop to the floor. Roll yourself or your client in a blanket or a throw rug to smother the fire more quickly. If no rug is available, just roll on the floor. Never run, because this makes the fire worse.
Trash can or wastebasket	Cover the can completely with a lid or a metal cookie sheet if one is handy.
Mattress or easy chair	If smoldering, pour water on it and call the fire department to remove it from the house.
Greasy broiler pan catches fire in the oven	Close the oven door and turn off the oven. Do not attempt to remove the pan if there are flames. Do not leave a greasy pan in the oven. Excess grease in a broiler pan can catch fire in a hot oven even after the oven has been turned off.
Grease fire in a pan on top of stove	Turn the heat off and cover the pan completely with the lid or a metal cookie sheet. Or, you can throw salt or baking soda at the base of the flame to smother it. Do not pick up the pan.

____ Are smoke alarms installed and checked monthly to make sure they are in good working condition?

____ Rags soaked in turpentine or paint thinner can catch fire spontaneously. They should be stored in a metal can or rinsed in water and thrown away.

____ If light switches or outlets are warm to the touch, the wiring may be faulty. Unplug the appliances.

____ A shock from an electrical appliance could mean the plug or wiring needs repair. The appliance should be unplugged and not used until it is fixed.

____ Do not overload electrical outlets.

____ Appliances and their cords should be in good repair. Check cords for fraying, especially if they are under rugs or furniture where the condition may not be noticed.

____ Do not operate electrical appliances with wet hands.

____ Keep ashtrays available for the client who smokes. Ashtrays should only be emptied when the ashes are cool. Pour a little water in the ashtray to be sure.

____ No one should smoke near oxygen equipment.

____ The client should not smoke unsupervised if he is confused or has taken a sleeping pill. He should not smoke in bed or when napping in a reclining chair.

General Safety

____ Are throw rugs secured to the floor?

____ Wipe up spills quickly to avoid accidents.

____ Keep stairways and hallways well lighted and free from clutter.

____ Does each stairway have a railing and is the railing secure?

____ Is furniture arranged to allow people to move around the room easily without bumping into it?

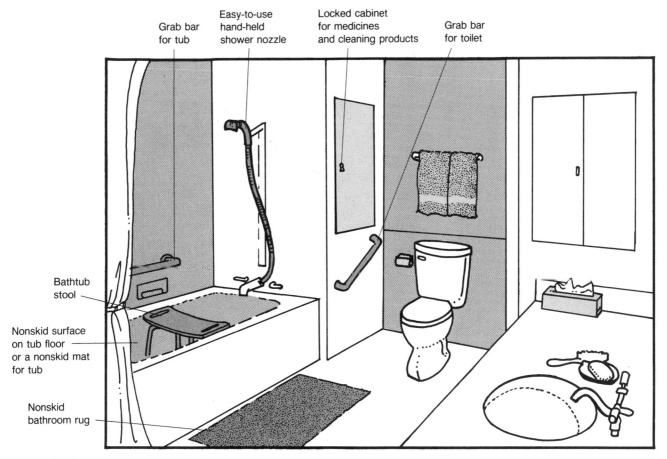

Figure 12-2
Bathroom safety.

___ Encourage the client to wear shoes or slippers to prevent falls, cuts, or bruises to his feet.

Special Equipment

___ Are the brakes on the client's wheelchair always locked when the client is getting in or out of the chair?

___ Do you always read the directions before using any equipment that you do not know how to use?

___ Do you always read labels before using any product or piece of equipment?

Bathroom Safety

See Figure 12-2.

___ Do the toilet and tub have secure handrails? (Towel racks will not support a person's weight.)

___ Does the tub or shower have a nonskid mat?

___ A weak client should use a shower/tub stool.

___ Does the client check the water temperature with his hand or a bath thermometer before getting into the tub or shower?

___ Does the hot water become too hot too quickly? (To protect children and older adults from scalds, the hot water heater temperature should be set between 120°F and 130°F.)

___ Do not leave young children or confused adults alone in the bathroom for even a minute.

The Safe Medicine Cabinet

___ Are medicines, cleaners, and other poisons kept in a locked cupboard or closet?

___ Medicines should be clearly labeled and kept in their original containers.

___ Are old medicines discarded?

___ Is there a first aid kit and is it well stocked?

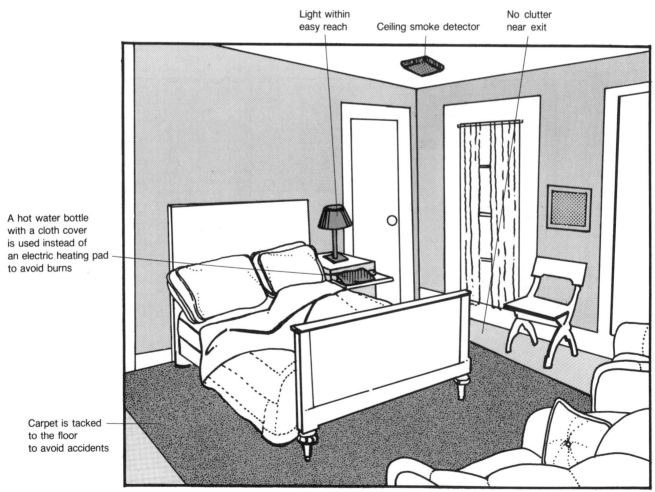

Light within easy reach

Ceiling smoke detector

No clutter near exit

A hot water bottle with a cloth cover is used instead of an electric heating pad to avoid burns

Carpet is tacked to the floor to avoid accidents

Figure 12-3
Bedroom safety.

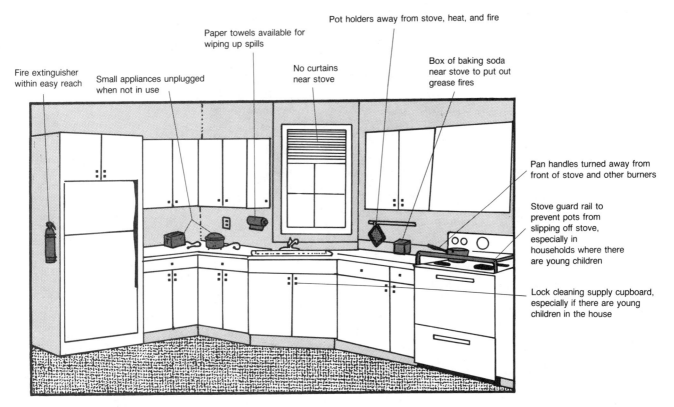

Fire extinguisher within easy reach

Small appliances unplugged when not in use

Paper towels available for wiping up spills

No curtains near stove

Pot holders away from stove, heat, and fire

Box of baking soda near stove to put out grease fires

Pan handles turned away from front of stove and other burners

Stove guard rail to prevent pots from slipping off stove, especially in households where there are young children

Lock cleaning supply cupboard, especially if there are young children in the house

Figure 12-4
Kitchen safety.

Bedroom Safety

See Figure 12-3.

____ Is there a light (and call bell if needed) within reach of the bed?

____ Does the client have an escape plan in case there is a fire at night?

____ If the client uses an electric blanket or heating pad, is the heat setting kept on low and turned off when not in use? (A hot water bottle is safer.)

Kitchen Safety

See Figure 12-4.

____ Are spills on the floor wiped up quickly?

____ Are small appliances (toaster, mixer, frying pan) unplugged when not in use?

____ Hands should be dry before plugging in an appliance.

____ Appliance cords should be kept in good condition.

____ Does everyone in the family know the toaster must be unplugged before removing toast with a knife or fork?

____ Keep pan handles turned away from the front of the stove so pans are not knocked over. Do not put the handles over another burner.

____ When lighting a gas stove, light the match before turning on the gas.

____ Lift the lid of a pan away from you to avoid a steam burn.

____ Curtains, dish towels, and pot holders should not hang near the stove.

____ Cut away from yourself when using a knife.

____ When handing a knife or scissors to another person, hand him the handle.

Review Questions

True or False

1. ____ A HM/HHA who wears a uniform and carries an agency bag never has to worry about safety.

2. ____ If a broiler pan catches fire in the oven, the safest thing to do is close the oven door and turn off the oven.

3. ____ To avoid scalds, the hot water thermostat should be set from 120°F to 130°F.

4. ____ It is not necessary to have the client wear shoes or slippers in his own house.

Multiple Choice

5. You and your client are alone in the house. Suddenly you see smoke filling the room. What is the safest thing to do?
   a. Scream for help.
   b. Put a wet cloth over your face, stay near the floor, and crawl to the closest exit. Have your client do the same.
   c. Open the hallway door quickly and run as fast as you can.
   d. Find the phone and call the fire department. Then leave the house with your client.

Questions for Discussion

6. A client is smoking in an overstuffed chair. He drops the burning cigarette and it makes a small fire in the chair. The client jumps up and puts out the flame with a glass of water. Should anything else be done?

7. Make a list of other safety guidelines that could be added to the Home Safety Checklist.

Chapter 13

Infection Control: Preventing the Spread of Disease

Objectives

At the conclusion of this chapter, the homemaker/home health aide will:

1. Understand and be able to explain how germs are spread.

2. Understand the importance of practicing medical asepsis and be able to give five examples of medical asepsis used in home care.

3. Be able to demonstrate how to wash the hands and explain the need for scrubbing the hands well.

4. Understand the terms medical asepsis, infection control, clean technique, contamination, sterilization, antiseptic, and disinfectant.

Preventing the spread of germs and disease is a goal in any household, but it is especially important for the HM/HHA. An ill client is usually more likely to pick up colds, infections, or other diseases than a healthy person who is strong enough to resist common germs. Using techniques to prevent the spread of germs and disease may take some time and effort, but in the long run it saves time and effort. It is much easier to *prevent* health problems by controlling germs and disease than to deal with the health problems after they have arrived.

When you care for clients, use good infection control techniques such as handwashing and keeping the house clean to keep from carrying germs between houses—and this includes your own house. You may also encourage the family to use the principles of infection control so they do not pass germs among themselves.

What Are Germs and How Are They Spread?

What Are Germs?

Germs are very small living plants and animals that can only be seen under a microscope. A more scientific term for a germ is *microorganism*. *Micro*- means "very small" and *-organism* means "living being." Most microorganisms are harmless. Some are even helpful, such as the ones found in the small intestine that help digest the food we eat. Others can cause disease and infection. The

harmful microorganisms are called *pathogens* or *germs*. Bacteria and viruses are pathogens. Some organisms are not harmful in one part of the body, but if they move to another part of the body, they can cause infections. *Infection* occurs when a harmful microorganism (pathogen) grows and develops within the body. A healthy person is better able to fight infection and disease than an ill person. Cleanliness is one of the best ways to prevent germs from spreading.

Where Do Germs Live?

Germs are everywhere. You will find germs on people, animals, flowers, food, bed linens, humidifiers—simply everywhere. Some pathogens can live in extreme conditions such as very hot or very cold environments, but most prefer medium temperatures.

The human body is an ideal home for germs because it has many warm, dark, moist places where germs can live (see box). Germs can live on old skin cells, the mucous membranes, open sores, and many other places. The human body is the perfect environment for germs to thrive.

Factors That Help Germs Grow
1. Moisture
2. Medium temperatures
3. Darkness
4. Oxygen
4. Nourishment

How Do Germs Enter and Leave the Body?

The skin is our first line of defense in preventing germs from entering the body. But even a small open sore can provide an entrance for a germ looking for a new home. Many microorganisms are found in the natural openings such as the ears, nose, mouth, throat, genitourinary tract, and anus. These areas have all the characteristics that microorganisms like: warmth, darkness, moisture, and nutrients. Germs leave the body when a person coughs or sneezes, or through body wastes such as stools, a runny nose, or a draining cut. That is why it is important to wash your hands well after using the toilet and after touching a client near any of these areas when you assist with personal care.

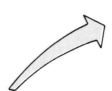

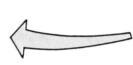

1. A place to live. Organisms need a place to live, grow, and reproduce. Usually that means a dark, moist, warm, and nourishing environment. The human body is perfect.

2. A way to escape. Germs need an escape route. An open sore or natural opening such as the mouth or nose works well.

3. A way to travel. Organisms need a way to travel, such as a cough or a runny nose, or an object like a bedpan or dust particle.

4. An entry to a new home. Organisms need a place where they can enter the body such as the mouth, nose, or urinary tract.

5. A person who is susceptible. Finally, organisms need a person who cannot fight the organism once it has entered the body.

Figure 13-1
How germs spread.

How Germs Are Spread

Organisms can easily travel from one person to another. They can be transported directly or indirectly. Although not all germs are pathogens, you need to be careful in situations where germs can easily be spread. Here are some examples:

1. When you assist with a bath or help a client use the toilet.
2. When someone sneezes or coughs without covering his mouth with a handkerchief, germs from that person's throat are released into the air. Even talking can release germs into the air.
3. Germs will cling to dust particles and the natural moisture in the air, and can travel easily in that way.
4. Spoiled food or contaminated water carry germs.
5. Personal care objects such as the bedpan, bed linens, hairbrushes, clothing, and tissues all carry germs. Wash these items regularly and dispose of tissues properly as soon as they are used.
6. Germs are spread when a person drops a pen on the floor, picks it up without washing it, and then puts it into his mouth while he is thinking about what to write.
7. The caregiver who changes a baby's diaper and then hands the baby a toy before he washes his hands may spread germs to the baby.

How the Body Fights Infection

The human body is often able to fight germs even if they have entered the body successfully. The ability of the body to fight germs depends upon the person's age, health, level of fatigue, nutrition, and natural resistance to that germ; and the strength of the invading pathogen.

If the person is not able to resist the infection, he is *susceptible.* The very young, the very old, and the very sick are most susceptible to infection and disease. Because they are the people you are most likely to have as clients, it is very important for you to use good infection control techniques.

Figure 13-1 shows how germs live and travel.

Preventing the Spread of Infection

Preventing the spread of infection is called *medical asepsis* or *infection control.* Handwashing, good personal hygiene, and keeping the house clean are all ways of practicing medical asepsis.

(*Text continues on page 124.*)

Purpose: Good handwashing is the single most important procedure you can do to prevent the spread of infection and disease.

Equipment:
- Bar soap and soap dish, or liquid soap
- Fingernail brush
- Clean, dry paper towels
- Warm running water

Safety: You will need to wash your hands even when they do not look dirty. Your hands need to be kept especially clean because clients who are ill may not be able to fight infection as easily as a healthy person. Be sure to wash your hands:
- when entering or leaving a client's home
- before preparing food
- after using the toilet
- after sneezing or touching your mouth or nose
- before and after every procedure and every time you touch or have contact with the client

Steps

1. Remove your watch and jewelry and put them in your pocket. Roll shirt sleeves up to the elbow.

2. Use a towel to turn the water faucet on and to adjust the temperature.

3. Rinse the hands and wrists under warm running water.

4. Lather well with soap.

5. Rub your hands together to lather the hands. Scrub for at least 10 to 30 seconds, and longer if you have touched blood, pus, stools, urine, and other body fluids. Scrub between the fingers and the entire surface of the hands and wrists. The forearms may also need to be scrubbed (Figure 13-2).

Reasons

1. Do not wear jewelry on the job because germs can get caught in the jewelry and be carried from one house to another.

2. The sink and faucets are always considered dirty. A paper towel is cleaner than a cloth towel because the cloth towel is often used several times by many people. Use the paper towels from your HM/HHA bag.

3. Warm water makes better soap lather than cold. Hot water dries the skin.

4. Soap lather removes germs and dirt particles. If using bar soap, rinse it off well before washing your hands.

5. Friction removes tiny germs and dirt particles that are deep within the skin, between the fingers and under the fingernails.

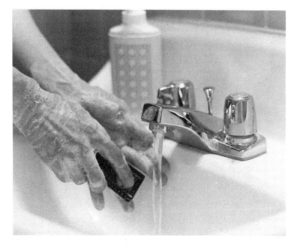

Figure 13-2

(continued)

HM/HHA Procedure:
Handwashing *(continued)*

6. Scrub under the fingernails with a fingernail brush or an orange stick. Lather and rinse (Figure 13-3).

6. Dirt particles and germs can lodge under the nails and spread to others if they are not cleaned regularly.

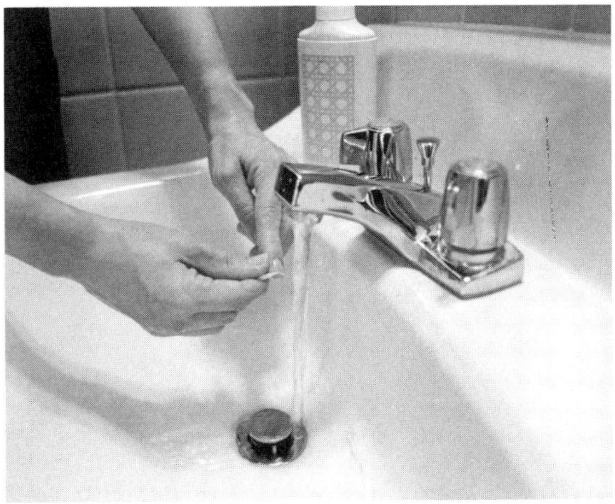

Figure 13-3

7. After washing, if you're using a bar of soap, rinse the soap and drop it in the soap dish without touching the dish.

7. Rinsing removes most of the dirt particles and germs from the bar of soap. This helps prevent organisms from being spread to the next user.

8. Rinse the hands from the wrist to the fingertips under warm running water (Figure 13-4).

8. This allows particles that were loosened by the soap and scrubbing to be washed down the drain.

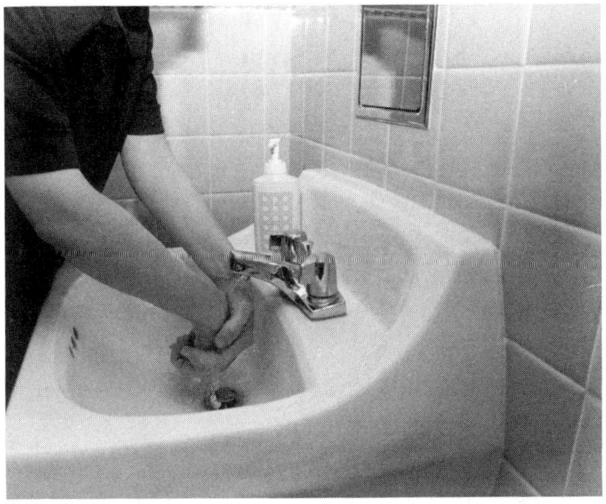

Figure 13-4

9. Rewash your hands if they are very dirty.

9. By washing a second time, you will remove germs that were loosened during the first handwashing.

(continued)

HM/HHA Procedure:
Handwashing *(continued)*

10. Dry the hands with a clean paper towel and use that towel to turn off the faucet (Figure 13-5). Pat the hands dry to avoid skin irritation.

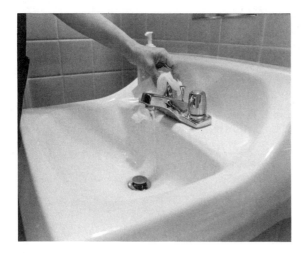

Figure 13-5

11. Apply hand lotion as needed.

11. Lotion keeps the hands soft and prevents chapping. Dirt particles and germs are easily caught in cracked skin.

Handwashing

The best way to prevent the spread of germs and disease is to wash your hands regularly using the method in this book. You can be a good example to the client and family when you wash your hands regularly with a good handwashing technique.

Simply rinsing the hands under a faucet is not effective handwashing. Soap, friction, and thorough rinsing are needed. Liquid soap is cleaner than bar soap, because germs can grow on the bar of soap, especially if the soap sits in a puddle of water. The outside of the dispenser of liquid soap should be kept clean. Under normal conditions, you will only need to use regular soap and a good handwashing technique instead of an antiseptic cleaning product. See HM/HHA Procedure: Handwashing on pages 122–124 for an explanation.

Other Ways to Prevent the Spread of Disease

Some areas of the house must be kept cleaner than others. The kitchen needs to be clean be-cause it is where meals are prepared and some-times eaten. The kitchen may be the gathering place in the house and that may make it harder to keep clean. Encourage your client and his family to wash or rinse out their dishes after a meal or snack. Countertops should be cleaned before and after preparing food. Spills should be wiped up right when they happen. See Chapter 14 for more details on cleaning the house.

Disposing of wastes properly and promptly prevents the spread of germs and also keeps pests away. The wastebasket should be emptied into a covered trashcan. Cockroaches, mice, flies, ants, and other pests carry diseases. Talk with the supervisor to find out how to handle these problems.

Disinfection and Sterilization

Useful Terms

Contamination

When an object has many germs on it, it is considered dirty or *contaminated*. Many things in the home will be contaminated. For example, a glass is

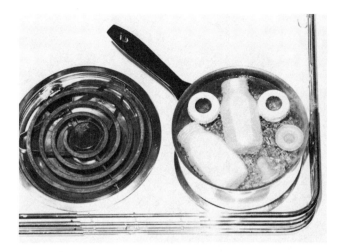

Figure 13-6
An example of wet heat sterilization is boiling baby bottles.

contaminated after a person has had a drink from it, and the floor is always contaminated. It is not necessary or possible to keep the house completely free from all germs, but you should know when things should be cleaned to prevent infections and disease. Use asepsis to prevent the germs from spreading.

Sterilization

To *sterilize* an object means that all organisms are completely removed from that object. Usually in home care, sterilization is not practical or necessary. For example, when you wash your hands they will be clean, but not sterile. Some equipment such as baby bottles may need sterilizing. If you need to sterilize an object, you can do so using wet or dry heat. Use the method recommended by your supervisor. Some pieces of equipment will not tolerate heat sterilization procedures, and will need to be cleaned using other methods.

Wet Heat Sterilization

Most organisms will be killed after boiling the object for 5 minutes, but they will all be removed after 20 minutes. Your supervisor will tell you exactly how much time is needed. Place the object in furiously boiling water so that the object is completely covered (Figure 13-6). Remove the object with sterile tongs after 20 minutes and place it in a sterile container. (A sterile container is a container that has been sterilized using wet or dry heat.)

Dry Heat Sterilization

Place the object in an oven preheated to 320°F for 1 full hour. A cloth dressing can be sterilized with dry heat by ironing it.

Antiseptic

Anti- means against and *-septic* means infection, so an antiseptic is a cleaning agent that is used to fight infection. Like the disinfectant, the antiseptic kills most of the germs and slows the growth of bacteria. In contrast to the disinfectant, the antiseptic can be used on people. For example, a person rinses his mouth out with an antiseptic, not a disinfectant. Alcohol is an antiseptic used to clean the skin. For practical purposes, the terms *disinfectant* and *antiseptic* are often used interchangeably, but technically they are different.

Review Questions

True or False

1. ____ Mouthwash is a disinfectant.
2. ____ Mouthwash is an antiseptic.
3. ____ When washing your hands, it is recommended that you rub them together with soap for at least 10 seconds and then rinse them under running water.

Questions for Discussion

4. Define *medical asepsis* in your own words. Give four examples of medical asepsis that you practice in your own home.

5. Think about the number of times and when you wash your hands in a normal workday. If you were the client, would you want your HM/HHA to have washed her hands more often? After which activities should a HM/HHA wash her hands?

Chapter 14

Keeping the Home and Laundry Clean

Objectives

At the conclusion of this chapter, the homemaker/home health aide will:

1. Understand the role of the HM/HHA when cleaning or teaching clients how to care for the home.

2. Be able to describe ways to help a family organize cleaning tasks.

3. Know how to organize your work schedule.

4. Understand how to clean each part of the house using inexpensive but effective cleaners.

5. Be able to explain how to do laundry and how to teach a client how to do the laundry.

Keeping the House Clean

Why Clean a Client's House?

Part of your job as a HM/HHA is to help the client live in a clean, healthy home. Studies have shown that people recover more quickly when their homes are neat and orderly. So a clean home is good for the client's physical and mental health.

The Role of the Homemaker/ Home Health Aide

There are two situations in which a HM/HHA might need to use home management skills. First, you will sometimes clean house for a client who is ill or injured and cannot clean his home by himself. Second, you may be asked to teach the client and family how to clean and how often certain cleaning needs to be done. In either situation, you will be able to rely on your home health agency for guidance.

Most HM/HHAs know basic home management because they take care of their own homes. But sometimes work habits that you use in your own home cannot be used when taking care of someone else's home. When you are working for another person in his home, you need to respect his wishes. Many clients like to use particular cleaning methods or products. And some clients have prized possessions that they don't want anyone else to touch. Try to put yourself in your client's position, and think about how you would react if you were unable to care for your home.

Usually, HM/HHAs are assigned only light housekeeping tasks such as washing the dishes, wiping spills, mopping a floor, emptying trash, or doing a load of laundry. Some cleaning tasks described in this chapter may be covered in more depth than you are asked to do in your work. This additional information will help you teach clients home management skills.

How Clean Is Clean?

Different people have their own ideas about how clean a house should be. Your supervisor will have visited the client and arranged which tasks you will do. Do only the tasks on your assignment sheet. In most cases, you will not be expected to clean as well as the client who keeps her home spotless, but you will need to do more than the client who lives in an absolute mess. For the client whose home needs a lot of work, you and your supervisor should work together to decide which tasks are most important for the client's health.

Teaching a Client How to Clean the House

Home management skills are fun to teach. Most clients appreciate the information and are glad to get your suggestions. But, some clients may be offended that you or people from the home health agency think they are not cleaning their homes well enough. You need to handle the situation delicately. For this reason, do not start a home cleaning teaching program without your supervisor's knowledge. For more specific information on how to teach, see Chapter 2 on communication and Chapter 5 on teaching older adults.

Some clients may be overwhelmed by a dirty house. They may not know where or how to start cleaning it. The sample cleaning schedule shown in Table 14-1 may help a family organize housekeeping tasks into daily and weekly chores. The family job assignment chart in Table 14-2 will help families divide the household chores fairly.

Your supervisor will probably encourage the family to have the children help with the housework. Even a 2-year-old can pick up her toys. When older children help decide what their jobs

Table 14-1
How Often to Clean

	Daily	Weekly	As Needed
Kitchen	Wash dishes Wipe spills from stove, counters, refrigerator, and floor Sweep floors Take out trash	Throw out old leftover food Clean stove burners and other appliances as needed Wet mop floor	Clean oven Defrost freezer and scrub refrigerator Clean closets, cupboards, and stored dishes
Living room	Straighten up room Throw out old newspapers and mail Encourage the family to dust tabletops and shelves as needed	Vacuum rugs and dust floors Dust corners of ceilings, baseboards by floors, and windowsills Dust furniture and lamps. Use a clean dust cloth and a vacuum with attachments, if available, for shelves and chairs. Empty wastebaskets	Clean rugs Wash lamps, pictures, shelves, and woodwork Polish floors
Bedroom	Make bed Hang clean clothes and put dirty clothes in hamper	Change sheets Dust and vacuum Straighten room Empty wastebaskets. (Rinse with hot water and household cleanser; wash with hot water and disinfectant as needed.)	Fluff pillows and blankets in dryer—no heat Wash mattress pad, bed skirt, bedspread, and blankets Turn mattress Store clothes out of season Clean and organize closets Clean windows, shelves, walls, and woodwork
Bathroom	Wash sink, tub, and shower Wipe wet floor	Scrub sink and tub/shower Clean toothbrush holder, soap dish, faucets, mirrors, tub mat, and wall tiles Scrub toilet Wash floor Empty wastebaskets Replace towels and bathmat with clean ones	Wash walls Wash floor rugs Clean and organize closets and medicine cabinet

Table 14-2
Family Job Assignments

Name	Job Assignments for July
Joe	Wash dishes (Mon, Wed, Fri, Sun)
Ann	Wash dishes (Tues, Thurs, Sat)
Judy	Empty wastebaskets
Dad	Pick up living room
Mom	Wash and sort clothes

will be, they are more likely to follow through with the work. This applies to others in the family, too. Rotating family jobs spreads the work more fairly.

Organizing Your Work Time

Organization is an important skill for the HM/HHA. When you are given an assignment you will be expected to get your work done on time. Each time you are assigned a new client, you will have to think about how to organize your day. Take a few minutes at the start of each workday and make a schedule. Most HM/HHAs find it helpful to write out a work plan. As things get done, items on the list are checked off.

When organizing your list, put things that absolutely need to be done at the top of the list. If you run out of time, you'll have the most important things done.

To Do List

1. Help Mrs. B get bathed and dressed.
2. Prepare and serve breakfast.
3. Straighten bedroom and bathroom.
4. Do one load of laundry.
5. Straighten living room.
6. Wipe refrigerator shelves.

Write out a work plan with a time schedule. This is especially helpful when you start working for a new client.

Work Plan

8:00 to 8:15 — Arrive and put in load of wash.

8:15 to 8:40 — Help Mrs. B with bath and dressing.

8:40 to 9:00 — Move clothes from washer to dryer while Mrs. B puts on make-up and fixes her hair. Prepare breakfast and set table.

9:00 to 9:15 — Help Mrs. B walk to the kitchen nook and serve her breakfast.

9:15 to 9:45 — While Mrs. B eats breakfast, make bed and straighten bedroom and bathroom. Fold and put away laundry.

9:45 to 10:00 — Help Mrs. B to living room chair.

If you visit the client several times a week, plan regular jobs for certain days of the week. For example:

Monday — vacuum, straighten rooms, wash floors

Wednesday — laundry and odd jobs

Friday — food shopping and other errands

Make good use of your time and free moments. In the above example, the HM/HHA started the load of wash before making the client's breakfast.

Preparing to Clean

- Gather the equipment you'll need and carry it with you in a bucket or basket (Figure 14-1).
- Start with clean equipment (dust cloths, mops, brooms, and water). You cannot clean a house with dirty tools.
- Do not have the client buy special cleaning products that you might buy for yourself at home. Use cleaners the client already owns or household cleaning products that you can mix yourself, as shown in Tables 14-3 and 14-4.

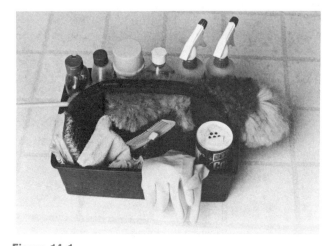

Figure 14-1
A well-organized cleaning carryall allows you to keep all your cleaning supplies in one place as you go from room to room.

Table 14-3
Household Products Used as Cleaners

Baking Soda	Vinegar	Ammonia
Gently scours appliances, countertops, bathtubs, sinks, plastic containers	Cleans lime off tile, water faucets, and chrome	Polishes mirrors/windows
	Removes soap scum	Cleans combs and hairbrushes
Removes odors from shoes, drains, and refrigerators	Polishes windows/mirrors	Set small bowl in oven overnight to chosen baked-on foods
	Cleans showerheads	Removes floor wax
	Removes smoke odors	

- Wear rubber gloves when cleaning to avoid skin irritation.
- Clean from top to bottom. Dust higher shelves before the lower ones because dust on the top shelves will fall to the lower shelves. Floors are always cleaned last.

Cleaning Different Parts of the House

The Kitchen

Cleaning the Stove

- Wipe stove daily after it is cool.
- Wipe sides and surfaces of stove with a window cleaner or soapy water. Baking soda on a damp cloth will remove baked-on food gently.

- Remove burners weekly for cleaning.

Cleaning the Refrigerator

- Wipe outside with window cleaning product or soapy water.
- Defrost when freezer coils are covered with ½ inch of ice. The job of the coils is to take heat out of the freezer. When ice builds up, it acts as an insulator and the coils cannot do their job. Coils at the back of the refrigerator should be vacuumed twice a year.
- A self-defrosting freezer or refrigerator still needs to be emptied and washed out regularly.
- Throw out food that is old or expired (with the client's permission).
- Clean the inside of the refrigerator with a solution of 2 tablespoons baking soda in 1 quart water to remove odors. Straight white vinegar will prevent mildew.

Table 14-4
Inexpensive Homemade Cleaning Products*

Windows/Mirrors	1 teaspoon rubbing alcohol + 1 cup water	or 1 tablespoon ammonia + 1 cup water	or 1 tablespoon vinegar + 1 cup water
Household cleaner	2 tablespoons ammonia, 2 tablespoons liquid detergent, and 1 quart water		
To remove water stains and lime	1 cup white vinegar and ½ teaspoon liquid soap; keep in a spray bottle and scrub with a soft toothbrush.		

*Store these products in labeled spray bottles.

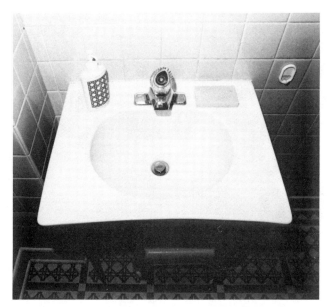

Figure 14-2
It is a good idea to keep a sponge on the sink to encourage people to wipe the sink after each use.

The Bathroom

Make cleaning simpler by teaching everyone in the house to rinse and wipe the sink and bathtub/shower after each use (Figure 14-2); to hang towels on the towel racks; to flush the toilet and wash their hands after using the toilet; and to wipe up spills and splashes when they happen.

Cleaning the Toilet

- Flush the toilet and raise the lid. Pour ⅔ cup of liquid bleach into toilet bowl. Bleach cleans and disinfects. (Or use toilet cleaner, but never mix bleach and toilet cleaner.) Let set while you clean the rest of the bathroom.

> Never mix toilet bowl cleaner and bleach. It can cause deadly fumes.

- After you have finished cleaning the rest of the bathroom, fill a bucket or pan with hot, sudsy water. Sponge the toilet seat and the outside of the toilet. Scrub inside the toilet bowl with a brush. Wear rubber gloves to prevent cleaner from splashing onto your hands.

> Once rags are used to clean the toilet, do not use them for any other cleaning job.

Cleaning the Sink, Tub, or Shower

- Remove drain stopper, clean, and replace.
- Fill sink or tub with 2 or 3 inches of water. Add cleanser and scrub. Rinse with hot water.

Cleaning the Mirrors, Soap Dish, Tiles, and Floor

- Use the mirror/window cleaner on mirrors and soap dishes.
- Wash wall tiles and floors with the homemade household cleaner or a product the client prefers.
- Clean the toothbrush holder with a cotton swab or an old toothbrush labeled "cleaning brush."

The Bedroom

A Quick Way to Make the Bed

- Pull back the covers to air the bed out each day for about 30 minutes.
- To make the bed, smooth wrinkles on bottom sheet first. To save steps, work on one side of the bed at a time. Pull the top sheet and blankets to the head of the bed. Then do the same on the other side of the bed. Smooth out wrinkles and fluff pillows last.
- Change and wash sheets weekly. Do this more often for the client who is bedridden or who soils the sheets more quickly.
- See Figure 14-3 for directions on how to make square corners.
- See the HM/HHA Procedure: Making an Occupied Bed on pages 133–135 if you have a client who is unable to get out of bed.

Washing the Laundry

Before using laundry appliances or products, read the instructions. Knowing how to use equipment saves time and avoids accidents.

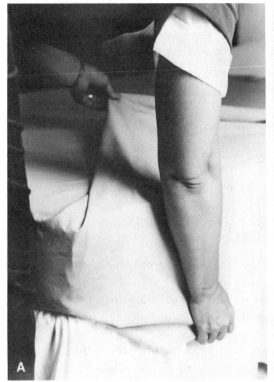
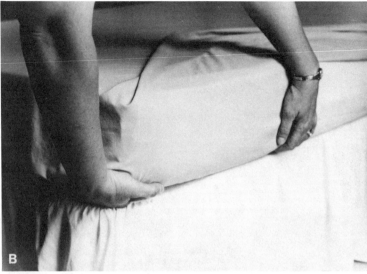
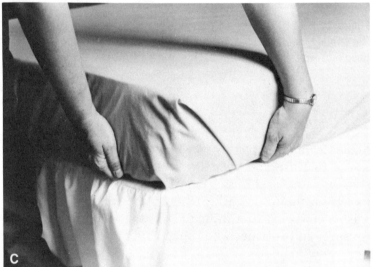

Figure 14-3
How to make mitered corners. (*A*) Step One: The top sheet should be tucked in at the foot of the bed. Hold the edge of the top sheet about a foot from the end of the bed and lift it up onto the bed, making a triangle as shown in the picture. (*B*) Step Two: Tuck in the edge of the sheet that hangs below the mattress. (*C*) Step Three: Bring the original triangle down over the edge of the mattress and tuck it in.

Laundry Equipment

The Washing Machine

There are many different brands of machines, but there are two basic types—front-loading and top-loading machines. All machines will have a choice of hot, warm, or cold water and a wash, rinse, and spin cycle. The deluxe machines have cycles for special fabrics. Read the instruction booklet before using the machine. Three elements are necessary for the washing machine to work properly. There must be:

1. Enough water to cover the clothes;
2. Enough room for the clothes to move freely in the water; and
3. Enough laundry detergent to clean the clothes. Use the amount recommended on the box of detergent.

The Dryer

Clean the lint screen before each load. A full lint screen is a fire hazard. Do not overload the machine. Clothes need room to move in order to dry.

A Word About Laundry Products

Read labels on laundry products carefully before using them. There are so many products in similar packages, it is easy to confuse them. Don't make the mistake one HM/HHA made when she put floor wax into the washing machine.

Soap

Laundry soaps clean the laundry well if the client has naturally soft water or a water softener, but most American homes have hard water. In hard

(*Text continues on page 135.*)

HM/HHA Procedure:
Making an Occupied Bed

Purpose:	To change the sheets on a bed when the client is unable to get out of the bed. You will make one side of the bed at a time.
Equipment:	• Chair (place at the foot of the bed) • Clean sheets • Laundry basket or bag (or use the pillow case) • Separate bag if sheets are soiled
Safety:	You can make an occupied bed by yourself, but you must always be sure the client is positioned so he will not fall out of bed. Think about how you will manage each step before you begin the procedure. To prevent the spread of infection, do not place any linens on the floor. Put soiled sheets in a laundry basket and keep clean linens folded on a nearby chair.

Steps

1. Gather your equipment, wash your hands, and tell the client what you are about to do. Find out how he can help.

2. Remove and fold the blankets, and place them on a nearby chair. If the blankets are not to be reused, put them in the laundry basket. Leave the top sheet so the client can stay covered.

3. How to position the client.
   a. Raise the side rail opposite the side where you will be working. If there are no side rails, use two straight chairs with the backs against the bed.
   b. Help the client turn toward the side rails or chairs. Then adjust the pillow for the client's comfort.

4. How to remove the soiled sheets from one side of the bed.
   a. Loosen the sheets and roll the soiled sheets to the center of the bed.
   b. Place the rolled log of soiled sheets close to the client's back as shown in Figure 14-4A. Now half of the bed is now ready for clean linens.

5. How to put clean sheets on one side of the bed.
   a. Fold the clean bottom sheet lengthwise and place the folded edge along the center of the bed.
   b. Roll the half that will go on the other side of the bed and place it along the client's back (Figure 14-4B).
   c. Tuck the bottom sheet under the mattress on the side where you are working.

Reasons

1. Listen to the client's suggestions and encourage him to assist as much as he can with this procedure.

(continued)

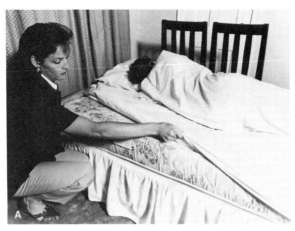

Figure 14-4

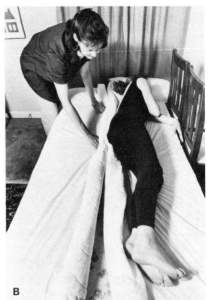

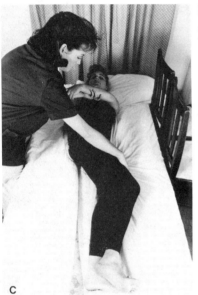

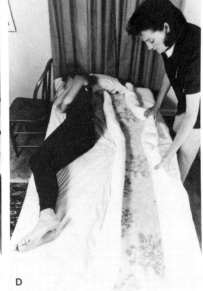

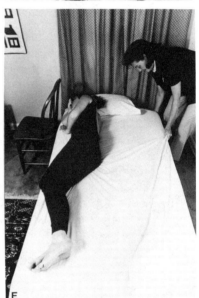

6. Preparing to make the other side of the bed.
   a. Raise the side rails or move the chairs to the side of the bed with the clean bottom sheet—the side that you have just made.
   b. Help the client roll to the side of the bed with the clean bottom sheet. The client will have to roll over the lump of sheets at the center of the bed. This may be very difficult for some clients (Figure 14-4C).
   c. Adjust the pillow and assist the client into a comfortable position facing the side rails.

(continued)

HM/HHA Procedure:
Making an Occupied Bed *(continued)*

7. Remove the soiled linens and put them in the laundry basket (Figure 14-4*D*).

8. Pull the clean bottom sheet tight and tuck it in (Figure 14-4*E*).

9. Finishing the bed.
   a. Place the clean top sheet on the bed and miter the corners of the top sheet as shown in Figure 14-3.
   b. Put the blankets and bedspread on the bed.
   c. Change the pillow cases.
   d. Position your client comfortably.

10. Put away the soiled laundry and wash your hands thoroughly when the procedure is completed. Record your observations and the client's tolerance of the procedure.

water, the soap combines with minerals in the water. This forms a sticky substance called scum that clings to the clothes, leaving them dull and gray. This is the same scum that makes a bathtub ring. It is difficult to remove scum whether it is in the bathtub or in the clothes.

Detergents

Detergents, like soap, loosen and remove dirt, but they may not create scum. Read the product label to find out how much detergent to use. For large or heavily soiled loads, you'll need to add more detergent according to the product label.

Water Softeners

Water softeners help detergents work more efficiently. When a client has a water softener, you may not need to use as much detergent.

Fabric Softeners

Fabric softeners make fabrics fluffier and more wrinkle-free, and take away static cling. Some go into the last rinse in the wash cycle, and others go into the dryer. Regulate the amount of fabric softener used by the size of the wash load, not the amount of water in the machine. When too much softener is used, clothes become discolored. Follow directions on the product label if you use fabric softeners.

Chlorine Bleach

Chlorine bleach is a strong product that disinfects and whitens. But, it can damage and discolor wool, silk, and man-made fabrics. Bleach may also reduce the effectiveness of detergents.

When using liquid bleach, dilute it in 1 quart of water and add it to the machine after the wash cycle has been going about 3 to 5 minutes. This lets the detergent work on the clothes before the bleach is added. Bleach can also be used by adding it and laundry detergent to the wash water before adding the clothes. This is a less effective way of using bleach. Never add more than the amount recommended on the product container.

Chlorine bleach can be used on:

Whites

Colorfast permanent press

Blends

Many colored fabrics

Chlorine bleach cannot be used on:

Silk

Wool

Spandex/elastic

Flame-resistant fabrics

Garments labeled "no bleach"

Prewash Treatments and Stain Removal

Why Use a Prewash Treatment

Prewash treatments are used to remove stains or brighten clothes. There are a number of products sold, but if regular detergent is getting the clothes clean, it is not necessary to use a prewash treatment.

Presoaks

To presoak clothes, fill the machine with the hottest water the fabric will tolerate, but do not add the clothes yet. Add detergent and turn the machine on. Stop the machine, add the clothes, and let them soak for 30 to 40 minutes before continuing the wash cycle.

Prewashing Formulas

- Test a small amount of any prewash treatment on an inside hem to make sure it does not discolor or harm the fabric.
- One of the best is plain soap. Apply a bar of strong soap, such as Fels-Naptha, to the stain. Rub the stained or spotted clothing together and wash normally.
- A detergent paste can be made by adding a few drops of water to some powdered laundry detergent. Rub it into the fabric.
- Liquid laundry detergent can also be applied directly onto clothing to remove stains or collar rings.
- To make prewash spray, mix ½ cup ammonia, ½ cup liquid detergent, and 1 cup water. Store in a spray bottle that you have labeled "prewash spray." Ammonia should not be used on silk or wool.

Stain Removal

Not all stains are removable, but if you get at the stain before it dries you will have a better chance of getting it out. (See the Stain Removal Chart.) A good rule of thumb is to wipe any stain with cold water. Hot water will set protein stains (such as milk, eggs, blood, juices from meat), making them difficult or impossible to remove. Treat unknown stains in the following way:

1. Sponge spot with cold water.
2. Rub with detergent paste or prewash

Stain Removal Chart

Protein stains (blood, milk, meat juices, ice cream, egg)	Rinse in cold water. Then soak in cold water and detergent. Launder using bleach if allowed.
Coffee, tea	Pour hot water through fabric. Launder as usual.
Chocolate	Rinse in cold water, and rub detergent paste on spot. Wash in hot water if fabric allows.
Mildew	Wash with detergent in hot water. Dry in the sun.
Urine	Soak in cold water for 20 minutes. Pretreat with detergent paste or stain remover. Rinse and launder.
Vomit	Rinse off particles in the toilet. Soak in a solution of ½ cup salt to 2 quarts water to remove odors. Rinse and launder.

product and rinse well. Do this several times if stain persists.
3. Wash in the hottest water the fabric can tolerate with liquid or powdered bleach and extra detergent.

The Five-Step Guide to Doing Laundry

Step One: Sort the Laundry

Sorting laundry prevents colors from fading and blending with other clothes. The dye in a new pair of blue jeans will run the first few times the jeans are washed. Anything in the machine with them is likely to turn blue. Below are some laundry sorting guidelines. Use these guidelines to sort the client's clothes into a few reasonably sized loads. Do not wash ten small loads when the clothes could have been washed safely in three normal loads.

Sort by color.
- Separate darks and lights. Dark colors washed

in hot water may fade, and whites washed with colors may pick up other colors or turn gray.

Sort by fabric and water temperature.

- Use hot water and a more vigorous wash cycle for cottons and linens.
- Use cool water and a shorter wash cycle for man-made fabrics (polyester, nylon).
- Use a cool rinse to prevent wrinkles in permanent press clothes.
- Washable wool sweaters need a short cycle with cool water and a mild soap to prevent fading and shrinking.

Sort by texture.

- Wash lint producers and lint collectors separately. Fuzzy socks and terry cloth towels give off lint. Corduroys collect lint.

Wash heavily soiled clothes separately.

- Separate lightly and heavily soiled clothes. Heavily soiled clothes need more wash time and more soap than lightly soiled clothes.

Step Two: Choose the Water Temperature

Read the labels on the clothes and on the laundry detergent to decide the water temperature for the wash. Table 14-5 is a general guide for choosing safe wash temperatures.

Step Three: Prepare Clothes for Washing

- Mend tears and loose buttons.
- Empty pockets.
- Zip zippers, snap snaps, hook hooks, tie apron or sweatshirt strings.
- Pretreat stains by soaking or use prewash treatments.

Step Four: Load the Washing Machine

Fill the machine with water and a measured amount of detergent before adding the clothes.

Table 14-5
Water Temperature Guide for Laundry

Hot Water	Warm or Cold Water
Whites	Permanent press clothes
Linens	Wools
Cottons that do not bleed	Delicates
Tennis shoes	Bright colors
Mattress pads	Dark or bright corduroys
Soiled work clothes	Fabrics that may bleed or shrink

Let the detergent mix with the wash water before adding the clothes to prevent spots. The wash water must cover the clothes completely for effective cleaning.

Step Five: Dry, Fold, and Put Away the Clothes

- Do not overload the dryer. Clothes need room to fluff.
- Remove clothes from the machine as soon as they are dry to avoid wrinkles and shrinkage. If the dryer does not have a timer, use a hand timer to remind yourself when they'll be done.
- Pillows, throw rugs, and coats can all be put in the dryer on a no-heat cycle to remove dust and lint.
- Instead of a dryer, your client may use a clothesline outside or inside the house.
- Fold and put away the clothes when they are dry.

Review Questions

True or False

1. ____ The care of the client's household is not very important for his health and well-being.

2. ____ It helps to broaden and sharpen your skills in home management because the HM/ HHA may be asked to teach clients and families about cleaning, preparing meals, and doing laundry.

3. ____ Taking a few moments at the start of your day to plan your workday will save time and energy later.

4. ____ If you cleaned the floor before cleaning a kitchen counter you would be following one of the basic rules of cleaning, that is, clean from top to bottom.

5. ____ All appliances are alike, so you really do not need to read the instructions.

6. ____ Never mix ammonia with household bleach or toilet bowl cleaner.

Chapter 15
Planning, Purchasing, and Serving Food

Objectives

At the conclusion of this chapter, the homemaker/ home health aide will:

1. Understand what a well-balanced diet is and why it is important.

2. Be able to list the Four Food Groups, give examples of foods from each groups, and state the recommended number of daily servings for an adult.

3. Understand the need for water and know how many glasses of water an average adult should drink in a day.

4. Be able to explain why a client might need a special diet and explain how to prepare foods in two special diets.

5. Be able to list some examples of foods and eating habits that relate to a client's culture.

6. Name four things to keep in mind when planning meals for a client.

7. Explain the need for using a receipt when handling a client's money and demonstrate how to make one.

8. Be able to describe some guidelines to follow when shopping for a client.

9. Understand the need for storing foods properly and know how to find out how long foods can be stored.

10. Know how to organize, prepare, and serve a meal for a client.

11. Describe how to feed a client and ways to help clients who have special eating problems.

Eating a well-balanced diet is one of the easiest and best ways to maintain health. *Nutrition* is the way the body uses food and fluids for growth and health. *Nutrients* are the parts of food that nourish the body. Proteins, carbohydrates, fats, vitamins, minerals, and water are all nutrients. Learning about nutrition also involves understanding different cultural eating patterns, learning how to shop for nutritious foods on a budget, how to prepare appetizing foods, and how to store foods safely. The HM/HHA can promote good nutrition by encouraging clients to eat well-balanced meals. Good nutrition influences physical and mental health and promotes a sense of well-being.

The Foods We Eat

The Four Food Groups

To get a balanced diet, a variety of foods from the Four Food Groups must be eaten daily. Foods have been divided into the Four Food Groups (milk, meat, fruit–vegetable, and grain) based on the nutrients that they contain. Each food within a group will contain other nutrients too, so it is important to eat different foods within the main groups to get the variety of nutrients needed to maintain health. For example, if a client decided to eat four oranges to meet his needed four servings of fruits–vegetables for the day, he would have satisfied an adult's need for the fruit–vegetable group. But his diet would be healthier if his fruit–vegetable choices were more varied. Study the Four Food Groups chart to learn the recommended number of daily servings from the milk, meat, fruit–vegetable, and grain groups needed for a particular person's age and condition. People who need more calories will need to eat more than the chart recommends.

Nutrients

Nutrients aid in the normal growth, development, and maintenance of body tissues and the normal functioning of body systems. There are about 50 nutrients needed by the body, but only the most common ones will be covered here. Most nutrients need to work with others in order to work effectively.

Proteins

Proteins are needed to build, maintain, and promote the healing of body tissues. They can also provide energy if carbohydrates and fats are not available. Proteins are often the most expensive foods we buy, but they are among the most important for good health and must be eaten daily. Proteins are either "complete" or "incomplete."

- A *complete protein* repairs and builds tissues.
- An *incomplete protein* maintains health but cannot build new tissues.

The easiest way to make sure a client is getting complete proteins is to serve an animal product such as meat, fish, poultry, eggs, cheese, or milk at every meal.

The Four Food Groups

Every day, be sure to eat the minimum recommended number of servings

Food Group	A serving is:		Minimum Recommended Number of Servings*				
			Children	Teenagers	Adults	Pregnant Women	Breast-feeding Women
Milk Group	1 cup	Milk	3	4	2	4	4
	1 cup	Yogurt					
	You can also get about the same amount of calcium by eating:						
	1½ oz	Cheese (1½ slices)					
	1 cup	Pudding					
	2 cups	Cottage cheese					
	1¾ cups	Ice cream					
Meat Group	2 oz	Cooked, lean meat, fish, poultry	2	2	2	3	2
	You can also get about the same amount of protein by eating:						
	2	Eggs					
	2 oz	Cheese					
	1 cup	Dried peas or beans					
	4 tbsp	Peanut butter					
Fruit–Vegetable Group	½ cup	Juice	4	4	4	4	4
	½ cup	Cooked vegetable or fruit	Dark green, leafy, or orange vegetables and fruit are recommended 3 or 4 times weekly for vitamin A. Citrus fruit is recommended daily for vitamin C.				
	1 cup	Raw vegetable or fruit					
	Medium	Apple, banana, or orange					
	½	Grapefruit					
	¼	Cantaloupe					
Grain Group	1 slice	Bread	4	4	4	4	4
	1 oz	Ready-to-eat cereal	Whole grain, fortified, or enriched grain products are recommended.				
	½ cup	Cooked cereal					
	½ cup	Pasta					
	½ cup	Rice					
	½ cup	Grits					
Combination Foods	1 cup	Soup	These count as servings (or partial servings) from the food groups from which they are made.				
	1 cup	Pasta dish (macaroni and cheese, lasagna)**					
	1 cup	Main course (stew, chili, casseroles)					
	¼ 14-in.	Pizza (thin crust)					
	1	Taco, sandwich					
"Others" Category	1 tsp	Butter, margarine	There are no recommended servings for foods in the "Others" category. Select these foods if you need additional calories, after you've met the recommended number of servings from the Four Food Groups.				
	1 tsp	Sugar					
	1 tbsp	Dressing, jelly, mayonnaise					
	1 cup	Soft drink					
	3½ oz	Wine					
	⅙ 9-in.	Pie					
	⅙ 9-in.	Layer cake					

*These servings are a basic foundation for good health. They supply about 1200 Calories and can provide a balance of the nutrients your body needs. However, most people need more than 1200 Calories. If you do, build upon this foundation by adding more servings from the Four Food Groups and the "Others" category.

**½ cup if used as a side dish.

(Courtesy of National Dairy Council: How to Eat for Good Health, 1987)

More About Complete and Incomplete Proteins

An amino acid is the building block of a protein. The body uses 22 amino acids. Fourteen of the amino acids are produced in the body naturally. There are eight that must be obtained from the foods we eat. When a protein food contains all eight amino acids, it is a *complete protein.* When a protein contains some, but not all, of the eight essential amino acids, it is an *incomplete protein.* Generally proteins that come from animals (milk, cheese, meat) are complete proteins. Proteins that come from vegetable sources (beans and grains) are incomplete. Clients who are vegetarians can eat a well-balanced diet without eating meat, but they need to make sure they are getting complete proteins in each meal. A strict vegetarian may also need to take vitamin B_{12} supplements because this vitamin is found only in foods from animal sources.

There are several ways to mix incomplete proteins together to make complete proteins (see chart, Completing Incomplete Proteins), but a dietitian should be consulted to make sure the client is getting the proper protein and vitamin combinations.

Carbohydrates

Carbohydrates provide an important source of nutrients and energy for the body and the brain. They make meals more flavorful and give a feeling of fullness. Some carbohydrates are a good source of fiber, which encourages better digestion and elimination. Sixty percent of the calories eaten in a day should come from carbohydrates such as rice, wheat, oats, cereals, pasta, breads, fruits, and vegetables.

Sugars are also carbohydrates. Americans now eat about 130 pounds of sugar per person per year. Much of that sugar is in soft drinks, processed foods, and other "hidden" sources. Sugar provides flavor and calories, but it does not provide any nutrients that help keep people healthy. Eating sugar also causes tooth decay.

Fats

Fats are needed in our diets for energy. Fats are high in flavor and tend to satisfy hunger longer because they leave the stomach slowly. Fats also provide essential fatty acids for infant growth and development, and they lubricate the intestinal

---

Completing Incomplete Proteins

Incomplete Proteins That Combine to Make a Complete Protein	Examples
Grains and legumes	Peanut butter on wheat bread
	Bean soup with wheat toast
	Pea soup with wheat roll
Grains and milk	Macaroni and cheese
	Toasted cheese on wheat bread
	Oatmeal with milk
Grains and eggs	French toast made from wheat bread
	Quiche with wheat pastry
	Egg salad sandwich with wheat bread

---

tract. A relatively small amount of fat is needed for good health. The American Heart Association recommends that less than 30% of an adult's daily calories should come from fat.

There are three major types of fats.

1. *Saturated fats* are generally found in animal products, and are usually solid fats. They raise the level of cholesterol in the blood, which can lead to heart and artery disease. Foods rich in saturated fats include butter, whole milk, cheese, egg yolks, ice cream, cakes, cookies, pies, and fatty meats such as pork, bacon, ham, beef, and lamb.

2. *Polyunsaturated fats* are found in vegetable products, and are either soft or in liquid form. They tend to lower cholesterol levels in the blood. Foods rich in polyunsaturated fats include vegetable oils (such as corn oil, safflower oil, and olive oil), and some margarines.

3. *Cholesterol* is found in animal products (egg yolks and rich cuts of pork and beef), but it is primarily produced in the liver when saturated fats are eaten. Cholesterol is a major ingredient in the fatty deposits that restrict blood flow in arteries. Clients with heart or circulatory diseases are often

advised to restrict the amount of cholesterol and saturated fat in their diets.

Vitamins and Minerals

Vitamins and minerals maintain normal growth, development, and health. Vitamins do not provide miracle cures or lessen the need for eating a well-balanced diet. They are only needed in small amounts. A well-balanced diet will provide the average person with all the vitamins and minerals needed for health. A client who is ill, pregnant or nursing, or physically active may need vitamin or mineral supplements, but only under a doctor's supervision. Overdosing on vitamins and minerals can cause serious health problems. Let your supervisor know if a client is taking vitamins.

Nutrients, vitamins, and minerals are summarized in the chart on pages 142–144.

Summary of Basic Nutrients, Vitamins, and Minerals

Nutrient	Why Needed	Food Sources
Protein	Builds, repairs, and maintains body tissues. Major component of all cells, enzymes, hormones, and fluids in the body. Also helps form antibodies to reduce infection. Provides energy if necessary.	Meat, fish, poultry, dried bean and peas, and dairy products such as milk and cheese
Carbohydrate	Provides energy for the brain and all the cells of the body. Allows protein to be used for growth and maintenance of the body cells instead of being used for energy.	Cereal, corn, potatoes, dried beans and peas, bread, and sugars
Fat	Provides a concentrated source of energy. Helps the body use the fat-soluble vitamins (vitamins A, D, E, and K) and supplies some essential fatty acids. Adds flavor to the diet and lubricates the intestinal tract.	Whole milk, cream, butter, lard, fried foods, cheese, bacon, meat fats, vegetable oils, salad dressing, nuts, avocados, chocolate, and peanut butter
Fiber	Helps digestion and aids elimination by absorbing water in the intestinal tract.	Fresh fruits and vegetables, especially in the skins and pulp; also dried fruits and whole grain bread
Water	Water is essential for survival. A person can live only a few days without it.	Adults need to drink the equivalent of 6–8 glasses per day. Sources of water include water, (continued)

Summary of Basic Nutrients, Vitamins, and Minerals *(continued)*

Nutrient	Why Needed	Food Sources
Water *(continued)*	Water makes up ½ to ¾ of the body weight. Most is found in the cells. The rest is in the blood, lymph, and secretions. Helps all organs and all body systems function.	juice, milk, and other beverages. Fruits, vegetables, and other foods also contain water.
Minerals		
Calcium and phosphorus	Forms teeth and bones. Helps muscles, heart, and nerves to function and aids blood clotting. Allows food and waste products to get in and out of cells. Needed throughout life. Vitamin D is needed to help calcium and phosphorus work effectively.	Milk and milk products such as yogurt and cheese; also green leafy vegetables
Iron	Needed in red blood cells to carry oxygen from the lungs to all the cells in the body. Prevents fatigue.	Organ meats such as liver and kidneys, lean meats, cereals, enriched breads, dry peas and beans, prune juice, dark yellow and green vegetables
Iodine	Need is increased during adolescence and pregnancy. Promotes normal growth. Lack of iodine causes goiters, but these are rare.	Iodized salt and seafoods
Vitamins		
Vitamin A (retinol)	Helps eyes adjust to the dark and prevents night blindness. Promotes normal growth. Maintains the skin and hair and the linings of the nose, mouth, throat, and digestive tract. Reduces infection in the mucous membranes.	Liver, carrots, sweet potatoes, dark green vegetables, and animal fats such as fortified butter, margarine, and milk

(continued)

Summary of Basic Nutrients, Vitamins, and Minerals *(continued)*

Nutrient	Why Needed	Food Sources
Vitamins		
Vitamin B_1 (thiamin)	Aids normal appetite and helps the body obtain energy from foods. Maintains nervous system.	Enriched cereals and breads, whole grains, dry beans and peas, pork, liver, and kidneys
Vitamin B_2 (riboflavin)	Helps cells use carbohydrates, fats, and proteins. Maintains health of eyes, skin, and mouth. Promotes general well-being.	Liver, milk, eggs, yogurt, cheese, and grain products
Vitamin B_3 (niacin)	Helps the cells of the body use oxygen. Builds brain cells and maintains the health of the skin, digestive, and nervous systems.	Whole grain foods, wheat germ, lean meats, liver, poultry, fish, and peanuts
Vitamin B_{12}	Helps the cells use protein. Aids red blood cell formation and prevents pernicious anemia. Maintains the nervous system.	Liver, kidneys, milk products, lean meats, and seafood
Vitamin C (ascorbic acid)	Strengthens blood vessels and holds cells together. Aids wound healing. Encourages resistance to infections.	Citrus fruits, tomatoes, strawberries, broccoli, cabbage and other green vegetables; is destroyed by overcooking.
Vitamin D	Helps the body use calcium and phosphorus to build strong bones and teeth. Needed throughout life, but especially in growing children and pregnant women.	Found in foods fortified with vitamin D, such as milk; also in oily fish and eggs. Sunshine promotes a substance in the skin to make vitamin D.

The Body's Need for Water

Water is essential to life. People can survive only a few days without it. The human body is made up of 45% to 75% water, depending upon a person's age. We need to maintain a particular amount of water in our systems to be healthy. The average adult should drink between six and eight glasses of water every day unless otherwise advised by his doctor. Some clients need to keep track of the amount of fluids that they drink. This is known as *intake.* See Chapter 20 to learn how to measure intake and output.

Special Diets

A *therapeutic diet* is one that is described by a doctor to improve or maintain health. All therapeutic diets are based upon the principles of normal nutrition and modified for a particular health problem. See the Special Diets chart on page 146 for a summary of therapeutic diets.

The HM/HHA needs to understand a client's therapeutic diet to make sure meals are prepared and followed correctly. Usually, diet instructions are taught by the dietitian, nurse, or doctor. The HM/HHA can help reinforce the teaching to the client and family if the home health supervisor approves.

Planning Meals

How to Plan a Meal for Your Client

Your supervisor will work with you when planning a client's meals. You will need to know:

- If the doctor has said the client cannot eat certain foods or that the client can only have a limited amount of certain foods.
- The client's cultural background, special eating practices (allergies, religious restrictions), and individual preferences.
- About how much money the client can spend on food.
- How to plan a nutritious meal based on the Four Food Groups

Follow Doctor's Orders

When a client's doctor has ordered a diet restriction, you must follow those orders.

The Client's Cultural Practices

Eating habits are learned from families and social groups. Some clients will eat their heavy meal at noon and others will have it in the evening. Some will eat three meals per day and others will eat five or six daily meals. Even though a client's family

has been in the United States for generations, that client may still enjoy the cultural foods of his ancestors. Some foods are associated with nationalities. Pasta is associated with Italians. Northern Europeans tend to eat more meat and dairy products than Italians. Hispanic people may prefer spicy Mexican foods, while people from the Far East may continue eating Oriental foods.

People from other countries may move to the United States and find that foods from their native countries are expensive or unavailable here. The family may not know how to eat a balanced diet using our foods. Or they may not like our foods or understand how to prepare them. The home health supervisor and dietitian will work closely with you so you can help your clients plan and prepare nutritious meals that are acceptable within their culture.

You may observe differences other than the type of foods. People who are Chinese or Japanese may continue to eat with chopsticks, while Arabs may prefer to use bread to scoop up their foods instead of using a knife, fork, or spoon. Many Moslems, Hindus, Mormans, and Jews do not eat pork for religious reasons. If your client is a vegetarian and will not eat meat, your supervisor will help you understand what foods can be eaten to obtain a balanced diet.

Ask the client about his eating habits.

What foods does the client especially like?
Are there any foods he does not like or finds hard to eat?
How many meals (including snacks) does he eat each day?
What time does he eat?
When does he eat his main meal?

If you understand and respect a client's reasons for his way of eating, you can help him maintain a balanced diet in a pleasant environment. One of the great advantages of home health care is that the client can continue his cultural practices without making changes to fit other people's expectations. Imagine how you would feel as a client if you were used to eating hot, spicy food for dinner and a HM/HHA from a different background prepared a bland meal of mashed potatoes, peas, and meat. If you work with your supervisor and listen closely to your client's requests, you should avoid this kind of mix-up.

Special Diets

Purpose	Foods Allowed	Foods Not Allowed
Bland Diet		
For clients who have stomach or intestinal problems such as ulcers	Unseasoned foods, dairy products, creamed soups, tender meats. Some doctors allow client to eat foods he can tolerate without discomfort.	Cola, coffee, alcohol, chocolate, curry powder, chili, hot peppers, and fried foods
Clear Liquid Diet		
For clients who are having tests, who have an upset stomach, or who have just had surgery	Water, ice, sodapop, coffee (black), tea, clear broth, apple juice, cranberry juice, gelatins (plain)	Any foods or drinks that are not clear liquids
Full Liquid Diet		
For clients with chewing problems	Clear liquid diet plus milk, custard, puddings, cream soups, yogurt, strained cooked cereals, ice cream	Solid foods
Soft Diet		
For clients who have trouble chewing or swallowing	Normal diet, but foods need to be blended, chopped, or strained	Foods that are not chopped, blended, or strained
Low Fiber Diet		
For clients who have inflammatory diseases of the colon	Ripe bananas and avocados, canned fruits, cooked vegetables, noodles, rice, white bread, and tender meats such as chicken and ground beef	High-fiber foods including whole-grain products, nuts, popcorn, and raw fruits and vegetables
High-Fiber Diet		
For clients who experience constipation or diverticulosis (an outpouching of the large intestine). Fiber absorbs water in the large intestine, which allows stools to soften and pass out of the body more easily.	Fiber is the undigestable part of the plant foods we eat. Examples include whole grain products such as bran and whole grain breads, nuts, popcorn, and raw fruits and vegetables with skins. Plenty of fluids are needed on a high-fiber diet.	
Diabetic Diet		
An individualized plan that balances protein, fats, and carbohydrates based on the insulin and nutritional needs of the client. Many follow an exchange list.	Regulated amounts of foods from a normal diet. Fruits and vegetables, meats, dairy products, breads, sugarless cereals, coffee, tea, and spices are all allowed.	Sugar is not allowed in any form or only in very small amounts. The client cannot have soft drinks or alcohol. Foods should not be eaten when the ingredients are not known.
Low-Fat Diet		
For clients with gallbladder, liver, or cardiovascular diseases	Skim milk; low-fat cottage cheese; decaffeinated beverages; dry cereals without nuts or oils; fruits and vegetables except avocados and olives; broiled, baked, or roasted lean meats; bread, potatoes, pasta, and rice served without butter, sour cream, or other fats. Often allowed 1 teaspoon of fat per meal.	Whole or low-fat milk, cream, and eggnog; sweet rolls, pancakes, waffles, and granola; all cheeses except mozzarella and others made from skim milk; ice cream, pies, chocolate, and cakes; peanut butter, mayonnaise, oils, or butter; breaded, fried, or fatty meats such as sausage; buttered popcorn, nuts, or potato chips

Food Fads

A *fad* is a short-lived, widespread interest. Clients may hear about fads from magazines, newspapers, television, and even friends and family. Unfortunately, there are no miracle diets. Many fads are not based on facts and they can cause harm if your client is not getting the foods he needs. With the home care team's assistance, you can help teach your clients about healthy eating patterns.

Food Costs

Your supervisor will help you decide how to buy and prepare foods so that you stay within the client's budget. Food costs and money-saving strategies are discussed later in this chapter.

The Four Food Groups

You will use the Four Food Groups on page 140 to plan well-balanced meals. Table 15-1 is a basic guide for preparing three meals. Table 15-2 shows other food combinations that follow the same recommendations. Both charts can be adapted for the client who eats smaller and more frequent meals. If the client prefers a heavier meal at noon

and a lighter meal in the evening, the noon and evening meals can be switched. Remember, when a casserole has only one cup of vegetables, another vegetable or salad must be served to meet the required need.

Other Factors in Planning Meals

There are some other important considerations when planning a meal for your client.

- *Variety.* Would you like to eat mashed potatoes, white fish, and applesauce all in one meal? Probably not. That meal would be dull because all the foods are so close in color and texture. A meal has greater appeal when there are contrasts in colors, temperatures, textures, flavors, and shapes.
- *Moderation.* Even with food restrictions, the client may not have to give up a favorite food completely. For example, a client who has been drinking ten cups of coffee a day may be asked to cut down to two or three cups. Ask your supervisor about specific food limits.

Table 15-1
Meal Planning Guide

Meal Suggestions	Examples
Morning Meal	
Fruit or fruit juice	Orange juice
Eggs or protein substitute	2 poached eggs
Cereal or bread	Bowl of oatmeal
Beverage	Milk and water
Noon Meal	
Fruit	Apple
Meat or protein substitute	2 oz. cheese sandwich
Bread or grain	Two slices of wheat bread (on sandwich)
Vegetable (may be in soup, salad, or casserole)	Tomato and lettuce on sandwich
Beverage	Milk
Evening Meal	
Meat or other protein substitute	Chicken
Potato, rice, or noodles	Brown rice
Green and yellow vegetable (may be in salad)	Broccoli and carrots
Beverage	Coffee and water
Dessert (optional)	

Table 15-2
Two Sample Menus That Meet the Minimum Food Requirements for an Adult*

Day One	Day Two
Breakfast	
Orange juice	½ grapefruit
2 eggs	oatmeal
2 slices of toast	8 oz. milk
Lunch	
¼ cantaloupe	Cheese sandwich with 2 slices of whole wheat bread
Cottage cheese	Apple
2 slices of wheat bread	Yogurt
Dinner	
Green beans	Fish
Potato	Rice
Chicken	Carrots
Ice cream	Spinach

*In these examples there is room for more food if extra calories are needed.

- *Avoid sudden changes.* Changes are easier to maintain if they are worked into the diet gradually. A client who is told not to eat butter may think he cannot adjust to eating margarine. If he mixes some margarine and butter in a bowl and over a period of time keeps adding more margarine until it is completely margarine, the adjustment will be easier. This mixing procedure can be done with whole milk and skim milk, and coffee and decaffeinated coffee too. Your supervisor will have other suggestions on how to help a client change his eating patterns gradually.

Buying Food for Your Client

Money and Receipts

Always keep close track of money that you handle for a client. When a client gives you money for groceries or any items that you will buy for him, fill out a cash receipt (Figure 15-1) as soon as he gives you the money. When you return, fill out another receipt (Figure 15-2). Most cash receipts have two copies. One copy goes to the client. The other copy is returned to the agency where it will be put in the client's chart as a record that you returned the correct change.

Cash Receipt 1

_____ received _____
(Homemaker/Home Health Aide)   (amount of money)

from _____
(client or family)

on _____ at _____
(date)   (time)

to buy _____
(list items or attach shopping list)

signed _____
(client's signature)

_____
(Homemaker/Home Health Aide's signature)

Figure 15-1
Use this receipt when the client gives you money for shopping.

Cash Receipt 2

On ______________________ (date and time), ______________________ (Homemaker/Home Health Aide) was given ______________________ (amount of money; refer to Cash Receipt 1) to buy items from store. Items cost ______________________.
(may attach store receipts)

______________________ (client) received ______________________ (amount of money) from ______________________ (Homemaker/Home Health Aide) on ______________________ (date) at ______________________ (time) as change from the original amount.

signed ______________________
(client's signature)

____
(Homemaker/Home Health Aide's signature)

Figure 15-2
Use this receipt when you are returning money to the client after doing his shopping.

Shopping Guidelines for Saving Money

Use a Shopping List

Your supervisor, the client, or the family will help you prepare the shopping list. Do not buy extras that are not on the list because you are spending your client's money. Find out what brands and sizes the client prefers.

Check Food Advertisements

Use the local newspapers to find the store with the best specials for the foods you plan to buy.

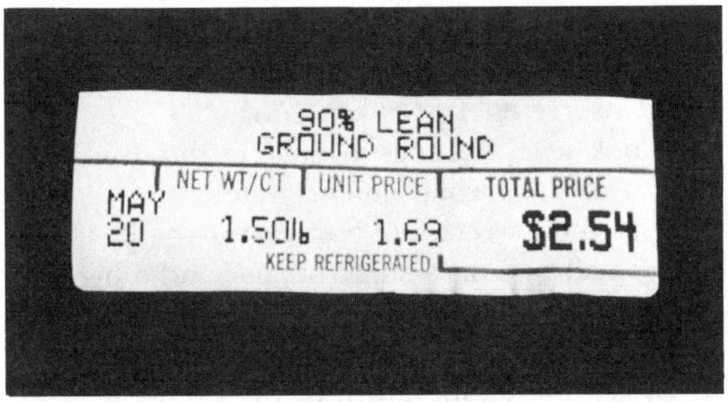
90% LEAN
GROUND ROUND
NET WT/CT
UNIT PRICE
TOTAL PRICE
MAY
20
1.50lb
1.69
$2.54
KEEP REFRIGERATED

Figure 15-3
Example of a unit price label. According to this label, the ground round costs $1.69 per pound. This package weighs 1.5 pounds. To get the total price for this package, multiply price per pound times weight ($1.69 × 1.5 = $2.54).

Use Unit Pricing to Compare Prices

Many grocery stores now have unit pricing labels on their shelves or on the product itself (Figure 15-3). The label will usually tell you the product name, the weight of the container, the total price, and the price per pound. This makes it fairly easy to compare various brands and containers. The largest container is often, but not always, the least expensive. If the store does not have unit pricing, you may want to figure out the price per unit yourself.

Store brands are often less expensive than nationally advertised brands. But you may not have saved any money if you buy a less expensive brand that the client will not use.

How to Determine Price per Pound

When an item is available in several sizes or brands, do you know how to tell which is the best buy? Let's say one jar of peanut butter contains 1 lb., 12 oz. (or 28 oz.) and costs $1.55. The second jar contains 12 oz. and costs 75 cents. Which is cheaper? First, determine the price per ounce by dividing the cost of the item by the number of ounces. Then compare your results.

$$\frac{\$1.55}{28\text{ oz.}} = 5.5 \text{ cents per ounce}$$

$$\frac{\$.75}{12\text{ oz.}} = 6.2 \text{ cents per ounce}$$

As you can see, the large jar of peanut butter is less expensive per ounce. If the client does not plan to use the item very much or does not have the room to store it, the smaller item may be the wiser choice even though it costs more.

Read the Food Labels

Food labels can give you information about contents, expiration dates, and servings per container.

- *The contents.* Foods are listed in the order of amount. The first ingredient on a label is the one that is the greatest amount. Some information about nutrients on the label is required by law (Figure 15-4).
- *Expiration dates.* Look for the expiration date on perishable food items such as dairy products. Dairy products can usually be used up to 1 week past the expiration date.
- *Servings per container.* You need to know how much you need and how much the client can store. Do not buy foods in large amounts if there is not room to store them properly or if the foods cannot be used while they are fresh.

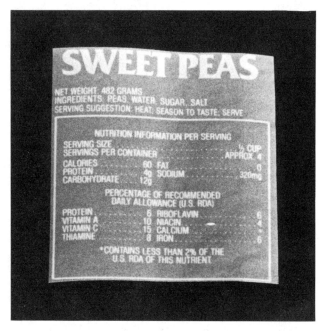

Figure 15-4
Example of a food label. Reading food labels is especially important when shopping or preparing food for someone who is on a special diet. If your client is on a low-salt diet, you would know from the label that this can of peas contains salt (320 mg of sodium per serving).

Other Money-Saving Ideas

- Buy fresh fruits and vegetables when they are in season.
- Buy the largest package of products that are used frequently, if the client has room to store it.
- Convenience foods and those wrapped in individual packages are expensive. Consider whether you or the client's family has the time and skill to make the same foods from scratch. Convenience foods might be the best buy for the one- or two-person household. Even though convenience foods are expensive, they may be worth it because of the time and effort they save the client.
- Chicken and turkey are usually the least expensive meats. Fish can also be a good buy. Look at the cuts of meat on special. If they have too much bone or fat on them, a more expensive cut may be a better buy.
- Consider the use for the foods. Fresh tomatoes make a salad more appealing, but a cheaper brand of canned tomatoes can be used in a casserole when appearance is not a factor.
- At the store, buy the meats, dairy products, and frozen foods last so they are out of the refrigerated case the shortest amount of time possible.

Food Preparation and Storage

Food Preparation Guidelines

- Work in a clean and safe kitchen.
- Never use food that you suspect may be spoiled. Do not use food from bulging or dented cans or from leaking containers.
- Conserve energy as you cook.
  Cook several things at once in the oven.
  Cover pans when boiling water.
  Use the correct size burner for the pan. Put a small pan on a small burner and a big pan on a big burner.
- If available, use an oven thermometer to check the temperature of the oven.

Food Storage Guidelines

- Read food labels to find out expiration dates and special storage directions.

- Rotate stocked foods. Put newer foods at the back and older foods at the front so they can be used first.
- The freezer and refrigerator should be kept clean and in good working condition. If available, use a freezer thermometer to check the temperatures in the refrigerator and freezer.

> Safe Temperatures for Food Storage
> Refrigerator   36°F to 40°F
> Freezer   0°F

- Frozen foods should not be stored in the ice cube compartment of a refrigerator for more than a week.
- Wrap foods securely for freezing with freezer paper or heavy-duty aluminum foil.
- Label frozen food with the food and the date.
- Do not refreeze foods after they have been thawed.
- Store meat in the coldest part of the refrigerator. Leave it in the store wrapping if it will be used within 2 days. Otherwise, rewrap in freezer paper or aluminum foil and freeze. Table 15-3 provides guidelines for safe storage times.
- Cool just-cooked meat and casseroles quickly by placing the meat dish in a bowl that is sitting in a pan of ice water (Figure 15-5). When cool, wrap tightly to keep out air and place in refrigerator or freezer. See Table 15-3.

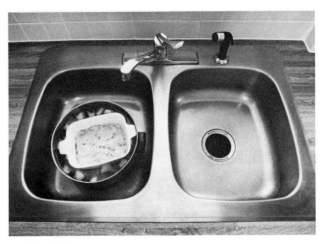

Figure 15-5
Food should be refrigerated as soon as possible to avoid spoilage. If you must cool a very hot casserole before refrigerating it, set the casserole in a pan of ice to cool it quickly before returning it to the refrigerator.

- Guidelines for storing staples at 70°F to maintain nutrients and flavor.
  Flour, sugar, salt, and pepper—2 years
  Most low-acid canned foods such as meats and vegetables—2 years
  Canned citrus fruits, fruit juices, and other high-acid foods—9–12 months

Serving Food

The Setting

Foods served in an attractive and relaxed setting stimulate the appetite. Meals are the highlight of the day for many people.

Table 15-3
Safe Storage Times for Refrigerated and Frozen Foods

Food	Time in Refrigerator	Time in Freezer
Beef		
Roasts and steaks	2–4 days	6–12 months
Ground beef and stews	1–2 days	2–4 months
Pork		
Ham and sausages	1–2 days	3–4 months
Bacon	1 week	3–4 months
Poultry		
Chicken and turkey	1–2 days	6–12 months
Lunch meats	1 week	1–2 months
Leftover cooked meat	3–4 days	2–3 months

- The room where the client eats should be clean and free from unpleasant odors and objects.
- Offer the client the chance to use the toilet before meals, and make sure there are supplies to wash his hands before and after meals.
- Arrange the food on an uncrowded plate. Use garnishes to make the plate more attractive.
- Try to steer the conversation away from unpleasant topics, such as health problems, during the meal.
- Food is easier to digest in a relaxed atmosphere. Sit and talk with the client for a few minutes during the meal.

Helping Clients Who Have Special Problems When Eating

1. Your client says he has no desire to eat.
   - There are a number of reasons a client may not feel like eating. Illness, depression, physical pain, emotional stress, or an unclean room can all make a person lose his appetite. Not eating is a problem because it starts a dangerous cycle. To help stimulate the client's appetite, follow the suggestions above for creating a relaxed setting for the client's meal.

Low appetite → weight loss → loss of strength and energy → nutritional problems and difficulty maintaining health

---

2. Your client complains of an upset stomach or nausea.
   - Serve small, frequent nutritious meals or snacks.
   - A glass of cool water before the meal may help.
   - Avoid serving the client's favorite food if he is feeling nauseated. You do not want him to associate his "sick feeling" with his favorite food.

3. Your client has chewing problems.
   - Milk is a good source of protein. Use it in soups, milkshakes, gravies, puddings, and custards.
   - Meats, poultry, and vegetables will become more tender if cooked slowly at a low temperature. Meat can be ground, shredded, or even blended in a creamy soup.
   - Fish will remain easy to chew when it is broiled, baked, or poached.
   - Eggs can be served any number of ways such as an omelet, poached, or scrambled.
4. Your client has mouth sores.
   - Cold foods like gelatin, yogurt, and milkshakes may be soothing.
   - Stay away from spicy, salty, and lemon-flavored foods.
   - A straw may make it easier to drink fluids.
5. Your client says his medication changes the way food tastes.
   - The food may need more seasoning (salt, pepper, lemon, herbs, and spices). Find out which seasonings are permitted by the doctor.
   - Wine adds flavor to gravies and the alcohol evaporates with cooking.
6. Your client needs help being fed.
   - Sit down with the client to let him know you have the time to help him. During the meal talk to the client as an adult, not as a child.
   - When you bring the plate, show the client the food and ask him what he'd like to eat first. If he cannot tell you, feed him in the order that you would like to eat the meal.
   - If the client cannot see the food, tell him what is on the plate. After the client has told you which foods he'd like to eat first, let him know what is on each spoonful. As you bring the spoon to the client's mouth, lightly touch the bottom lip to let the client know where the spoon is. Don't forget to let him know whether the food is hot or cold for the first few bites of food.
   - Feed the client *slowly*. Take a deep breath and relax while you are helping with the meal. A rushed meal is not pleasant.
   - When the meal is over, record the amount of food eaten. An entry that states "client ate well" does not tell others on the home health care team much.

Step One: List the Tasks and the Time They Will Take

Task	Cooking Time	Preparation Time
Set table		5 minutes
Help client to table		10 minutes
Frozen peas on stove	10 minutes	
Broiled hamburger patty	5 minutes	10 minutes
Tomato and lettuce salad	5 minutes	
Serve the meal		5 minutes
Ice cream		
Instant coffee		5 minutes

Step Two: Put the Tasks in Order

Mealtime: Noon

1. Set table (11:25 AM).
2. Boil water for peas and instant mashed potatoes and have everything ready to start them later. Make hamburger patty (11:35 AM).
3. Help client to the dining table (11:45 AM).
4. Put hamburger in broiler and start peas and potatoes. Prepare salad and take it to the client. Or chill the salad and serve it with the rest of the meal (11:55 AM).
5. Flip hamburger and stir the peas and potatoes.
6. Serve hamburger, potatoes, peas, and salad (noon).
7. Serve coffee and ice cream when client is finished with the meal.

Saving Time While Preparing and Serving Meals

How to Get Organized When Preparing Meals

1. Make a list of all the tasks that need to be done and include an approximate amount of time for each task, including cooking time and preparation and serving time. See the above chart for Step One for an example.
2. Put the tasks in order according to when they need to be done. An example is given above in the chart for Step Two.
3. Decide what time the meal will be served and work backwards. If the meal will be at noon and the preparation time is about 35 minutes, start fixing the meal about 11:25 AM or a little earlier.

Review Questions

True or False

1. ____ Proteins help build, maintain, and heal body tissues. They should be eaten every day.

2. ____ Carbohydrates are a poor source of energy.

3. ____ Polyunsaturated fats found in vegetable products are lower in cholesterol.

4. ____ It is impossible to take too many vitamins.

5. ____ The average adult should drink six to eight glasses of water each day unless otherwise advised by his doctor.

6. ____ A fluid intake and output record must be kept for every client.

7. ____ Buying the largest container available always saves money when shopping for food.

8. ___ Hamburger should not be stored in the refrigerator for more than 2 days, but lunch meats will stay fresh for a week.

9. ___ Before starting a meal or any task in a client's home, form a work plan so that you know how long each step will take.

Meal Planning Exercise

Can you plan two days of nutritious meals that follow the Four Food Group recommendations? First, fill in the number of servings that an adult needs from each group. Then, using the chart below, plan a breakfast, lunch, and dinner to meet the Four Food Group needs. When you fill out the second day, use different food items than you used for the first day.

Fill in the number of servings an adult needs each day:
___ Milk Group
___ Fruit – Vegetable Group
___ Meat Group
___ Grain Group

Meals	First Day	Second Day
Breakfast		
Lunch		
Dinner		

The Feeding Exercise

You will need a partner and you will both take turns posing as the client. Prepare a small dish of food for you and your partner. Then take turns feeding each other. The one who is being fed should not help the server by guiding the spoon. Try having the client drink water from a cup. To make this exercise more challenging, the person who is being fed should be blindfolded as though the client were blind. Or pretend the client cannot talk, as might happen if your client has had a stroke.

After doing the feeding exercise you will have a better understanding of how it feels to be fed. Then answer the following questions.

1. How did it feel to have someone feed you? Did you want to help or give the server directions?

2. Did your server feed you at a pace that was comfortable for you? Did you ever feel he was in a hurry?

3. Did your server ask you about the order that you wanted to eat the different foods on the plate?

4. If you were blindfolded, did your server tell you what was being served and warn you about the temperature of the food?

5. When serving, were you tempted to talk in a sing-song tone as though the client were a child? ("Alrighty, now you better eat all your peas.")

Part Six

Personal Care and Medical Procedures

Chapter 16

Lifting, Positioning, and Exercise

Objectives

At the conclusion of this chapter, the homemaker/home health aide will:

1. Be able to demonstrate and explain the benefits of good body posture for standing, sitting, and lying down.

2. Be able to list and demonstrate the rules of lifting.

3. Know how to reposition a client using all of the techniques taught in this chapter.

4. Know when a client is not using a walker or cane safely, and know how to explain to the client how to use the walker or cane properly.

5. Be able to demonstrate range-of-motion exercises.

> This chapter contains several procedures. You must practice them on well clients under the supervision of a qualified health professional before trying them on your clients.

Body Mechanics

Body mechanics is the study of how to use the body as an efficient machine without causing injury. It involves learning good posture and how to coordinate the body when moving and lifting. HM/HHAs lose more time off work from back injuries than from any other health problem. Learning good body mechanics will help you lift and assist clients in ways that will ensure the client's safety and yours. You will also find these rules useful in your daily life.

Good Body Posture

Posture refers to the way a person holds his body. Using good body posture will reduce fatigue, prevent sore muscles, lessen the chance of bedsores, give the internal organs room to work effectively, and allow the client to be more comfortable. Good posture positions for standing and sitting are explained below. In all cases, the back is kept straight. Remember these examples of good posture when you are positioning a client.

When *standing*, the back is straight and the hips are tucked under (Figure 16-1). Shoulders

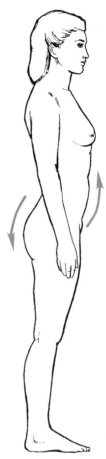

Figure 16-1
Good posture for standing.

are directly over the hips and the arms are at the sides. The feet are about 12 inches apart with the knees slightly bent.

While *sitting*, the head is erect and the back is straight (Figure 16-2). Body weight is evenly held by both thighs and the bottom. (This prevents pressure and strain to one hip and reduces the chance of bedsores.) The heels and toes touch the floor. (A shorter client may need a footstool to keep his ankles flexed.)

Useful Terms

Base of support is the area of your body that is in contact with the ground. When standing, your feet are the base of support. A wide base of support is more stable than a narrow base. The following exercise demonstrates the need for a wide base of support. Try standing with your feet together and have someone give you a slight push to one side. It is likely that you will stumble. Now place your feet 12 inches apart. Have your friend give you another slight push. You can see that

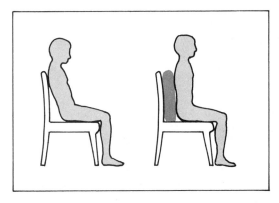

If the chair is deep, use a pillow to support the client's back.

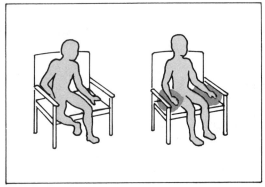

If the chair is too wide, use pillows or small cushions to keep the client from slipping to one side.

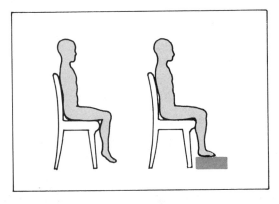

If the seat of the chair is too high, use a footstool to keep pressure off the client's back and legs.

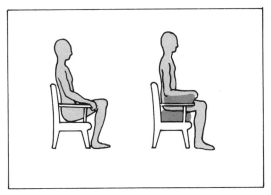

If the chair is too low, use a pillow or cushion on the seat and the chair arms.

Figure 16-2
Adjusting the chair to fit the client. (Adapted with permission from Talbot D: Principles of Therapeutic Positioning: A Guide to Nursing Action, p 12. Copyright 1981, Sister Kenny Institute, 800 East 28th Street, Minneapolis, MN 55407. Figures redrawn.)

when your base of support widened, you were much more stable.

A person's *center of gravity* is the point in the body where an equal amount of weight is above, below, and to each side of that point. When a person stands with good posture, the center of gravity is just below the navel.

Lifting Rules

When lifting and carrying a heavy object, you will feel more stable and use less energy when you carry it close to your center of gravity. For example, if you lift a heavy book and hold it at your waist, you can manage it without too much trouble. If you take the same book and hold it out to the side at arm's length, the book feels much heavier and you may have to lean to the side in order to balance yourself.

To lift a heavy object safely, follow these rules:

1. Keep your back straight.
2. Squat, instead of bending from the waist. This is shown in Figure 16-3.
3. Keep the object close to your body.
4. Lift with your legs, not your back. After taking hold of the object, stand up by straightening your legs. Tighten your abdominal and bottom muscles to help with the lift. Do not bend up from the waist, because this will use your weaker back muscles.
5. Do not twist from the waist when lifting. Twisting puts strain on the back. When moving a client up to the head of the bed, your feet should face the direction you are moving the client to prevent twisting.
6. Pivot instead of twisting to face your work

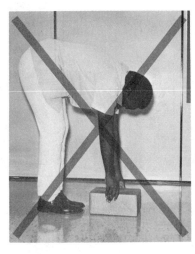 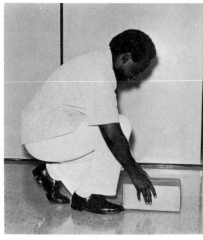

Figure 16-3
(*Left*) The wrong way to lift an object from the floor. (*Right*) The safe way to lift an object from the floor. The homemaker/home health aide has kept his back straight, placed his feet about 12 inches apart, and bent his knees to squat. He holds the object close to his body and will lift by straightening his legs. (After Lewis LW: Fundamental Skills in Patient Care, 3rd ed, p 72. Philadelphia, JB Lippincott, 1984)

area. To pivot, lean forward on the balls of your feet, raise your heels, and turn, keeping your body straight.

7. Whenever possible, push, or pull instead of lifting.
8. Work at waist level.

These rules are especially important to remember when you are repositioning a client and when teaching lifting techniques to the family.

Positioning

Guidelines for Moving a Client

1. Wash your hands as you would before starting any procedure.
2. Before starting, explain to the client what you are about to do and how he can help.
3. When you need to lift or reposition a client who cannot help, ask capable family members to assist you. It is always easier to lift and reposition a client if you have two people. This also allows the family to participate in the care and to learn to move, lift, and reposition the client using good body mechanics.
4. Follow the rules of good body mechanics. Avoid lifting whenever possible. Slide, roll, or pivot instead. Point your toes in the direction that you are moving. Keep your back straight. Lift with your legs and keep the weight close to your body.
6. Before you actually move a client, count out loud to three (1, 2, 3, lift). This lets the client know exactly when he'll be moved so he can prepare himself.
7. *Stop right away* if you are hurting a client.

Equipment for Positioning

Be familiar with the following equipment. Your supervisor will let you know when to use any of it for a particular client. Most of these supplies can be found in the client's home.

Pillows. Pillows are frequently used when positioning a client. If you run out of pillows, use folded sheets, blankets, towels, or cloth diapers.

Trochanter Roll. A trochanter roll prevents the hips and legs from turning out as shown in Figure 16-4. To make a trochanter roll, fold a large bath towel lengthwise and roll it, leaving about 12 inches unrolled. Place the unrolled flap under the client's hips and upper thighs so that the roll is turned under. Roll the towel under to fit snugly against the client's hips and upper thighs as shown in Figure 16-5.

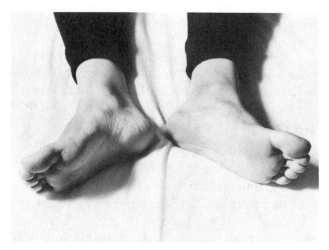

Figure 16-4
The hips and legs normally turn out and the feet drop down when a person is in bed. If a client is confined to bed for a long time, serious muscle problems can develop. A trochanter roll and footboard will help prevent these problems.

Figure 16-5
How to make a trochanter roll to prevent the legs from turning out. (Lewis LW: Fundamental Skills in Patient Care, 3rd ed, p 346. Philadelphia, JB Lippincott, 1984)

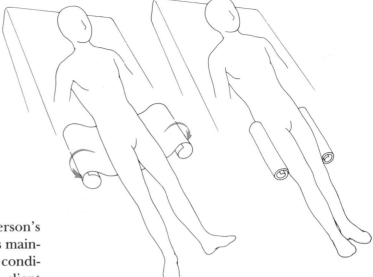

Footboard. When lying on the back, a person's feet naturally fall forward. If this position is maintained, the foot muscles are affected by a condition called *footdrop*. With footdrop, the client would have trouble pointing his toes up and may have difficulty walking. A footboard helps prevent footdrop (Figure 16-6). A temporary footboard can be made by rolling a pillow in a large sheet, twisting the ends of the sheet, and then tucking the ends under the mattress.

Drawsheet. A drawsheet is a folded sheet that goes under the client's torso. It is used to help move the client to the top of the bed.

Bed Cradle. The doctor, nurse, or physical therapist may want the client to have a bed cradle to keep the top sheets off the client's legs. Top linens can irritate the skin of some clients. Cradles can be made from a large cardboard box as shown in Figure 16-7.

Siderails. Siderails are most often used to remind a client not to get out of bed without calling for assistance. They may also be used to prevent a client from falling out of bed or to help the client support himself while repositioning himself in bed. Temporary siderails can be made by putting two chairs with their backs against the bed.

Figure 16-6
How to position the feet with a footboard when the client is on prolonged bedrest. (Walsh J, Persons CB, Wieck L: Manual of Home Health Care Nursing, p 240. Philadelphia, JB Lippincott, 1987)

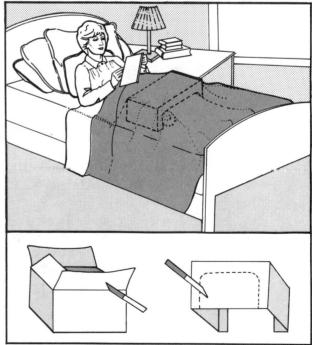

Figure 16-7
A bed cradle keeps the weight of the blankets and sheets off the client's legs.

Procedures to Help Your Client Lie in Bed Comfortably

HM/HHA Procedure:
Positioning the Client on his Side

Purpose:	To give the weak or elderly client extra support when lying on her side
Equipment:	• Four pillows (folded towels and blankets can replace some of the pillows) • Two washcloths
Safety:	If the client has a weak or paralyzed side, she should only be positioned on her strong side or her back unless you are instructed otherwise by your supervisor. Reposition a client who cannot move himself every 2 hours.

Steps

1. Help the client roll onto her side. (See page 165 for HM/HHA Procedure: Turning the Client From his Back to his Side.) If one side is weak, the stronger leg should be on the bottom. Bend the knee of the bottom leg slightly.

2. Use a small pillow to support the head and to keep it in line with the back.

3. Bring the top leg forward and bend the knee. The top leg should not rest on the bottom leg. Support the knee on a folded pillow (Figure 16-8).

Illustrations

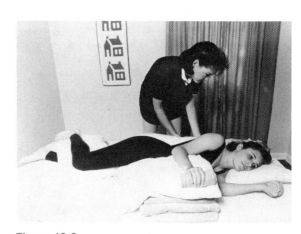

Figure 16-8
The sidelying position.

4. Pull the hips out to straighten the back. Tuck a pillow behind the back to keep it straight and stable.

5. Bring the top arm forward and support it on a pillow. The bottom arm can be placed as shown in Figure 16-8. A rolled washcloth in each hand keeps the hands in a comfortable position.

HM/HHA Procedure:
Positioning the Client on his Back

Purpose: To give the weak or elderly client extra support while lying on her back

Equipment:
- Two pillows
- Two washcloths
- Two folded towels
- Trochanter roll

Safety: Reposition a client who cannot move himself every 2 hours.

Steps

1. Have the client lie down on her back. Place a pillow under her head to support her head and neck.

2. A small pillow or folded towel under the small of the back above the hips gives support to the lower back (Figure 16-9).

3. Another small towel under the knees gives them a slight bend, which allows the blood to circulate more freely.

4. The arms can be positioned as shown in Figure 16-9. The elbows, like the knees, should be slightly bent.

5. A rolled washcloth as a hand grip will prevent the hand from becoming stiff.

6. The trochanter roll may be placed under the hips to prevent the hips from turning out. If the client is on extended bedrest, a footboard may be needed at the end of the bed to prevent footdrop.

Illustrations

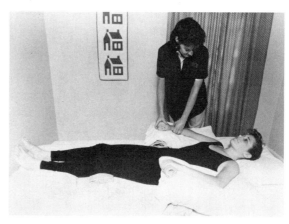

Figure 16-9
Positioning the client on her back.

HM/HHA Procedure:
Moving the Client to the Side of the Bed

Purpose: Before helping a client turn or reposition, you need to move her to one side of the bed to make sure she will not roll out of bed when turning. The client should always be encouraged to do all that she can to assist. In this procedure, you will learn to move the client to the side of the bed safely by yourself if you need to.

Steps

1. Have the client on her back with her arms across her chest and her legs straight. Stand on the side of the bed so that the client will turn toward you.

2. Place your feet 12 inches apart with one foot ahead of the other. Place your arms (palm up) under the client's knees and lower legs. Slide the lower legs towards you by rocking backwards (Figure 16-10A).

Illustrations

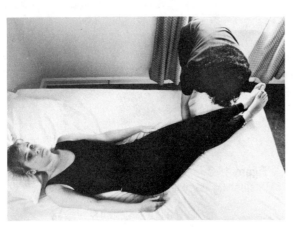

A

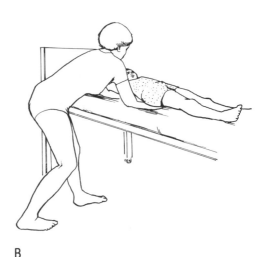

B

Figure 16-10
(*A*) Support the client's knees and ankles as you move the feet. (*B*) Use good body mechanics to slide the client. Face the client, keep one foot ahead of the other, slide your hands under the hips, and keep your back straight as you rock backwards. (*B*: Wolff L, Weitzel MH, Zornow RA et al: Fundamentals of Nursing, 7th ed, p 423. Philadelphia, JB Lippincott, 1983)

3. Place your hands palm up under the client's hips and rock backwards to move them towards you to the edge of the bed (Figure 16-10B).

4. Slide your arms under the client's shoulders. Her head should rest on your arm. Move the shoulders as you moved her in steps 2 and 3.

Purpose: This technique will allow you to roll a client from her back to her side by having the client roll towards you.

Steps

1. Stand on the side of the bed that you want the client to face. Place the client's hand closest to you under her hip, palm up, to prevent her from hurting that arm when she rolls.

2. Place the client's far leg over the near leg and bend it at the knee.

3. Have the client look away from you so that she will not roll on her face when turning over.

4. Hold the client's far shoulder with one hand and her hips with the other as shown in Figure 16-11. Your knees should be bent and your feet should be 12 inches apart with one foot in front of the other. On the count of three, rock backwards and pull the client onto her side.

Illustrations

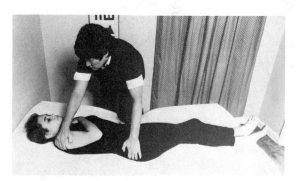

Figure 16-11
Turn the client towards you for better control.

HM/HHA Procedure:
Assisting the Client With a One-Sided Weakness to Move to One Side of the Bed

Purpose: This technique can be used to instruct the client with weakness on one side of the body (such as a stroke victim) how to move herself safely.

Safety: You should encourage this technique only if it has been taught to the client by the supervisor and the supervisor has instructed you to use it.

Steps

1. Have the client put her weak arm on her abdomen. The strong hand can hold the siderail or the edge of the bed.

2. The strong foot should be placed under the weak ankle. This can be done by putting the foot directly under the ankle or by putting it under the knee and sliding it down to the ankle.

3. Lift the weak ankle with the strong leg and move it toward the weak side of the bed (Figure 16-12A).

Illustrations

(continued)

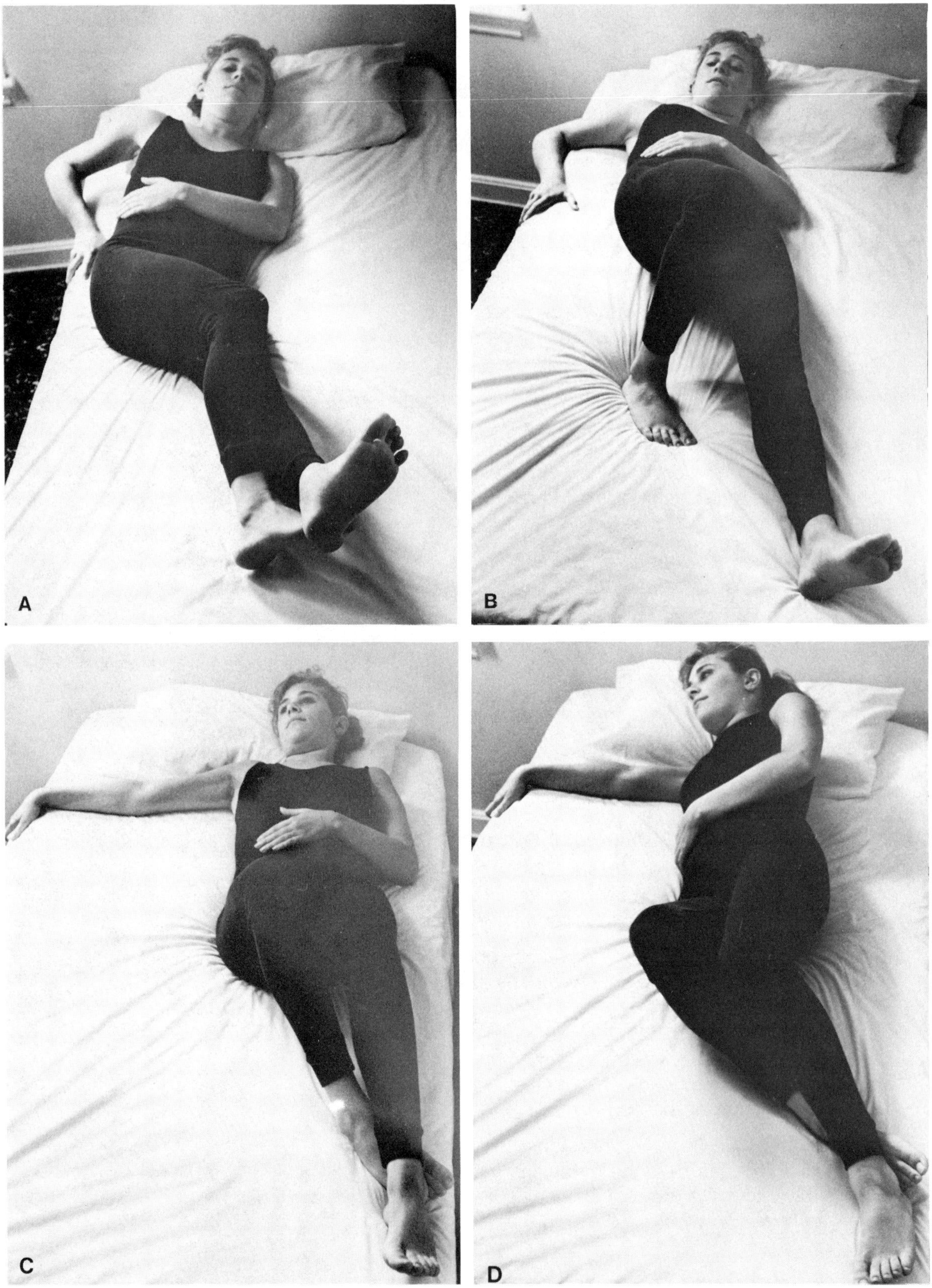
A
B
C
D

Figure 16-12

(continued)

Steps

4. Place the strong foot on the bed opposite the other knee. Bend the knee and push down on the bed to lift the hips and move the midsection to the weak side of the bed (Figure 16-12B).

5. Raise the head and shoulders and push against the mattress or siderail with the strong hand to move the top part of the body toward the strong side.

6. Now the client is ready to turn onto her strong side.

7. Place the weak arm on the abdomen.

8. Place the strong foot under the weak ankle. Lift the weak leg and bend the knees so both feet are on the bed (Figure 16-12C).

9. With the strong hand, pull on the siderail or the edge of the mattress towards the strong side (Figure 16-12D). At the same time roll the legs and body onto the strong side.

10. Straighten the client's position with pillows.

Illustrations

HM/HHA Procedure:

Assisting the Client Who Can Help to Move to the Head of the Bed

Steps

1. Place one pillow against the headboard and remove any others. The pillow on the headboard prevents the client from hurting her head if she accidentally hits the headboard while moving up in bed.

2. Have the client bend her knees.

3. Stand at the side of the bed. Place one of your arms under the client's hips and the other one under her shoulders (Figure 16-13). Her head will rest on your arm.

Illustrations

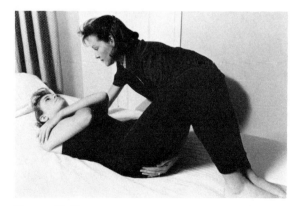

Figure 16-13
The client will push with her legs as you rock forward to help slide her to the head of the bed.

(continued)

HM/HHA Procedure:
Assisting the Client Who Can Help to Move to the Head of the Bed *(continued)*

Steps

4. Bend your knees, and keep your feet 12 inches apart with one foot ahead of the other. Point your feet towards the head of the bed. Keep your back straight as you stoop to place your arms under the client's hips and shoulders.

5. On the count of three, rock towards the head of the bed, holding the client's weight with your arms and legs. The client should push down on the bed with her feet to assist. If the bed has siderails, some clients can hold the rails and use their arms to assist.

Illustrations

HM/HHA Procedure:
Sliding the Client to the Head of the Bed With a Drawsheet — One Person

Purpose: This method can be used if the bed is pulled away from the wall and the bed does not have a headboard.

Steps

1. Have the client lie flat on her back. Place the drawsheet under the client with some extra sheeting at her head.

2. Stand at the head of the bed with one foot ahead of the other. Have the client bend her knees and push with her legs if she can (Figure 16-14).

Illustrations

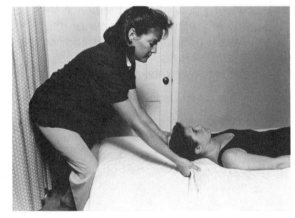

Figure 16-14
Keep your back straight as you rock backward to pull the client up in bed.

3. On the count of three, pull the drawsheet and the client to the top of the bed.

HM/HHA Procedure:
Sliding the Client to the Head of the Bed With a Drawsheet—Two Persons

Steps   **Illustrations**

1. The two persons who are lifting should stand on either side of the client's bed. Place a pillow on the headboard.

2. Put the drawsheet (a regular sheet folded in half) under the client so that it can support her head, back, and hips. Roll the edges of the drawsheet so they are close to the sides of the client's body (Figure 16-15).

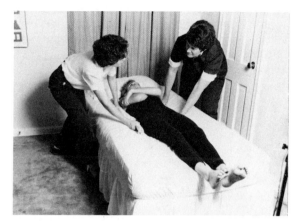

Figure 16-15
Note that the lifters' feet are pointed toward the foot of the bed as they rock backwards to pull the client to the head of the bed.

3. The two lifters should stand opposite each other at the client's chest and face the foot of the bed. This position encourages the use of arm muscles when lifting.

4. Place feet 12 inches apart with the leg closest to the bed behind. Bend both knees slightly. Each person must hold the rolled edge of the drawsheet firmly.

5. On the count of three, the two lifters can rock backwards using their body weight to move the client to the head of the bed. While rocking, keep the knees bent, back straight, and hold the rolled edge close to your center of gravity (your hip bones).

Procedures to Help Your Client Sit Up and Transfer

HM/HHA Procedure:
Assisting the Client to Sit up in Bed Using the Arm Lock

Steps   **Illustrations**

1. Stand so that you are facing the head of the bed. For demonstration purposes, we'll assume you are on the client's right side.

(continued)

HM/HHA Procedure:

Assisting the Client to Sit up in Bed Using the Arm Lock *(continued)*

Steps

2. Put your right hand through the client's armpit and hold onto her right shoulder. Have the client hold onto your right shoulder in the same manner so your arms are locked (Figure 16-16).

Illustrations

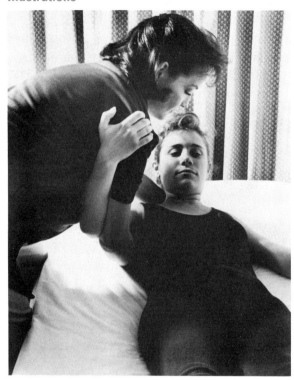

Figure 16-16
The arm lock

3. Then put your left arm around the client's far shoulder. On the count of three, lift the client to a sitting position by rocking backwards.

HM/HHA Procedure:

Assisting the Client to Move From the Bed to a Chair

Steps

1. Place a chair or wheelchair parallel to the bed. If using a wheelchair, make sure the brakes are locked and the footrests are up.

2. Help the client to a sitting position using the arm lock hold. Let her dangle her feet from the edge of the bed for a few minutes to avoid dizziness.

3. Stand facing the client with your feet 12 inches apart and your knees bent. Place your feet around the client's feet to prevent them from slipping, as shown in Figure 16-17A.

Illustrations

(continued)

HM/HHA Procedure:
Assisting the Client to Move From the Bed to a Chair *(continued)*

Steps

4. Have the client place her hands on your shoulders while you put your hands under the client's arms.

5. Bend your knees, and on the count of three, support the client as she stands and pivots to the chair (Figure 16-17*B*). Keep your back straight as you lift and pivot.

6. Make sure the client is seated comfortably.

Illustrations

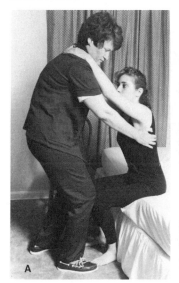
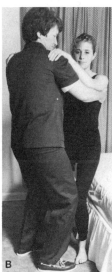

Figure 16-17

Helping the Client With Walking and Assistive Devices

Wheelchairs

Some wheelchairs are operated manually and others are electric. If your client has a wheelchair, learn how to operate it. You should always know how to work the brakes and how to work any special parts such as footrests, removable sides, and any other special parts of the chair. Wheelchair transfers are shown in Figure 16-18.

Assisting With Walking

The following techniques should be used when walking with any unstable or older client, even when they are not using an assistive device.

- Stand on the affected or weaker side and a little behind the client. Keep one arm ready by the client's waist and use your other arm to hold the client's upper arm closest to you. If the client begins to fall, you are in a good position to support the client and ease her to the floor.

- Encourage all clients to look up when walking. Accidents are more likely to occur when the client is looking down.

Guidelines for Walking With a Cane or Walker

- Encourage the client to look up when walking with a cane or walker.
- Stand on the weaker side of the client and a little behind her. Keep one arm ready by the client's waist, and your other arm by the client's upper arm that is closest to you. This position will allow you to ease the client to the floor if she begins to fall.
- Walkers, canes, and crutches should not be used to help the client rise from a chair. The assistive device can be used after the client has come to a standing position.
- There are several different ways of walking with crutches that depend upon the client's strength and condition. If you have a client who is learning to walk with crutches, your supervisor will review the method that is appropriate for that client.

(Text continues on page 177.)

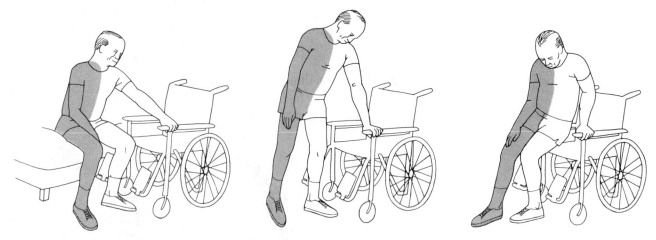

(A) Weight-bearing transfer from bed to chair. The client stands, pivots, and does not begin to sit until his back is to the chair.

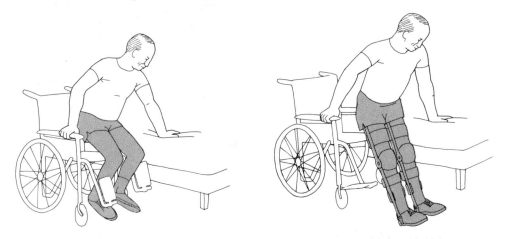

(B) (Left) Non-weight–bearing transfer from wheelchair to bed. (Right) Non-weight–bearing transfer with braces.

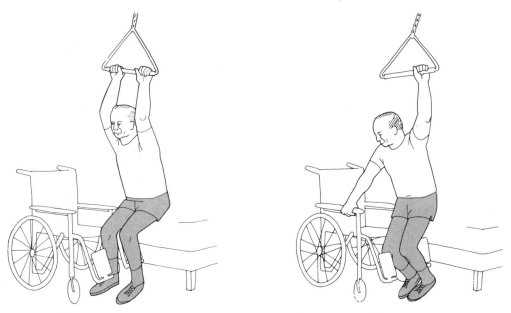

(C) Non-weight–bearing transfer with trapeze.

Figure 16-18

Wheelchair transfers. The shaded areas represent the non-weight–bearing (weak) part of the body. (After Hirschberg GG, Lewis L, Vaughan P: Rehabilitation, pp 74–75. Philadelphia, JB Lippincott, 1976)

HM/HHA Procedure:
Using a Walker

Steps

1. *Holding the walker.* Have the client hold both handgrips of the walker. Remind the client to look up and to pick up the walker instead of pushing it (Figure 16-19).

Illustrations

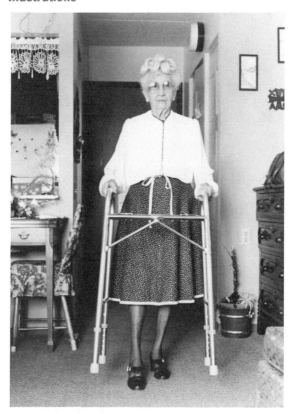

Figure 16-19
This client is looking up and lifting the walker as she prepares to take her next step.

2. *Walking.* The client should lift the walker and move it about 6 inches forward. Then she should take a step, first with the weak leg and then with the strong leg. Remember, it is always in this order: walker/weak/strong.

HM/HHA Procedure:
Using a Cane

Steps

1. Have the client hold the cane on his strong side.

2. *Walking.* Have the client take the first step with the strong leg (Figure 16-20). Then the client should move the cane and the weak leg at the same time for the next step. Remember: strong/weak and cane.

Illustrations

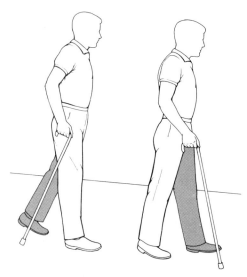

Figure 16-20
The cane is always held on the client's strong side. The shaded area is the non-weight–bearing side. (Walsh J, Persons CB, Wieck L: Manual of Home Health Care Nursing, p 333. Philadelphia, JB Lippincott, 1987)

3. *Climbing up stairs.* Have the client take the first step with the strong leg. Then the client can move the cane and the weaker leg at the same time to go up the step. Remember: strong/weak and cane.

4. *Climbing down stairs.* Have the client take the first step with the weak leg and cane together. Then the strong leg can follow. Remember: weak and cane/strong.

HM/HHA Procedure:
Rising From a Chair With a Walker or Cane

Steps

Illustrations

1. Have client sit on the edge of the chair and hold onto the armrests. The cane or walker can lean against the chair.

2. The client should lean forward slightly and use the armrests to lift herself up (Figure 16-21). The client should not hold the walker when rising because it may tip over.

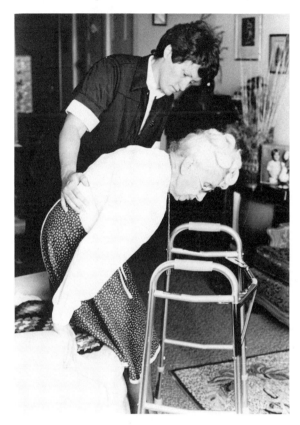

Figure 16-21
The client should hold onto the chair, not the walker, when rising from a chair.

3. Once she is standing, the client can start using the cane or walker.

HM/HHA Procedure:
Sitting With a Walker or Cane

Steps

1. Have the client stand with her back to the chair. The back of her legs should touch the edge of the seat (Figure 16-22).

Illustrations

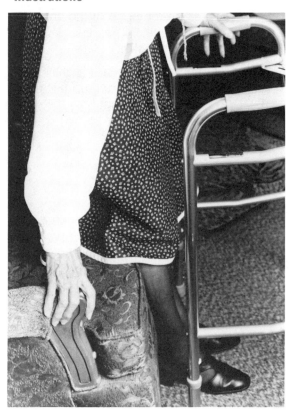

Figure 16-22
With the back of her legs touching the chair and her hands on the chair arms, this client is ready to lower herself into the chair.

2. The client should reach behind her to hold the armrests.

3. Then she should lean forward and lower herself into the chair by bending her legs. She can then scoot to the back of the chair to a comfortable position.

Range-of-Motion Exercises

Without use, muscles quickly lose their ability to work. This is because when muscles are not used, they quickly become shorter and more difficult to move. Range-of-motion (ROM) exercises are prescribed by the doctor for the client whose muscles are not getting enough movement. These exercises take each joint through every motion possible. This maintains and strengthens the client's muscles and allows the client to do more for himself as he gets stronger. Most clients can take an active role in doing ROM exercises. Do not have the client do ROM exercises unless you are instructed to do so by your supervisor.

There are three kinds of ROM exercises: passive, active, and active/assist. In *passive* ROM, a physical therapist, nurse, or family member takes the client through all the range-of-motion exercises. The client cannot help at all. Many home health agencies do not allow the HM/HHA to do passive ROM without further training and supervision.

Active ROM exercises are done by the client without any assistance.

In *active/assist* ROM, most of the exercises are done by client without help, but he may need assistance with some exercises.

Guidelines for Range-of-Motion Exercises

1. Do not start ROM exercises unless they have been ordered by the doctor and you have been instructed and supervised for your particular client.
2. When the client feels discomfort or pain, stop the exercises. Let your supervisor know if the client finds the exercises harder than usual.
3. Follow a logical sequence for the exercises. Do one side of the body at a time. Do each exercise smoothly and gently to prevent muscle spasms.
4. Repeat each exercise five times unless other instructions are given by your supervisor.
5. Support joints adequately with a firm, comfortable grip.
6. The exercises that your physical therapist or nurse supervisor has you perform may be slightly different than the exercises shown on pages 178 to 187, depending on the client's condition. Follow the advice of your supervisor.

Steps

1. Wash your hands. Explain to the client what you are about to do, and how she can help. Have the client lie on her back.

2. Neck
   • Have the client move her head forward and try to touch her chin to her chest (Figure 16-23A). Hold head erect. Then move head all the way back (Figure 16-23B).

Illustrations

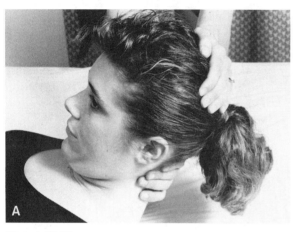
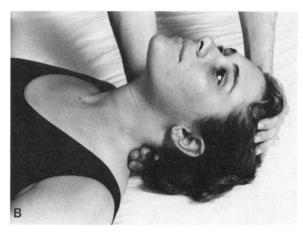

Figure 16-23

   • Have client start with her head erect. Bring her right ear to the right shoulder. Head erect. Then bring her left ear to left shoulder (Figure 16-24).

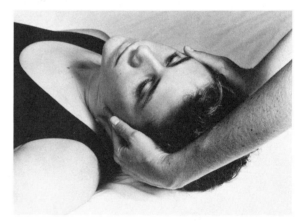

Figure 16-24

   • Rotate head in one direction, and then switch directions (Figure 16-25).

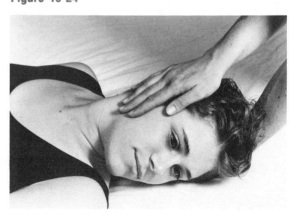

Figure 16-25

(continued)

Steps

Illustrations

3. Shoulders
  • Arms at sides. Straighten elbow (Figure 16-26*A*) and raise arm over the head (Figure 16-26*B*) and back to the side.

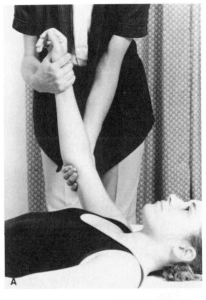
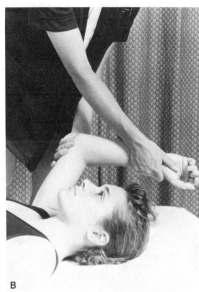

Figure 16-26 A B

  • Arms at sides. Straighten elbow. Move straight arm behind body and back to the side (Figure 16-27).

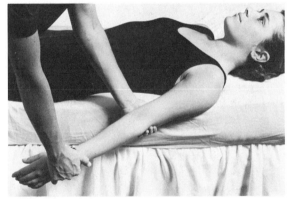

Figure 16-27

  • Arms at sides. Straighten elbow and move arm out to the side, above the shoulder, and back to the side (Figure 16-28).

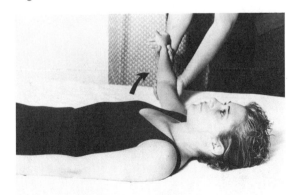

Figure 16-28

(continued)

HM/HHA Procedure:
Range-of-Motion Exercises *(continued)*

Steps   **Illustrations**

4. Elbows
   • Arms at sides. Bend elbow so lower arm
     moves toward shoulder and back to side
     (Figure 16-29A and B).

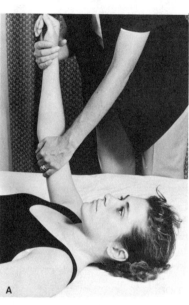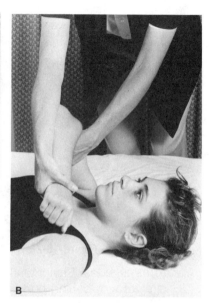

Figure 16-29

5. Forearms
   • Hands at sides, palms down. Turn hand
     over so palm is up and then back so palm
     is down (Figure 16-30A and B).

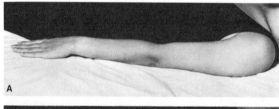
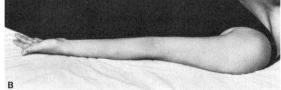

Figure 16-30

(continued)

HM/HHA Procedure:
Range-of-Motion Exercises *(continued)*

Steps

6. Hands and wrists.
   - Wrist in neutral position (Figure 16-31*A*). Bend palm towards inner arm (Figure 16-31*B*) and back to neutral position. Then bend hand back (Figure 16-31*C*) and return to neutral position.

Illustrations

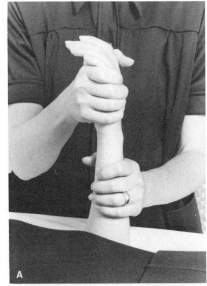

Figure 16-31

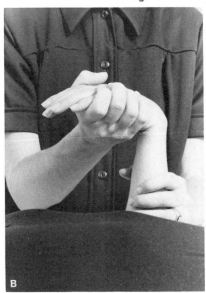
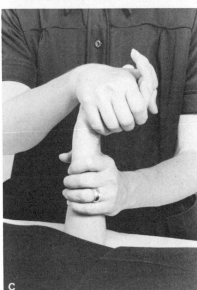

(continued)

HM/HHA Procedure:
Range-of-Motion Exercises *(continued)*

Steps   Illustrations

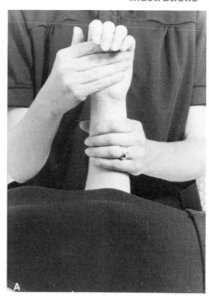 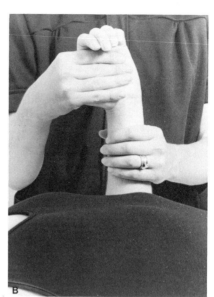

Figure 16-32

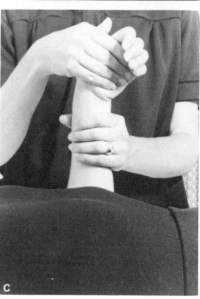

- Wrist in neutral position (Figure 16-32*A*).
  Bend hand towards body in the direction
  of the thumb (Figure 16-32*B*) and back to
  neutral position. Then bend hand away
  from body in the direction of the last finger
  (Figure 16-32*C*).

(continued)

HM/HHA Procedure:
Range-of-Motion Exercises *(continued)*

Steps

- Make circles with hand in one direction and then reverse the direction of rotation (Figure 16-33).

Illustrations

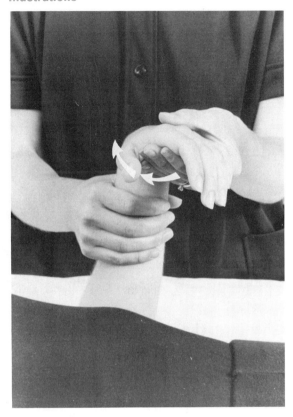

Figure 16-33

7. Fingers
- Make a fist and open it, bending the fingers back as far as comfortably possible (Figure 16-34*A* and *B*).

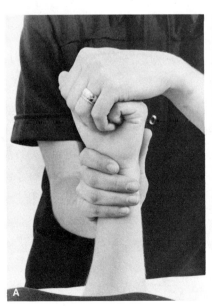 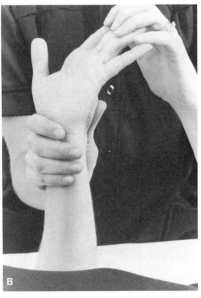

Figure 16-34

(continued)

HM/HHA Procedure:
Range-of-Motion Exercises *(continued)*

Steps   **Illustrations**

• Spread fingers apart and bring them
  together again (Figure 16-35A and B).

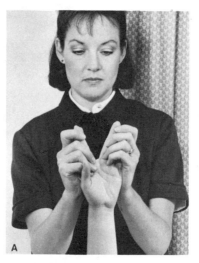 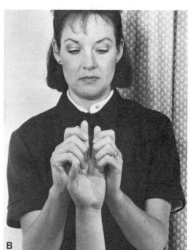

Figure 16-35

• Touch the tip of the thumb with each
  finger, and open the hand fully between
  each touch (Figure 16-36).

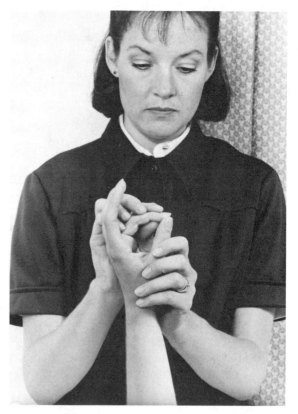

Figure 16-36

(continued)

HM/HHA Procedure:
Range-of-Motion Exercises *(continued)*

Steps	Illustrations
8. Hips • Raise and lower the leg slowly, keeping the knee straight (Figure 16-37).	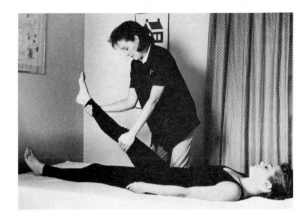 **Figure 16-37**
• Move the leg out to the side and then back into the neutral position, keeping the knee straight (Figure 16-38).	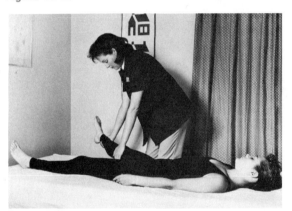 **Figure 16-38**
9. Knees • Have client standing, or lying on her side. Bend the knee so the heel of the foot moves toward the back of the thigh (Figure 16-39).	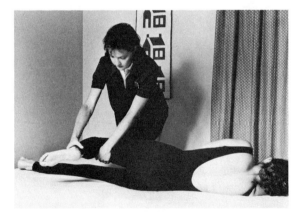 **Figure 16-39**

(continued)

Steps

Illustrations

10. Ankles
    - Move the foot so the toes point up and then down (Figure 16-40).
    - Rotate the foot in one direction and then switch directions.

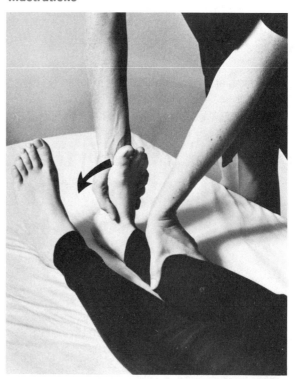

Figure 16-40

11. Toes
    - Curl and uncurl toes (Figure 16-41).

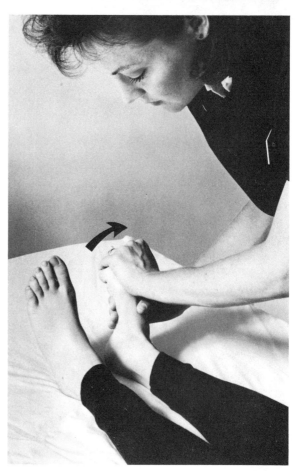

Figure 16-41

(continued)

HM/HHA Procedure:
Range-of-Motion Exercises (*continued*)

Steps	Illustrations
12. Wash your hands and record your observations about how the client tolerated the procedure.	

Review Questions

True or False

1. _____ Using good body mechanics can prevent injuries for yourself and your client.

2. _____ Whenever a client is about to rise from a wheelchair, he should check to make sure the brakes are locked.

3. _____ It is not necessary to remind a client what you are about to do before starting a procedure.

4. _____ To help prevent dizziness when the client is getting out of bed, have him get up very quickly.

5. _____ When helping a client move to the top of the bed, keep your feet about 12 inches apart and point them towards the top of the bed to make a stable base of support.

6. _____ After you have read the procedures in this chapter, you must practice them on well people under the supervision of a qualified professional before you attempt to try them on one of your clients.

7. _____ When done properly, range-of-motion exercises may occasionally hurt the client.

Multiple Choice

8. Tom, a HM/HHA, has been asked by his supervisor to remind Mr. Gold how to use his cane. Which one of the following statements is not correct?
   a. When going downstairs, take your first step with your weaker leg and your cane, and then follow with your stronger leg.
   b. Hold your cane on your stronger side, so you can use it to balance yourself when your stronger leg is taking a step.
   c. When you are climbing up the stairs, take your first step with your strong leg and then follow with your cane and weaker leg.
   d. To avoid an accident, look down and watch your feet when you are using your cane.

9. You need to lift an 18-pound child who has been playing on the floor. Knowing that you should use good body mechanics to avoid back injuries, how would you lift the child?
   a. Keep your back straight and twist from the waist as you bend down to reach the child. Keep your legs straight as you lift.
   b. Bend over from the waist to reach the child. Then straighten your back as you lift the child.
   c. Squat down to lift the child. Keep your back straight as you hold the child close to your body at about waist level. Rise by straightening your legs.
   d. Keep your back straight as you lean over to pick up the child. Hold the child out at arm's length as you straighten your legs and lift.

Chapter 17
Measuring the Vital Signs

Objectives

At the conclusion of this chapter, the homemaker/home health aide will:

1. Understand what vital signs are and why they are measured.

2. Be able to state the normal range for an adult's temperature, pulse, respiration, and blood pressure.

3. Describe how the following equipment is used and cared for: the glass thermometer, the electronic thermometer, the stethoscope, the blood pressure cuff, the mercury manometer, and the aneroid manometer.

4. Describe how the vital signs are measured, including three sites for measuring the temperature; three ways to describe the pulse; how to find the radial, carotid, and apical pulses, ways to describe the respirations; how to estimate the systolic blood pressure; and how to measure the actual blood pressure.

What Are Vital Signs?

There are four *vital signs* that tell us about the health or vitality of the human body. They include temperature (T), pulse (P), respiration (R), and blood pressure (BP). The vital signs may be abbreviated as VS or TPRBP.

What Do the Vital Signs Measure?

- Temperature (T) measures the amount of heat in the body.
- Pulse (P) measures how fast the heart is beating.
- Respiration (R) measures how fast the client is breathing.
- Blood pressure (BP) measures how effectively the heart and blood vessels are working.

When to Take Vital Signs

Generally, the vital signs are only taken once during a home visit, because visits do not usually last more than a couple of hours. Vital signs may need to be taken more often if a client is ill and his vital signs are unstable. For example, a person with a high temperature should have his temperature rechecked every 4 hours. Family members can recheck the temperature and report to the home care nurse or doctor when the HM/HHA is not working. Some home care agencies do not allow the HM/HHA to take the blood pressure because this skill needs much training to be done accurately.

Normal Values for Vital Signs

This chapter will discuss the normal values for each of the vital signs. You must remember that each client is different and that normal values may vary for individuals. Your supervisor will let you know if he expects a client's vital signs to fall outside of the normal ranges.

Temperature

What Is Temperature?

The body produces heat during exercise, when food is used by the cells, and when fighting disease during illness. The body releases excess heat through the skin by sweating and through the lungs and the circulatory system. When more heat is produced than is released, the body temperature rises. Normally, the body temperature remains fairly constant. Temperatures that are either too high or too low can endanger the health of a person.

Thermometers

A thermometer is an instrument used to measure body heat. There are several types. The glass thermometer is most common because it is the least expensive and most accurate thermometer available. Glass thermometers contain a liquid metal called *mercury* that expands and rises in the stem of the thermometer when heated. Some home health care agencies may use digital or electronic thermometers (Figure 17-1). These are quicker, but they need to be checked frequently against a glass thermometer for accuracy. Heat-sensitive strips indicate body temperature by changing color when they are pressed against the skin. These strips are the least accurate method of taking a temperature, but they can be useful in approximating the body temperature. If the temper-

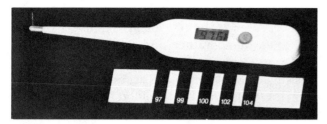

Figure 17-1
The digital thermometer and the temperature strip. Always use a plastic probe cover when using the digital thermometer. The temperature strip is applied to the forehead.

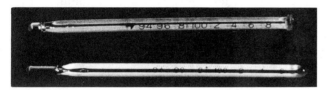

Figure 17-2
The rectal/stubby/safety thermometer is on top, and the oral thermometer with the long thin bulb is below it.

ature appears higher or lower than normal when using a strip, recheck the temperature with a glass thermometer.

There are two types of glass thermometers.

1. The *oral thermometer* has a long, thin bulb and can be used either in the mouth or under the arm. It should never be used

rectally because the long bulb can damage rectal tissue (Figure 17-2).

2. The *rectal thermometer* may also be called the *stubby thermometer* or the *safety thermometer*. It has a rounded bulb and can be used in the mouth, under the arm, or in the rectum. If the thermometer is used in the rectum it should never be used in the mouth.

Safety Precautions for Glass Mercury Thermometers

Glass thermometers should never be put into hot or even warm water, because the mercury will expand and break the thermometer. If a thermometer does break, do not touch the mercury because it is a poisonous substance that can be absorbed into the body through the skin. Call a pharmacist for advice on cleaning up mercury. Mercury will adhere to gold rings and can be absorbed into the skin if it sticks to a ring. If you happen to get mercury on gold jewelry, a jeweler will need to clean the ring.

How to Read a Thermometer

The glass thermometer should be held by the stem at eye level and turned slowly until the mercury and numbers can be seen as shown in Figure 17-2. See Figure 17-3 to learn how to read the Fahrenheit and centigrade scales.

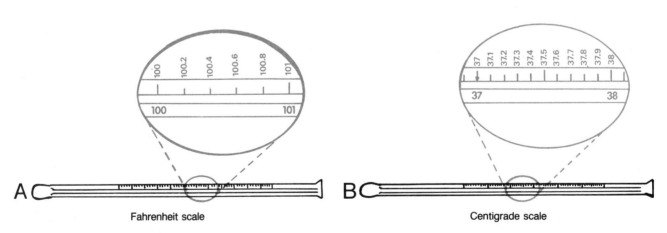

Fahrenheit scale

Centigrade scale

Figure 17-3
Reading the Fahrenheit and centigrade thermometers. (*A*) The Fahrenheit scale. There are only five small lines between each degree on the Fahrenheit scale. Each small line is equal to 0.2 degree. Always double-check the decimal points carefully because there is a great difference between 100.4°F and 104.0°F. (*B*) The centigrade scale. There are ten small lines between each degree on the centigrade scale. Each small line is equal to 0.1 degree.

Table 17-1
Average Normal Temperatures in Well Adults

Site	Amount of Time Needed	Normal Fahrenheit Temperature	Normal Centigrade Temperature
Oral	8 minutes	98.6°	37.0°
Axillary	10 minutes	97.6°	36.4°
Rectal	3 minutes	99.6°	37.5°

The Fahrenheit and Centigrade Temperature Scales

There are two scales for measuring temperature. The most commonly used scale is called *Fahrenheit*. On this scale, water boils at 212 degrees, water freezes at 32 degrees, and normal body temperature is 98.6 degrees. The other scale is called *centigrade* and is part of the metric system. On this scale, water boils at 100 degrees, water freezes at 0 degrees, and normal body temperature is 37 degrees. You may never have to use the centigrade scale, but you should be able to recognize a centigrade thermometer in case your client owns one.

Selecting the Site for Taking the Temperature

There are three places on the body where you can take a temperature reading. Your supervisor will tell you where to take the temperature on your particular client. The mouth is used when taking an *oral* temperature. The *axillary* temperature measures the amount of body heat in the armpit, which is also known as the *axilla*. This method is useful for clients who cannot use an oral thermometer. The HM/HHA should not use the *rectal* method unless approved by the supervisor. Advantages and disadvantages of each location are summarized in Sites to Use When Measuring Temperatures. Normal temperatures are listed in Table 17-1.

(Text continues on page 197.)

Sites to Use When Measuring Temperatures

Location	Advantages	Disadvantages
Oral	Most convenient and comfortable for most clients	Oral temperatures should never be taken on young children, people who can breathe only through their mouths, or confused adults.
Axillary	Safest method for young children or people who cannot cooperate, such as a stroke victim or a client who is confused	This method takes the longest and is the least accurate.
Rectal	Most accurate method	This is the least comfortable method for the client and can be dangerous if a client has rectal problems such as hemorrhoids or diarrhea. The rectal tissue of an infant is especially sensitive. This method should be used only if your supervisor has given prior approval.

HM/HHA Procedure:
Cleaning the Glass Thermometer

Purpose: The thermometer should be cleaned carefully after every use to prevent the spread of germs that might cause disease.

Equipment:
- Thermometer
- Soap
- Cool running water
- A clean soft tissue or cotton ball

Safety:
- Even if you are using a plastic sheath, the thermometer needs to be cleaned well before and after every use. Plastic sheaths often have small tears.
- A thermometer that has been used rectally should never be used orally.
- A thermometer should be used for only one person. If a thermometer is used for more than one person, it must be sterilized between uses.

Steps

1. Gather your equipment and wash your hands before you begin the procedure.

2. Hold the thermometer by the stem and wipe it with a clean damp tissue from the stem to the bulb (Figure 17-4).

Reasons

1. Having all your equipment ready saves you time.

2. Wash from the cleanest area to the dirtiest area.

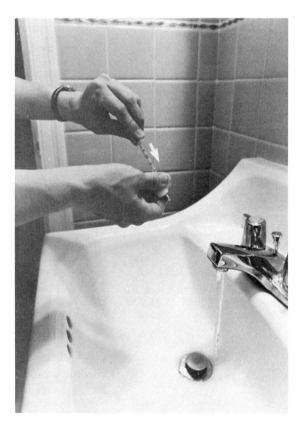

Figure 17-4
Wipe the thermometer from stem to bulb (*arrow*) when cleaning.

(continued)

HM/HHA Procedure:
Cleaning the Glass Thermometer *(continued)*

Steps	Reasons
3. Put soap on the tissue. Rotating the tissue, clean the thermometer from the stem to the bulb.	3. Soap and friction will help loosen germs and particles.
4. Rinse the thermometer in cool running water using a clean tissue and friction to remove the soap.	4. Always use cool water because the thermometer may break if the water is too hot.
5. Dry the thermometer from stem to bulb using a clean tissue.	5. Drying the thermometer helps prevent germs from growing during storage.
6. Place the thermometer in the case.	6. Store the thermometer in a sturdy case to prevent it from breaking.
7. Clean the area and return all equipment to its proper place.	
8. Wash your hands.	

HM/HHA Procedure:
Taking the Temperature Orally

Purpose: To measure the body temperature by mouth

Equipment:
- One clean oral or safety thermometer
- A clean cotton ball or tissue
- A watch with a sweep hand to time the procedure
- Paper and pen to record the temperature

Safety: The oral thermometer should not be used:
- on an infant or young child.
- on any person who cannot cooperate or is confused.
- if oxygen is being given by mask.
- on a person who cannot breathe through his nose while his mouth is closed.

Steps	Reasons
1. Tell the client that you are about to take his temperature by mouth. Gather your equipment and wash your hands.	1. Never assume the client knows what you are about to do. The client has a right to be informed.
2. Make sure the client has not eaten, smoked, or had anything to drink for the last 15 minutes.	2. A temperature reading will not be accurate if the person has smoked, eaten, or had something to drink within 15 minutes.
3. Remove the thermometer from the case. Hold the thermometer up to the light to make sure that it is not cracked or chipped.	3. Never use a cracked or chipped thermometer because it may injure your client.
4. Stand over a bed or soft surface and hold the thermometer firmly by the stem using your forefinger and thumb. Shake the	4. Always hold the thermometer securely. Do not stand near a hard surface such as a countertop when shaking the thermometer.

(continued)

HM/HHA Procedure:
Taking the Temperature Orally *(continued)*

Steps

mercury in the thermometer down below the lowest number on the scale by snapping your wrist several times.

5. Rinse the thermometer in cool water and recheck the reading to make sure the mercury is below the lowest number on the scale.

6. Have the client open his mouth and lift his tongue. Place the thermometer under the client's tongue and have the client hold it in place with his lips closed (Figure 17-5).

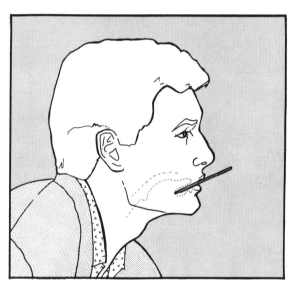

Figure 17-5
Placement of the oral thermometer.

7. The thermometer should be left in place for 8 minutes to get an accurate reading.

8. Remove the thermometer. Hold it by the stem and wipe it with a tissue from stem to bulb so that it is easy to read.

9. Hold the thermometer at eye level and twist it until the mercury can be read accurately. Record the results.

10. Shake the thermometer down. Clean it using the procedure on page 192 and then store it in its case.

11. Wash your hands.

Reasons

If it falls on a soft surface, the thermometer may not break.

5. Rinsing the thermometer will make it easier to slide into the client's mouth.

6. If the thermometer is not placed correctly, the reading will not be accurate.

7. Eight minutes is most accurate, but many agencies only require 3 minutes. Follow the policy of your agency.

8. Never hold the thermometer by the mercury end or it may register the temperature of your hands. Remove saliva with a tissue before reading.

Purpose: To measure the body temperature under the arm

Equipment:
- One clean oral or safety thermometer
- A clean cotton ball or tissue
- A watch with a sweep hand to time the procedure
- Paper and pen to record the temperature

Safety: The axillary temperature is the safest and most comfortable method of measuring the temperature for:
- an infant or young child.
- any person who cannot cooperate or is confused.
- a person who is being given oxygen by mask.
- a person who cannot breathe through his nose while his mouth is closed.

Steps

1. Tell the client what you are about to do and have him either sit or lie down comfortably. Gather your equipment and wash your hands before beginning the procedure.

2. To shake down the thermometer and check for cracks, follow steps 3 and 4 on oral temperatures page 193.

3. Have the client unbutton his shirt so that you can place the bulb of the thermometer in the center of the armpit.

4. Take the client's arm that has the thermometer under it and place it on the opposite shoulder (Figure 17-6).

Reasons

1. Never assume the client knows what you are about to do. The client has a right to be informed.

3. You may need to assist the client in unbuttoning his shirt.

4. This position allows the thermometer to touch the surface of the armpit. This provides an accurate reading by avoiding air pockets.

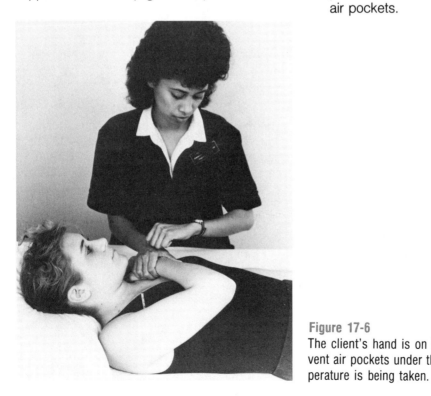

Figure 17-6
The client's hand is on her opposite shoulder to prevent air pockets under the arm while the axillary temperature is being taken.

(continued)

HM/HHA Procedure:
Taking the Axillary Temperature *(continued)*

Steps	Reasons
5. Leave the thermometer in place for at least 10 minutes. Stay with the client so that the thermometer remains in place properly.	5. Because the axillary temperature measures the temperature on the surface of the skin, more time is needed for an accurate reading. Oral and rectal readings take less time because they are internal measures of temperature.
6. Remove the thermometer and hold it by the stem as you wipe it with a tissue before reading it.	6. Wipe any perspiration away by holding the stem securely and wiping from the stem to the bulb (from clean to dirty).
7. Hold the thermometer at eye level and turn it until you can see the mercury line for the temperature reading. Record the results.	
8. Shake the thermometer down and follow the procedure on pages 192 and 193 for cleaning and storing the thermometer.	
9. Wash your hands following the procedure.	

HM/HHA Procedure:
Taking the Rectal Temperature

Purpose: To measure the body temperature in the rectum

Equipment:
- One rectal or safety thermometer
- Lubricating jelly
- A clean cotton ball or tissue
- A watch with a sweep hand to time the procedure
- Paper and pen to record the temperature
- Disposable gloves

Safety: The rectal method can be harmful to people with sensitive rectal tissue, such as infants or people who have hemorrhoids, diarrhea, or recent rectal surgery. The HM/HHA should not perform this procedure on clients unless approved by the home care supervisor in your home care agency.

Steps	Reasons
1. Tell the client what you are about to do. Gather your equipment and wash your hands before beginning the procedure.	1. Never assume the client knows what you are about to do. The client has a right to be informed.
2. To shake down the thermometer and check for cracks, follow steps 3 and 4 on oral temperatures on page 192. Remember to rinse and dry the thermometer if it has been stored in a chemical disinfectant.	
3. Place some lubricating jelly on the mercury bulb and about a half inch above the bulb.	3. Lubricating jelly allows for easier insertion of the thermometer and also reduces the chances of irritating the rectal tissue.

(continued)

HM/HHA Procedure:
Taking the Rectal Temperature *(continued)*

Steps	Reasons
4. Have the client remove his pants, cover himself with a blanket, and lie on his side.	4. You may need to assist, but it is best to allow your client to do as much for himself as he can.
5. Pull back the covers and separate his buttocks so you can see the anal opening. Insert the thermometer an inch into the rectum as shown in Figure 17-7.	5. Proper placement avoids an inaccurate reading and prevents damage to the rectal tissue.

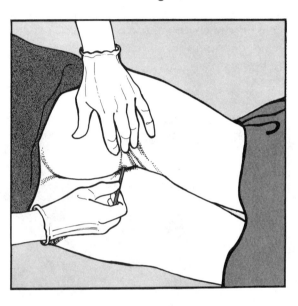

Figure 17-7
Placement of the rectal thermometer. Never leave a client alone when a rectal thermometer is in place.

6. Cover the client with the blanket while you hold the thermometer in place for 3 minutes. Never leave a client alone with a rectal thermometer in place.	6. If you leave the client, he may not realize the thermometer is still inserted. If he moves, the thermometer may injure him. Holding the thermometer prevents it from sliding out and ensures an accurate reading.
7. Remove the thermometer and wipe it with a tissue from the stem to the bulb before taking the reading. Record the results.	7. Hold the thermometer at eye level for an accurate reading.
8. Shake the thermometer down and follow the procedure on pages 192 and 193 for cleaning and storing the thermometer.	
9. Wash your hands.	

Pulse

What Is the Pulse?

Each time the heart beats, it pumps blood through *arteries*, which carry blood to cells throughout the body. The arteries expand and contract as the blood is pushed through the circulatory system. There are several places on the body where you can feel the arteries expanding and contracting. This feeling is called the pulse. So, the *pulse* is a way of measuring the number of times that the heart pumps in a single minute. This is one way of determining how well the heart is doing its job.

How to Find the Pulse

The *radial* pulse is the most common and convenient place to measure the pulse. The radial artery is located right on the bend of the inner wrist just below the thumb as shown in Figure 17-8*A*. Place the tips of your first three fingers on the radial pulse and press gently. Never use your thumb to feel a client's pulse because you have an artery in your thumb and you might count your own pulse instead of your client's. If you have never felt your radial pulse, it will take some practice. Practice on several people. You may find that the pulse is easier to find on some people than on others.

Figure 17-8 also shows other places on the body where the pulse can be found. If you ever have trouble finding the radial pulse, try using the *carotid* pulse, which is located on the neck. This pulse is strong and easy to find.

Three Ways to Describe the Pulse

Rate, rhythm, and strength or force are three ways of describing the pulse.

The *rate* of the pulse describes the number of times the heart beats in 1 minute. The normal pulse rate for adults is 60 to 100 beats per minute. Table 17-2 lists normal pulse rates for persons of various ages. The home care supervisor should be called if the client's pulse is under 60 or over 100 beats per minute, unless you have been told otherwise.

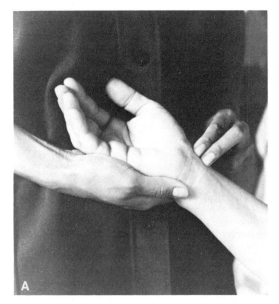

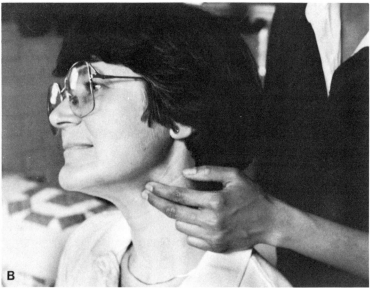

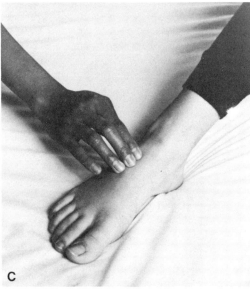

Figure 17-8
(*A*) The radial pulse. (*B*) The carotid pulse. (*C*) The pedal pulse.

HM/HHA Procedure:
Measuring the Radial Pulse

Purpose: To count the number of times the heart beats per minute

Equipment: • A watch with a second hand to time the procedure
                    • Pen and paper to record your observations

Safety: • Report pulses under 60 and over 100 beats per minute to the home care supervisor immediately.
                    • Always count an irregular or abnormal pulse for a full minute.

Steps	Reasons
1. Tell the client that you are about to take his pulse and have him sit or lie down comfortably. Gather your equipment and wash your hands before beginning the procedure.	1. The client should be relaxed. If he has exercised recently, his pulse will probably be higher than normal.
2. If the client is sitting, have him support his arm on an armrest or table. If he is lying down, he can rest his arm on his abdomen.	2. The position should be comfortable for the client and the HM/HHA who is measuring the pulse.
3. Place your first three fingers on the radial pulse and apply gentle pressure until you can feel the pulse.	3. Apply enough pressure to the wrist so that you can feel each beat, but not so much that you cut off the pulse.
4. Use the sweep hand of your watch to count the number of beats in 30 seconds. Try to glance at the time without watching the sweep hand throughout the 30-second period. Remember, if the pulse is irregular, count for 60 seconds.	4. Glance at the sweep hand to avoid counting the movements of the sweep hand instead of the client's pulse.
5. After counting the number of beats in 30 seconds, multiply that number by 2. If the pulse is irregular and you counted the number of beats in 60 seconds, then that is the number of beats in a full minute.	5. Counting the beats for 30 seconds and multiplying that number by 2 will give you the number of beats per minute. For example, if you count 36 beats in 30 seconds, then the pulse rate is 72 ($36 \times 2 = 72$).
6. Record your observations according to your agency's policy.	
7. Wash your hands.	

Table 17-2
Normal Pulse Rates for Well Persons at Various Ages

Age	Pulse Rate/Minute
Birth	120–160
1 year	80–140
2 to 6 years	75–130
6 to 12 years	75–110
Teenagers	60–100
Adults	60–100

Normally the pulse should have a steady *rhythm*. Rhythm describes the amount of time between the beats of the heart. The pulse is described as regular or irregular. A pulse is described as *regular* when there is a steady beat and an even amount of time between beats. Here is an example:

Regular: X X X X X X X X X X X X

A pulse is described as *irregular* when the beat is unsteady. An irregular pulse should be taken for

(*Text continues on page 202.*)

HM/HHA Procedure:
Measuring the Apical Pulse

Purpose: To count the number of times the heart beats. This method should be used only if you have special approval from your home care supervisor.

Equipment: • A stethoscope
    • A watch with a second hand to time the procedure
    • Pen and paper to record your observations

Safety: Report pulses under 60 and over 100 beats per minute to the home care supervisor immediately.
    Always count the apical pulse for a full minute.
    This procedure should be done only with special approval from your home care supervisor.

Steps

1. Gather your equipment and wash your hands before beginning the procedure. Be sure to clean the earplugs and diaphragm of the stethoscope with an alcohol swab before beginning the procedure.

2. Tell the client that you are about to listen to his heart, and have him sit or lie down comfortably. Then have the client unbutton his shirt to expose his chest.

3. Place the stethoscope directly on the skin just under the left nipple where you can hear the loudest heart sounds (Figure 17-9).

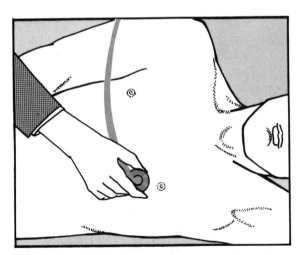

4. Take the pulse for a full minute and record your observations according to your home care agency's policy.

5. Clean the earpieces and diaphragm of the stethoscope and put away the equipment. Then wash your hands.

Reasons

1. Clean the stethoscope well each time you use it to prevent germs from spreading from one client to another.

2. Explain that to listen to the heart you need to have the stethoscope right on the skin over his heart. The client will need to pull up or unbutton his shirt. Maintain privacy by keeping the client's chest covered with his shirt or a blanket.

3. The stethoscope should be placed under the left nipple because the sounds of the heart are the loudest and clearest in this position. Instead of feeling for the pulse, you will be listening to the pulse.

Figure 17-9
The apical pulse must be taken for a full minute.

4. The apical pulse is always taken for a full minute to ensure accuracy.

HM/HHA Procedure:
Measuring the Respirations With the Pulse

Purpose: To count the number of times a person breathes in and out in 1 minute and to count the number of times the heart beats per minute

Equipment:
- A watch or clock with a sweep hand to time the procedure
- Pen and paper to record your observations

Safety: Do not let the client know you are counting the respirations because this will make it difficult for him to breathe normally.

Steps

1. Gather your equipment and wash your hands before the procedure.

2. Explain to the client that you are about to take his vital signs, or tell him you are going to take his pulse.

3. Hold the client's arm across his chest and measure the radial pulse as described in steps 3, 4, and 5 of the procedure on page 199. Then without letting your client know, count the respirations by watching his chest rise and fall (Figure 17-10).

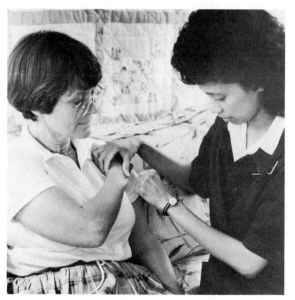

Reasons

2. Do not tell the client that you are going to count his respirations or he may have difficulty breathing normally.

3. The client's arm is placed across his chest to make it easier to see the chest rise and fall with each respiration.

Figure 17-10
Measuring the pulse and respirations together.

4. Note the rate and character of the respirations and the rate, rhythm, and force of the pulse. Record your observations according to your agency's policy.

5. Put away the equipment and wash your hands.

4. If the pulse or respirations are irregular, then you need to count them for a full minute. If they are regular, count for 30 seconds and multiply by 2.

a full minute to make sure that you are getting an accurate count of all the beats. An irregular pulse should always be recorded in your progress notes. Here is an example:

Irregular: X X X X   X X X X X

The *strength* or *force* of the pulse can also be described. The *normal pulse* is full and strong. The *weak pulse* may be hard to find and feels very light or faint. The *bounding pulse* is very forceful.

Respirations

What Are Respirations?

A *respiration* is the act of breathing in (inhaling) and breathing out (exhaling). Respirations allow fresh oxygen to be taken into the lungs during inhalation, and the cell waste products to be released from the lungs during exhalation. Normally, the brain controls breathing automatically so that we do not have to think about each breath that we take. But we can also control breathing voluntarily to an extent when we laugh, talk, or hold our breath for a short time. A young child sometimes frightens his parents when he tries to hold his breath during a temper tantrum. You can assure them that before long, the child will breathe automatically whether he wants to or not.

It may be difficult for a client to breathe normally if he knows you are counting his respirations. For this reason, respirations are usually counted during the same minute that you are counting the pulse. Simply hold the client's wrist to count his radial pulse for 30 seconds, and continue to hold the wrist while you are watching the client's chest rise and fall for the next 30 seconds. This way the client will think you are taking his pulse and will continue to breathe normally.

How to Describe Respirations

The *rate* describes the number of respirations per minute. One complete respiration equals one inhalation and one exhalation. The normal respiratory rate for adults is 14 to 20 breaths per minute. The home care supervisor should be called if the rate is higher or lower than normal, unless you have been told otherwise.

You will also want to describe the *character* of the respirations. Some terms you may use to de-

scribe respirations are quiet or noisy, labored or unlabored, shallow or deep, and regular or irregular. Normal respirations are automatic, quiet, even, regular, and without effort. Call the home care supervisor if there is a change in the rate or character of a client's respirations.

Blood Pressure

What Is Blood Pressure?

The *blood pressure* (BP) is the measurement of the force of the blood against the walls of the arteries as the blood flows to all the cells of the body.

Two numbers are used to describe the blood pressure. The *systolic* (or top number) measures the pressure in the arteries when the heart contracts and pushes blood through the arteries. The *diastolic* (or bottom number) reflects the pressure in the arteries when the heart relaxes and the arteries are at rest. So, the systolic reading reflects the highest amount of pressure in the arteries and the diastolic reading reflects the lowest amount of pressure in the arteries.

There are two ways to record the blood pressure:

1. systolic/diastolic or 120/72

2. $\dfrac{\text{systolic}}{\text{diastolic}}$ or $\dfrac{120}{72}$

Accurate measurement of the blood pressure helps medical professionals understand many things about the condition of the circulatory system. Measuring the blood pressure accurately is a skill that takes a tremendous amount of practice to learn. Unfortunately, many think it is an easy skill, so it is often done quickly and incorrectly.

What Is a Normal Blood Pressure?

Unlike temperature, there is no standard blood pressure that is considered a normal blood pressure. Instead, a range of blood pressures can be considered "normal." There are so many individual differences that one client's normal blood pressure could be very different from another client's normal, even if they are the same age and have the same health problem. Table 17-3 gives the American Heart Association's guidelines for reporting high blood pressure. Your supervisor will tell you the normal range for your individual

Table 17-3
The American Heart Association's Guidelines
for Reporting High Blood Pressure

Age	Blood Pressure
20–40 years	Over 140/90
Over 40 years	Over 160/95

client and when the supervisor should be notified. Guidelines for notifying the supervisor are in the accompanying chart. The supervisor will give you a normal range instead of a fixed number, because the blood pressure changes constantly. If you take a client's blood pressure now and again in 10 minutes, you will find that the blood pressure reading will be slightly, but not significantly, different.

High Blood Pressure

High blood pressure is also called *hypertension*. It is a serious health problem and can lead to kidney disorders, a stroke, or a heart attack. High blood pressure is sometimes called the "silent killer," because people who have it often feel fine. The only sure way to tell if the blood pressure is elevated is to have it checked by someone who has been trained to measure the blood pressure accurately. For this reason, people who have high blood pressure or those at risk for getting high blood pressure need to have their blood pressure taken regularly. If it appears elevated, then a doctor should be seen to determine if the person does indeed have hypertension. You may suspect that a client has hypertension, but only a doctor is licensed to diagnose an illness. The client's blood pressure may be elevated temporarily for any number of reasons.

Guidelines on When to Call the Home Care Supervisor About Blood Pressure

1. When either the systolic or diastolic readings are higher than the blood pressure figures on the American Heart Association chart,
   or
2. When the blood pressure is above or below guidelines provided by your supervisor for that individual client.

High blood pressure cannot be cured, but the symptoms can be treated with diet and medication. This means that while the blood pressure is kept in control, no further damage will be done to the body. When a doctor prescribes medication or diet restrictions, the orders must be followed. Sometimes people who have kept their blood pressure in control through medication for years may think they do not need to take the medication any longer. Usually they do not realize that the blood pressure has stayed within normal limits *because* they are taking the medication. Most people who need medication must take it for life. Only a doctor can determine the *rare* circumstances when medication is no longer needed.

Low Blood Pressure

A consistently low blood pressure, such as 98/60, is not considered a health problem. In fact, it seems to indicate that the heart and blood vessels are operating efficiently. However, if your client's blood pressure suddenly drops more than 30 mm HG, there may be a problem. The blood pressure drops because of poor circulation when a person is in shock. Certain illnesses and medications can also cause the blood pressure to drop. A sudden drop in blood pressure should be reported.

A common condition called *orthostatic hypotension* or *postural hypotension* is characterized by a drop in the blood pressure when a person gets up too quickly after lying down or sitting. The person will experience dizziness and could lose his balance. To avoid this problem, encourage the client to sit on the edge of the bed for a few minutes after lying down and then have the client rise slowly.

Factors That Influence the Blood Pressure

1. Age—The blood pressure rises with aging.
2. Sex—Women generally have lower blood pressures than men of the same age.
3. Race—Blacks are more prone to hypertension than whites.
4. Position—The blood pressure is usually lower when lying than when sitting or standing.
5. The blood pressure rises: during activity; after smoking; when the bladder is full; when the legs are crossed; after drinking a caffeinated beverage; when a person experiences pain or strong emotions; and late in the day and in the early evening.

Blood Pressure Equipment

Electronic or Coin-Operated Blood Pressure Monitors

Your client may have his own electronic blood pressure cuff or perhaps has his blood pressure taken with a coin-operated monitor in a drug store. These devices can be helpful for someone who wants to keep track of his own blood pressure, but they should not replace a regular blood pressure checkup done by a properly trained person.

These machines may not be kept in good working order, or the client may not use them correctly. Sometimes problems occur when the microphones in the stethoscopes interpret room noises as blood pressure sounds, or when the cuff is not applied correctly. Even if the machine measures blood pressure accurately, many people do not know what their normal blood pressure should be, so they may not recognize an abnormal blood pressure reading. In such a situation, that person may fail to notify his doctor when he should.

Stethoscope

The stethoscope is used to make the sounds of the blood pressure loud enough to be heard. Figure 17-11 has the parts of the stethoscope labeled. The *chestpiece* is at the end of the stethoscope's long tube (marked *A* in both pictures). There are two kinds of chestpieces, the diaphragm and the bell. Either kind can be used to listen for the blood pressure. The *diaphragm* or *disk* is flat and round. It is usually used to measure the blood pressure because it is best at detecting high-pitched sounds. The *bell* is smaller, and is usually used for listening to low-pitched sounds.

Some stethoscopes have both a bell and a diaphragm with a chestpiece that rotates so only one side will work at a time. To make sure the correct side is rotated, put the earpieces in your ears and tap the chestpiece lightly. If you cannot hear anything, rotate the chestpiece so you can hear.

The *tubing* (marked *B* in both pictures) is usually made of plastic. The tubing should not be longer than 20 inches from the brace to the chestpiece so the sound can travel well.

The metal *braces* (marked *C* on both pictures) connect the tubing and the earpieces. They are movable so you can adjust the earpieces to a comfortable position.

The *earpieces* (marked *D* on both pictures) are made of soft rubber or plastic. They are removable for cleaning and can be replaced with others if the ones you have are not comfortable. Position the ear pieces so they are turned down and forward toward the tip of your nose, as shown in Figure 17-12. If the earpieces are not positioned correctly, you will not hear the sounds of blood pressure.

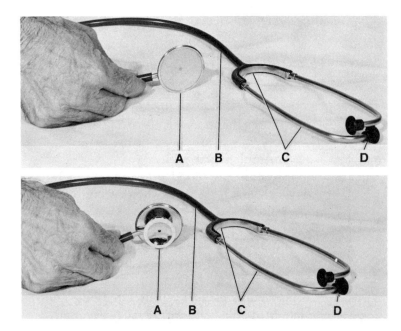

Figure 17-11
The stethoscope. (*A*) The chestpiece. (*B*) The tubing. (*C*) The metal brace. (*D*) The earpieces. (Lewis LW: Fundamental Skills in Patient Care, 3rd ed, p 151. Philadelphia, JB Lippincott, 1984)

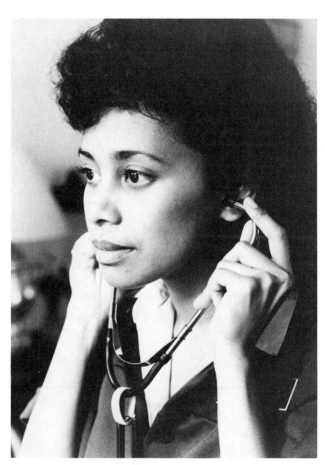

Figure 17-12
Place the earpieces of the stethoscope slightly forward in your ears to help you hear better.

General Care of the Stethoscope

To avoid carrying germs from one client's house to another, the stethoscope (especially the chestpiece and earpiece) should be cleaned with an alcohol swab every time you enter and leave a client's home.

Before you use the stethoscope, always tap the chestpiece lightly to make sure the chestpiece and earpieces are positioned correctly in your ears.

Sphygmomanometer

The sphygmomanometer is used to measure the blood pressure. Figure 17-13 shows the parts of the sphygmomanometer. The *sphygmomanometer* is often called the *blood pressure cuff*, even though it consists of the cuff, the bladder, and the gauge. The *cuff* (marked *A*) contains an inflatable rubber bladder that holds air when measuring the blood pressure. The bladder has two tubes that lead from it. One tube leads to the *bulb* (marked *B*), which fills the bladder with air when squeezed. The bulb has an *air release valve* (marked *C*) that is tricky to control when you are first learning.

The second tube from the cuff leads to a *manometer*, which is the instrument where the blood pressure is read. There are two kinds of manometers: the mercury manometer (marked *D*) and the aneroid manometer (marked *E*). Both are accu-

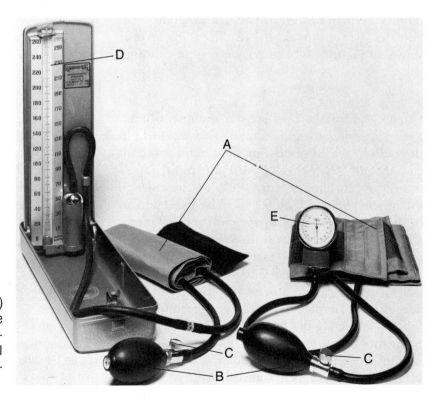

Figure 17-13
The sphygmomanometer. (*A*) The cuff. (*B*) The bulb. (*C*) The air release valve. (*D*) The mercury manometer. (*E*) The aneroid manometer. (After Lewis LW: Fundamental Skills in Patient Care, 3rd ed, p 150. Philadelphia, JB Lippincott, 1984)

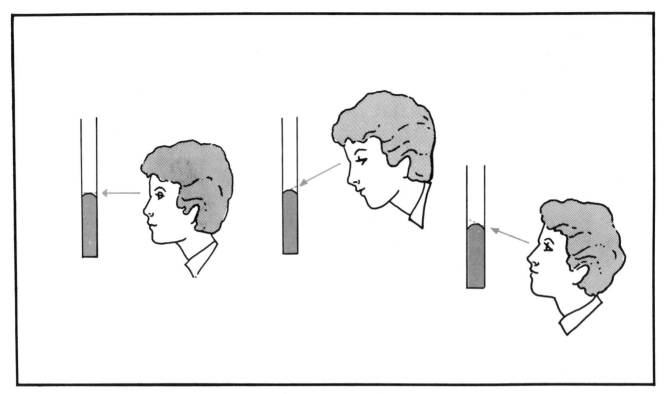

Figure 17-14
When using a mercury manometer, the reading should be taken at eye level as shown in the left picture. The other two pictures demonstrate how the reading could be interpreted to be too high or too low if not read at eye level. For some clients, a slight variance in the reading makes a difference.

rate and do the same job. But, because the aneroid type is lighter and easier to carry, it is used for home visits more often. If you use a mercury manometer, be sure to take the reading at eye level as shown in Figure 17-14 to get an accurate reading.

How to Operate the Air Release Valve
Usually the bulb is held in your dominant hand. Let's say you are right-handed. You would hold the bulb in the palm of your right hand and control the air release valve with the right hand's thumb and forefinger. Turn the knob clockwise to inflate the cuff and counterclockwise to let air out of the cuff. When inflating the cuff, you will pump with your right hand's last three fingers, as shown in Figure 17-15. This takes some practice and coordination. The object is to pump the cuff up as quickly as you can and then to let the air out very, very slowly. The needle on the gauge should only fall 2 to 3 mm Hg per heartbeat. Many health care professionals do not take the time to do this part of the procedure slowly enough, so many HM/HHAs may think it is not necessary. If you let the

air out too quickly, you can easily miss several heartbeats in the top or bottom range of the blood pressure scale. The needle may bounce as you let air out of the manometer, but the bouncing needle does not correspond to the actual blood pressure reading. You cannot measure blood pressure by watching the needle or mercury gauge bounce.

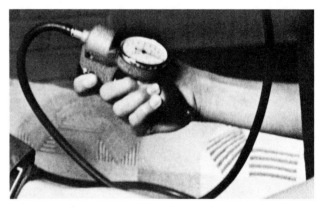

Figure 17-15
Operating the air release valve. Use your last three fingers to pump the bulb and your thumb and forefinger to manipulate the air release valve.

Selecting the Correct Cuff Size

One of the most important factors that affects blood pressure readings is the cuff size. If the cuff is too big, the reading will be lower than it should be. If the cuff is too small, the reading will be too high. One easy way to check is to hold the width of the bladder up to the middle of the client's upper arm. The width of the bladder should be 40% of the upper arm's circumference (the width around the arm). So, the bladder's width should go almost halfway around the upper arm, as shown in Figure 17-16. If the cuff in your bag does not fit a particular client, let the supervisor know and use another cuff that fits.

Placing the Cuff on the Upper Arm

In order to place the cuff correctly, you will need to know how to find the center of the cuff's bladder and how to find the brachial artery on your client.

1. To find the center of the cuff's bladder:
   - Figure 17-17 shows the bladder inside the cuff. Find the bladder inside the cuff.
   - Fold the bladder in half and mark the

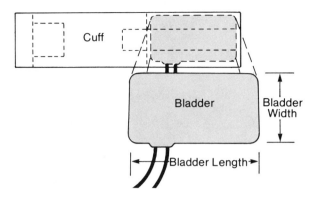

Figure 17-17
This sketch illustrates how the bladder fits inside the blood pressure cuff. (Report of the Subcommittee of the Postgraduate Education Committee: Recommendation for Human Blood Pressure Determination by Sphygmomanometers. Dallas, American Heart Association, © 1980. Reprinted with permission of the American Heart Association.)

   center of the bladder on the outside of the cuff with sturdy tape or a marker. (Some cuffs are marked on the outside of the cuff to show the center of the bladder, but the mark is often not accurate.)
   - The center of the bladder that you have marked will go right over the brachial artery when you are taking the blood pressure.
2. To find the brachial artery pulse, place three fingertips an inch or two above the bend of the elbow on your inner arm. You should feel the pulse about a third of the way in, straight up from your little finger, as shown in Figure 17-18.

(*Text continues on page 211.*)

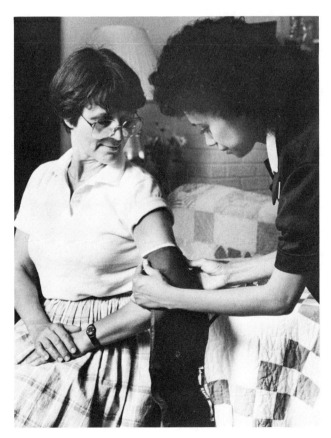

Figure 17-16
Measuring the cuff size.

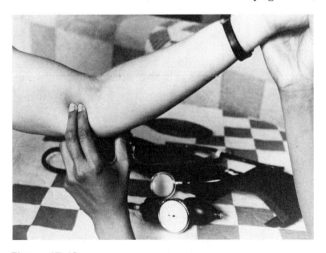

Figure 17-18
Locating the brachial artery. The stethoscope goes over this artery when taking the blood pressure.

Purpose: Estimating the blood pressure before taking an actual measurement allows you to know how much air to pump into the cuff for that individual client. Without estimating, the actual reading may be inaccurate and the client could experience unnecessary discomfort if the blood pressure cuff is pumped too high.

Equipment: A blood pressure cuff that fits properly

Safety: This method should be used on clients when you have never taken their blood pressure or on those whose blood pressure fluctuates between visits. If you know a client's blood pressure is fairly constant, you may only need to use this method the first time you care for him or as often as your home care supervisor requests.

Steps

1. Gather your equipment and wash your hands before beginning the procedure.

2. Explain to the client that you are about to estimate his blood pressure so that you can avoid inflating the blood pressure cuff higher than necessary when you measure the actual blood pressure. Encourage the client to relax.

3. Have the client sit comfortably. He should have his back straight, legs uncrossed, feet flat on the floor, shirt sleeve rolled to expose his upper arm, and arm resting on a table or cushion at heart level with the palm up, as shown in Figure 17-19.

Reasons

2. Emotional stress, recent exercise, and pain can all cause the blood pressure to register higher than normal.

3. This is the best sitting position for measuring the blood pressure accurately. The shirt sleeve should be rolled so the arm is bare to avoid muffling the first and last sound of the blood pressure. The blood pressure should not be taken over a shirt sleeve.

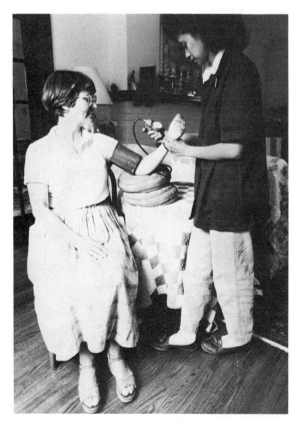

Figure 17-19
Estimating the blood pressure. Note the client's correct sitting position.

(continued)

HM/HHA Procedure:
Estimating the Blood Pressure *(continued)*

Steps	Reasons
4. Find the brachial pulse and the center of the cuff's bladder using the directions on page 207.	4. The sounds of blood pressure are heard best when the cuff is placed correctly.
5. Place the blood pressure cuff on the upper left arm so that the center of the bladder is right over the brachial artery. The cuff should be about an inch or two above the bend in the elbow.	5. The blood pressure should always be measured on the same arm because the blood pressure varies between arms. Usually the left arm is used, but your supervisor may have a reason for you to use the right arm instead.
6. Find the radial pulse on the left wrist.	6. The radial pulse is found at the base of the thumb on the inner wrist as described on page 198.
7. Close the air release valve on the blood pressure cuff. While feeling the radial pulse, watch the gauge as you steadily pump air into the cuff. When you feel the pulse disappear, note the number on the gauge and continue to inflate the cuff another 30 points.	7. Be sure to let the air out very slowly so you can know exactly when the pulse disappears. When the pulse disappears, this is your estimated systolic or top number.
8. After you've pumped the gauge up 30 points above the estimated systolic, slowly let the air out by twisting the air release valve while still watching the gauge. Note the number on the gauge when you feel the radial pulse start beating again.	8. The pulse reappears at the estimated systolic or top number again. This allows you to double check the number you got in step 7. Remember, you can only estimate the systolic number, *not* the diastolic number.
9. The pulse should disappear and reappear at about the same number. Add 40 points to this number to get your estimated systolic (top) blood pressure. If the pulse disappeared and reappeared at different numbers, add 40 points to the higher number.	9. For example: Imagine the pulse appeared when inflating and disappeared while deflating at about 120 mm Hg on the gauge. Add 40 to this number to get the estimated top number (120 + 40 = 160). So, when taking the actual blood pressure, you know that the systolic or top number is between 120 and 160. Therefore, you only need to pump up the cuff just above 160.
10. Wait at least 30 seconds before taking the actual blood pressure or repeating this procedure.	10. The arteries need to rest to get back to their normal condition. If you take the blood pressure too soon, it will be higher than normal.

HM/HHA Procedure:
Measuring the Blood Pressure

Purpose: To measure the blood pressure accurately

Equipment:
- A stethoscope
- A sphygmomanometer (blood pressure cuff)
- Alcohol swabs or cotton-soaked alcohol
- Pen and paper to record your observations

(continued)

Steps

1. Gather your equipment and wash your hands before beginning the procedure.

2. Tell the client what you are about to do and encourage him to relax.

3. Have the client sit comfortably. He should have his back straight, legs uncrossed, feet flat on the floor, shirt sleeve rolled to expose his upper arm, and arm resting on a table or cushion at heart level with the palm up, as shown in Figure 17-19.

4. Find the brachial pulse and the center of the cuff's bladder using the directions on page 207.

5. Place the blood pressure cuff on the upper left arm so that the center of the bladder is right over the brachial artery. The cuff should be about 1 or 2 inches above the bend in the elbow. Secure the cuff snugly and smoothly to the arm.

6. Ask the client not to talk while you do the procedure. Put the stethoscope in your ears so the earpieces are pointed down and forward.

7. Feel the client's brachial pulse. Place the diaphragm of the stethoscope directly over the brachial pulse on the bend of the arm.

8. Close the air release valve. Inflate the bladder by pumping the bulb quickly until the gauge is just above the estimated systolic number (see page 208). While inflating the cuff, keep the stethoscope flat against the skin where you felt the brachial pulse. Make sure the stethoscope does not touch the cuff or tubing (Figure 17-20).

Reasons

1. Be sure the cuff fits the client correctly because a cuff that is too large or too small will give an inaccurate reading.

2. Emotional stress, recent exercise, and pain can all cause the blood pressure to register higher than normal.

3. This is the best sitting position for measuring the blood pressure accurately. If the client is lying down, have him keep his arm straight at his side so that the upper arm is at the same level as the heart.

4. The sounds of blood pressure are heard best when the cuff is placed correctly.

5. Blood pressure should always be measured on the same arm because the blood pressure varies between arms. Usually the left arm is used, but your supervisor may have a reason for you to use the right arm instead.

6. The first and last sounds of blood pressure can be very quiet. If the client is talking, you may not hear the blood pressure sounds.

8. Inflate the cuff quickly to make the sounds of blood pressure louder and easier to hear. This will help you get a more accurate reading. If the stethoscope touches the cuff or tubing, rubbing noises could easily be mistaken for blood pressure sounds.

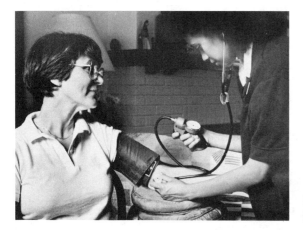

Figure 17-20
Measuring the blood pressure.

(continued)

HM/HHA Procedure:
Measuring the Blood Pressure *(continued)*

Steps	Reasons
9. Prepare to open the valve to let the air out of the cuff. The needle on the gauge should fall slowly, 2–3 mm per heartbeat. It should also fall steadily. Do not reinflate the cuff once you have started to let the air out without letting the client rest for at least 30 seconds.	9. Letting the air out slowly and steadily is the skill that takes the most practice when learning to take blood pressures. If the air is let out of the cuff too quickly, it is very easy to miss the first tapping sound. Reinflating the cuff once it has started to deflate causes the blood pressure to rise.
10. Open the air valve slowly and deflate the cuff. At first you should not hear any noises, but soon you will hear a faint tapping sound. Note the number on the gauge for the first tapping sound you hear and continue to release the air very slowly. This is the actual systolic number.	10. You can recognize the first tapping sound because it will be followed by other sounds at regular intervals. One isolated sound is probably room noise or the stethoscope hitting the cuff. The first tapping sound occurs when the blood begins to flow into the artery after it has been cut off by the blood pressure cuff.
11. Continue to let the air out of the cuff slowly until the last muffled sound is heard. Note this number on the gauge. This is the diastolic number.	11. The last sound may be faint. You can tell the last sound from an isolated noise because it is the last regular, steady beat. An isolated noise is not a blood pressure sound.
12. Let the air out slowly for another 20 mm Hg after the last sound is heard to make sure it was the last sound. Then open up the valve fully and release the rest of the air quickly.	12. Let the air out slowly after the last sound is heard to make sure you did hear the last sound. Then deflate the cuff quickly for the client's comfort.
13. The blood pressure is recorded in even numbers. If a reading appears to fall between two numbers, record the higher number.	13. Therefore, if the top number seems to be between 110 and 112, record 112, not 111.
14. Record your observations, clean your stethoscope with an alcohol swab, and put away your equipment. Wash your hands.	14. In your record also note which arm the blood pressure was taken—(LA) for left arm; (RA) for right arm.

3. To place the cuff correctly, place the cuff securely around the upper arm so that the center of the bladder mark touches the place where you felt the brachial artery. The cuff should be about an inch or two above the bend in the elbow. It should be secure enough so that it will not slide, yet you should be able to put two fingers under the cuff.

Blood Pressure Procedures

Two procedures are shown on pages 208 to 211. The first explains how to estimate the blood pressure and the second tells how to measure the actual blood pressure. The next section discusses how to make the sounds of blood pressure louder. Perfecting blood pressure skills takes many hours of training. Before taking a client's blood pressure, your technique should be measured by a professional.

How to Make the Sounds of Blood Pressure Louder

Sometimes it is very difficult to hear a client's blood pressure because of room noises or just a quiet blood pressure. If you ever have trouble hearing the blood pressure, try it two more times using the following technique to make the sounds of blood pressure louder. If you still cannot hear the blood pressure, simply tell your supervisor.

Never pretend you can hear the blood pressure sounds when you do not.

1. Have the client seated comfortably and apply the blood pressure cuff securely.
2. Estimate the systolic blood pressure for a new client or one whose blood pressure fluctuates (see HM/HHA Procedure: Estimating the Blood Pressure on page 208).
3. Lift the arm above the heart and support it for 15 seconds.
4. Quickly inflate the cuff 40 points above the estimated systolic level.
5. Lower the client's arm.
6. Have the client open and close his hand rapidly five to ten times.
7. Take the blood pressure reading (see HM/HHA Procedure: Measuring the Blood Pressure on pages 209 to 211).

Review Questions

1. ____ The client should know when you are counting his respirations.

2. ____ If you ever have trouble finding the radial pulse in the wrist, you can use the carotid pulse in the neck instead.

3. ____ Only 120/80 is considered a normal blood pressure.

4. ____ Call your supervisor if the diastolic (bottom number) of the blood pressure is 90 or over.

5. ____ A client can always tell if his blood pressure is higher than normal.

6. ____ When the blood pressure is taken too quickly, it will not be accurate.

Matching

Match the vital sign with the appropriate function.

7. ____ Temperature   A. Measures how fast the heart pumps in one minute.
8. ____ Pulse   B. Measures how many times the client breathes in one minute.
9. ____ Respirations   C. Measures the amount of body heat.
10. ____ Blood pressure   D. Measures how well the heart and blood vessels are working.

Match the answers on the right with the column on the left. Each question has just one answer.

11. ____ oral temperature   A. Keep in place 3 minutes for an accurate reading.
12. ____ axillary temperature   B. Keep in place 10 minutes for an accurate reading.
13. ____ rectal temperature   C. Keep in place 8 minutes for an accurate reading.
14. ____ oral thermometer   D. Do not use this site on a small child or a client who is using oxygen.
15. ____ axillary thermometer   E. This site is the least accurate, but is a good one to use on babies, young children, or a person who cannot hold a thermometer in his mouth.
16. ____ rectal thermometer   F. Do not use this method unless specifically instructed to do so by your supervisor.

Thermometer Exercise

On the blank thermometers, fill in the mercury to show how the Fahrenheit and centigrade thermometers would look at the temperature reading shown to the left. See the examples on numbers 17 and 24. Have your class instructor or supervisor check your answers.

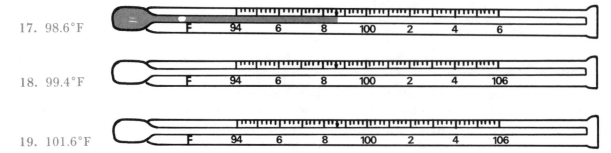

The Fahrenheit Scale

17. 98.6°F

18. 99.4°F

19. 101.6°F

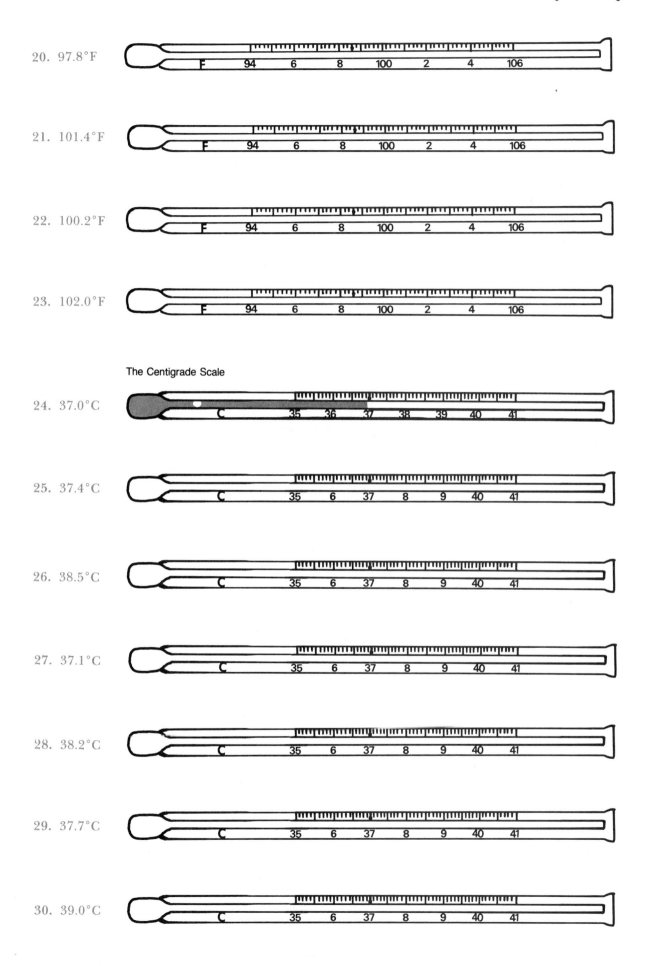

20. 97.8°F

21. 101.4°F

22. 100.2°F

23. 102.0°F

The Centigrade Scale

24. 37.0°C

25. 37.4°C

26. 38.5°C

27. 37.1°C

28. 38.2°C

29. 37.7°C

30. 39.0°C

Chapter 18
Personal Care Skills

Objectives

At the conclusion of this chapter, the homemaker/ home health aide will:

1. Understand the need for oral hygiene.

2. Be able to describe how to floss and brush the teeth and how to take care of dentures.

3. Be able to describe how to assist a client with a bedpan, urinal, and commode.

4. Understand how a catheter works, what kinds of care the HM/HHA is permitted to do for a client with a catheter, and what to do if the catheter is not working.

5. Will know how to show understanding and support for an incontinent client and measures that can be taken to prevent incontinence.

6. Will be able to state three reasons for bathing and explain why a client may not need a daily bath. The HM/HHA will be able to explain how to give a bed bath and a safe tub bath.

7. Will be able to explain the need for careful foot care and why the HM/HHA may not cut a client's toenails.

8. Understanding why and how the HM/HHA provides hair care.

9. Know how to shave a client's beard.

10. Know how to give an effective backrub.

11. Will be able to describe how to assist a client who has a one-sided weakness to dress and undress.

It is often difficult for clients to accept assistance with personal care practices that have been done privately and independently all their lives. The HM/HHA who shows understanding and respect and encourages the client to do all he can, will make it easier for the client to accept assistance. Before providing services to a client, the HM/HHA should demonstrate each procedure before a qualified health professional to ensure that the procedures are being performed safely.

Assisting With Oral Hygiene

The Need for Oral Hygiene

Good daily mouth care is important for several reasons.

1. Clean, well-cared-for teeth help a client look and feel better.
2. A clean mouth helps food taste better and improves the appetite.
3. Oral hygiene preserves the teeth by preventing cavities and infections in the mouth.
4. Oral hygiene helps prevent bad breath.

Daily brushing and flossing help prevent cavities. When the teeth are not brushed after eating, food particles mix with saliva and create an acid. This acid can quickly form a film called *plaque*. The plaque can eat right through the hard covering on the teeth known as *enamel*. Once the enamel has been penetrated, cavities form. The best way to avoid cavities is to avoid eating sweets between meals and to brush the teeth after eating. At the very least, the mouth should be rinsed out after eating meals and snacks. Flossing helps remove food caught between the teeth. Most dentists recommend flossing the teeth daily.

(*Text continues on page 221.*)

HM/HHA Procedure:
Flossing the Teeth

Purpose: To remove food particles from between the teeth that cannot be removed with a toothbrush

Equipment:
- Cup with water (and straw if necessary)
- Dental floss
- Basin or bowl
- Towel
- Disposable gloves

Safety:
- Use the method below unless the client's dentist or the home health agency recommends another method.
- To avoid awkwardness, practice flossing your own teeth using this method.

Steps

1. Gather your equipment, wash your hands, put on gloves, and tell the client what you are about to do before beginning the procedure.

2. Cut an 18-inch strand of dental floss. Wrap the floss around the two middle fingers as shown in Figure 18-1A.

3. To floss the upper teeth, hold the floss as shown in Figure 18-1B. Gently insert the floss between two upper teeth. Bring the floss to the gum, but do not force it because this will cause bleeding.

4. Move the floss up and down six times so that the back, side, and front edges of each tooth are cleaned.

Illustrations*

1. Gloves will not be needed if the client flosses his own teeth.

2.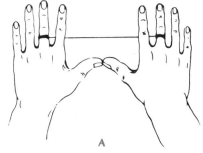

A

3.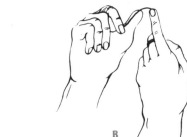

B

4.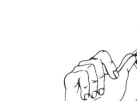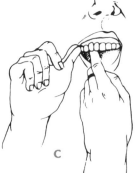

C

*(Effective Oral Hygiene. Developed by USAF School of Aerospace Medicine, Brooks Air Force Base, TX. Courtesy of The Academy of Periodontology, Chicago, IL.)

(continued)

Steps

5. Repeat steps 3 and 4 until all the upper teeth are cleaned. Then rinse the mouth well to clear away the loosened food particles.

6. To floss the lower teeth, hold the floss as shown in Figure 18-1*D*.

7. Gently insert the floss between two lower teeth. Again, bring the floss to the gum, but do not force it. After flossing between all the lower teeth, allow the client to rinse his mouth.

8. Clean up the area and put away all the equipment. Wash your hands and make a note in the client's record.

Illustrations

6.

7.

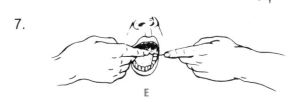

Figure 18-1

Purpose: To remove food particles from the teeth, to prevent cavities, to preserve the teeth and gums, and to refresh the client

Equipment:
- Cup with water (and straw if necessary)
- Toothbrush and toothpaste
- Basin or bowl
- Towel
- Disposable gloves

Safety: Use the method below unless the client's dentist or the home health agency recommends another method.

Steps

1. Gather your equipment, wash your hands, put on gloves, and tell the client what you are about to do before beginning the procedure.

2. Have the client sit up in bed or sit on the side of the bed if he is able. Put a towel over his chest and shoulders to protect his clothing. If the bristles on the toothbrush are stiff, run the brush under hot water to soften them. Place all the equipment within reach, and allow the client to brush his own teeth if he needs no further assistance.

Reasons

1. Always let the client know what you are about to do before you begin a procedure.

2. The client could easily choke if he tries to brush his teeth while lying on his back. If the client is able to brush his own teeth, give him some privacy by looking away if he does not need your assistance. Stay in the room so you can assist if necessary and so you can remove the equipment quickly when he is done.

(continued)

HM/HHA Procedure:
Assisting the Client With Mouth Care *(continued)*

Steps	Reasons
3. If the client is not able to sit up to brush his teeth, have him lie on his side with his head at the edge of a pillow. Place a towel under his head so that it covers the pillow and bed linens. Then place a low spit basin by his mouth (Figure 18-2). The client may find it easier to use a straw to rinse his mouth out. If the client is not able to hold his mouth open, use a padded tongue blade to keep the mouth open. Never try to open the client's mouth with your fingers.	3. The side-lying position allows fluids to drain out of the mouth so the client is less likely to choke. In this position the client may need assistance brushing his teeth. Wrap some gauze around the top of a tongue depressor to make a tongue blade for the client who is not able to keep his mouth open.

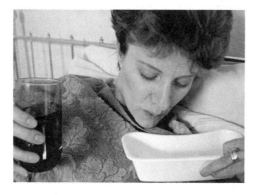

Figure 18-2
Hold the basin close when the client is rinsing her mouth. (Walsh J, Persons CB, Wieck L: Manual of Home Health Care Nursing, p 259. Philadelphia, JB Lippincott, 1987)

4. If you are brushing the client's teeth, follow the method shown in Figure 18-3.	4. The method of cleaning the teeth is more important than the brand of toothpaste.

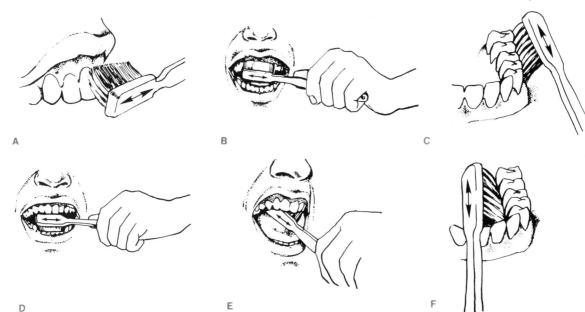

Figure 18-3
This figure illustrates how to brush the teeth. (Effective Oral Hygiene. Developed by USAF School of Aerospace Medicine, Brooks Air Force Base, TX. Courtesy of The Academy of Periodontology, Chicago, IL.)

(continued)

HM/HHA Procedure:
Assisting the Client With Mouth Care *(continued)*

Steps   **Reasons**

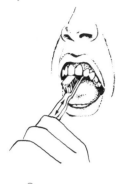
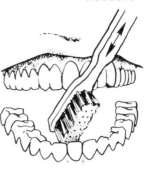
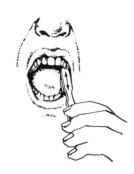

G   H   I

Figure 18-3 *(continued)*

5. Allow the client to rinse his mouth. Some may want to use mouthwash. The client may find it easiest to use a straw to drink.

6. Clean up the area and put away all the equipment. Wash your hands and make a note in the client's record.

5. Unless instructed otherwise, use the brand of mouthwash and toothpaste the client prefers.

HM/HHA Procedure:
Care of Dentures

Purpose: Dentures should be cleaned at least once a day and good mouth care should be provided for the client at the same time.

Equipment:
- Denture cup
- Small basin or sink
- Cool water
- Denture brush or toothbrush
- Denture cleaner or toothpaste
- Denture soaking solution
- Denture adhesive
- Small towel and washcloth
- Disposable gloves

Safety:
- Dentures are fragile and expensive so they need to be handled carefully.
- The denture cup should be clearly labeled so that it is not thrown away by mistake.

Steps   **Reasons**

1. Gather your equipment, wash your hands, put on gloves, and let the client know what you are about to do before beginning the procedure. Check with your supervisor if the client wants his dentures cleaned using a different method.

1. The client has a right to know what you are about to do before a procedure is started. Do not use the client's method unless your supervisor approves it because you and the home health agency could be responsible if the dentures are damaged.

(continued)

HM/HHA Procedure:
Care of Dentures (*continued*)

Steps

2. Ask the client to remove his dentures and have him place them in the denture cup. If the client needs assistance, use a tissue to handle the dentures.

3. After the dentures have been placed in a denture cup filled with cool water, carry the cup to the sink.

4. Line the sink with a small towel or washcloth. Then fill the sink with lukewarm water.

5. Hold the dentures securely in the palm of your hand and clean them thoroughly with a toothbrush and toothpaste or a denture cleaner (Figure 18-4). *Never* use bleach or abrasive cleaners on dentures.

Reasons

2. Make sure the client is standing over a soft surface if he is unsteady so the dentures do not break if they drop. Some clients may want privacy while they remove their dentures.

3. A plastic margarine dish can be used for a denture cup. Try not to use a clear glass because most people do not like to see their teeth sitting in a glass.

4. The towel will cushion a fall if the dentures slip. Hot water may warp the dentures and then they will not fit the client.

5. Dentures are slippery when wet so hold them carefully. Use only the cleaning products recommended by the home care supervisor. Bleach and abrasive cleaners will destroy dentures.

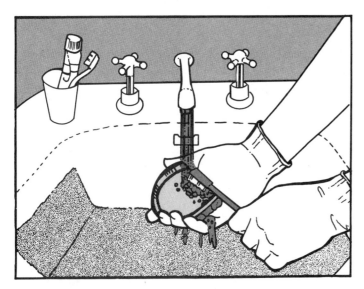

Figure 18-4
Hold the dentures securely when cleaning them.

6. Rinse the dentures thoroughly in cool water and then set them in the denture cup with cool water or a soaking solution. If using a soaking solution, follow the directions on the package.

7. Before inserting the dentures, the client's mouth should be cleaned and rinsed well. Check the mouth for redness and mouth sores.

6. If the dentures are soaked, be sure they are rinsed well before they are inserted again.

7. Dentures are easier to insert if the mouth and dentures are moist.

(continued)

HM/HHA Procedure:
Care of Dentures *(continued)*

Steps	Reasons
8. The client's mouth and dentures should be well rinsed so they are moist. If the client uses a denture adhesive, apply it as directed on the package.	8. Most will not need assistance to reinsert the dentures, but some clients may need help.
9. Keep the denture cup within reach in case the client wants to remove his dentures.	9. Dentists usually want clients to keep their dentures in as much as possible. Your client should always have a safe place to store them if he wants to remove them before a nap or for any other reason.
10. Clean up the area and put away all the equipment. Wash your hands and make a note in the client's record.	

Assisting With Elimination (Toilet Care)

Some clients may not be able to get out of bed to go to the toilet or may need help in the bathroom. Women who are confined to bed will need to use a bedpan and men will need to use a urinal and bedpan. Some clients may use a commode if they cannot walk all the way to the bathroom. When assisting a client with toileting, always consider his dignity, his need for cleanliness, and his right to privacy. If you need to keep records of your client's input and output, see Chapter 20.

Terms

There are many words for emptying the bladder: urination, voiding, passing water, and micturition are just a few. Emptying the bowels is known as having a bowel movement, a BM, or a stool. Many people have their own terms for these body functions and it is important that you understand and use the terms the client uses. This will make it easier for both of you to understand what is being said. A client who would say he needs to "pass water" may not understand what you mean if you ask if he needs to urinate.

Assisting With Bedpans and Urinals

Bedpans come in several sizes to fit adults and children. Sometimes a thin adult may find that a child's bedpan is more comfortable than the full-size bedpan. The *fracture pan* is a lower and smaller bedpan that many find easier to use than the regular bedpan (Figure 18-5).

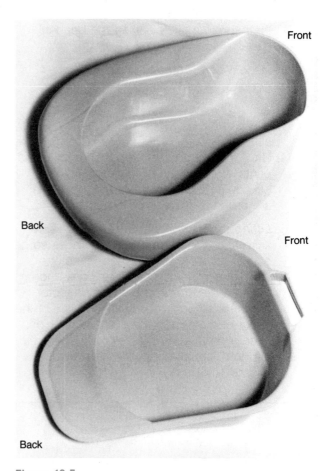

Figure 18-5
(Top) The traditional bedpan *(bottom)* the fracture pan. Note that the handle is at the front of the fracture pan.

HM/HHA Procedure:
Assisting With the Bedpan

Purpose: To help the bedridden client on and off the bedpan

Equipment:
- Bedpan
- Toilet tissue
- Supplies for handwashing
- Bed protector such as newspaper or plastic-covered cloth to go under the bedpan
- Disposable gloves

Steps	Reasons
1. Before beginning, find out which kind of bedpan the client uses and whether the client will lift his hips or roll onto the bedpan. Explain to the client what you are about to do and how he can help. Gather your supplies, wash your hands and put on gloves before beginning the procedure.	
2. Prepare the bedpan by rinsing it with warm water. Dry it and apply a small amount of lotion along the seat where the bedpan touches the skin. Talcum powder or corn starch can be used instead of lotion. If the client is going to empty his bowels, place a few sheets of toilet tissue or a little water in the bedpan make cleaning the bedpan easier.	2. A cold bedpan is unpleasant and may make it more difficult for the client to void. Lotion and powder on the rim of the bedpan make it easier to get on and off the bedpan and prevent skin irritations.
3. Place a bed protector under the hips.	3. Spills will be easier to clean up and the linen will not have to be changed as often with a bed protector. A bed protector can easily be made from newspaper or plastic under a towel.
4. Have the client raise the gown or lower his pants. A towel can be used to provide privacy for the client while the top linens are pulled to the end of the bed.	4. To ensure the client's dignity, privacy must be maintained.
5. *Lifting the hips.* If the client needs assistance, have him bend his knees so he can lift his hips with his feet. Place one hand under the client's lower back and use the other hand to slip the bed protector and bedpan under the client's hips. On the count of three, help the client lift his hips. Then slide the bed protector under the hips and the bedpan on top of the protector (Figure 18-6).	5. It takes less energy for the client and the HM/HHA if both people help each other. Be sure to keep your back straight, and lift with your legs.

(continued)

HM/HHA Procedure:
Assisting With the Bedpan *(continued)*

Steps

Reasons

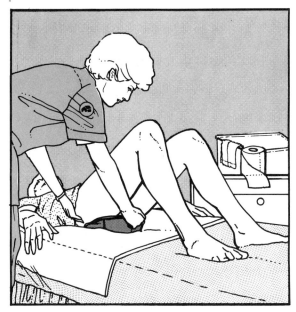

Figure 18-6
When using the fracture pan, hold the handle to slide the pan under the client's hips.

6. *Rolling.* If the client needs assistance, have him roll away from you onto his side. Then place the bed protector on the bed and the bedpan firmly on his bottom and help him to roll onto his back (Figure 18-7). To make rolling back easier, you can push the bedpan into the bed while keeping it in place on the client's bottom.

6. Many find it easier to roll onto a fracture pan than a standard bedpan because the fracture pan has lower sides.

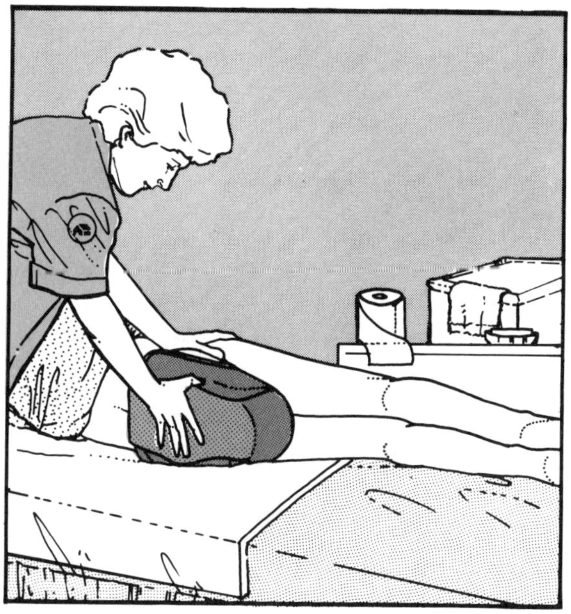

Figure 18-7
Hold the bedpan firmly to the client's body when helping him roll onto the bedpan. When helping the client roll off the bedpan, hold the bedpan level with the bed to avoid spills.

(continued)

HM/HHA Procedure:
Assisting With the Bedpan *(continued)*

Steps

7. Use pillows to prop the client into a sitting position. Bending the knees may help the position seem more natural. A weaker client may need to have you help hold him up in a sitting position. Ask the client to tell you if the bedpan is adjusted properly.

8. Replace the top linens and give the client a bell to signal when he is finished if you are permitted to leave the room. Be sure to leave toilet tissue and handwashing supplies nearby. If the client has trouble voiding, the sound of running water in a nearby bathroom may help.

9. Help the client raise his hips and remove the bedpan. If the client prefers to roll off the bedpan, keep a firm hand on the bedpan to prevent spills (see Figure 18-7).

10. Cover the bedpan with a paper towel and help the client clean himself if needed. To assist, wrap plenty of toilet paper around your gloved hand and wipe from the urinary area to the anal area in a single stroke. Dispose of the tissue. Repeat until clean. If necessary, a washcloth may be used.

11. Offer the client supplies to wash and dry his hands.

12. When the client is comfortable, take the bedpan and supplies to the bathroom. Measure the urine if necessary and note any unusual appearances. Then dispose of the waste products in the toilet.

13. Clean the equipment as recommended by your home care agency and put all the supplies away. Wash your hands well after removing your gloves and record your observations.

Reasons

7. The sitting position makes it easier to void and to move the bowels. If the client needs support to maintain a sitting position, use the arm lock as shown in Figure 16-16 on p. 170. This allows you to face away from the client to give him some privacy.

8. Never leave the room if the client is unsteady. A simple call signal such as a whistle or marbles in a jar can be used if a bell is not available.

9. Removing the bedpan without spilling it can be tricky. Practice on a well person with supervision before ever trying this on a person who is weak or ill.

10. Cover the bedpan to save the client embarrassment and to reduce odors. The client must be cleaned properly to prevent skin irritation, infections, and odors. Clean from the less soiled to the most soiled areas: front to back.

11. Washing the hands after toileting is often forgotten, yet it is one of the best ways to prevent the spread of germs.

12. Most clients will not need to have their intake and output measured. If the urine or feces have blood or pus, or are unusual in any other way, phone the home care supervisor before disposing of them. They may need to be tested.

13. Rinsing the bedpan with water is not enough. It needs to be cleaned with a disinfectant.

A bedpan never fits anyone perfectly and some people find them hard to get used to. Do not leave anyone on the bedpan for very long. If someone wants more time, suggest taking the bedpan away and then bringing it back in 10 to 15 minutes for another try.

Women usually find it easiest to void in a sitting position. Men generally like to stand while voiding into the urinal. Both sexes find it simplest to empty their bowels in a sitting position. These positions are recommended only if allowed by the doctor.

Rules for Assisting the Client to the Bathroom

1. If a client is unsteady, offer to take him to the bathroom regularly. Clients who are confused or unsteady may try to walk to the bathroom alone and could easily fall simply because they do not want to bother others for assistance. For more on how to walk with an unsteady client, see Assisting With Walking in Chapter 16.
2. If you leave the bathroom after the client has been helped to the toilet, leave the door to the bathroom unlocked and stay close to the door so you are available to assist if needed. Let the client know you are there.
3. You may need to assist cleaning the genital area. Lack of proper cleaning leads to skin irritation and unpleasant odors. Women should clean themselves from front to back to avoid urinary tract infections.
4. Blood in the urine or stools, pain upon urination, or any other problems should be reported to your supervisor promptly.
5. Encourage the client to wash his hands thoroughly after using the toilet.

Assisting With a Commode

A *commode* is a chair with a toilet seat and a removable container below to catch the waste products (Figure 18-8). Usually it is used for the client who can get out of bed, but cannot walk to the bathroom. The commode is convenient in a home where the toilet is upstairs and the client's bedroom is downstairs. The commode should always be emptied and cleaned well after every use to prevent the spread of infection and to reduce odors. Keep toilet paper and handwashing supplies next to the commode for easy access. Some commodes have wheels so the client can sit on the commode and be wheeled to the toilet.

Care of Catheters

A *urinary catheter* is used to drain urine from the bladder. Your client may need a catheter if he is not able to urinate normally. It consists of a long plastic tube that is inserted into the bladder. The tube leads to a plastic bag, which is kept below the level of the bladder so the urine can drain (Figure 18-9).

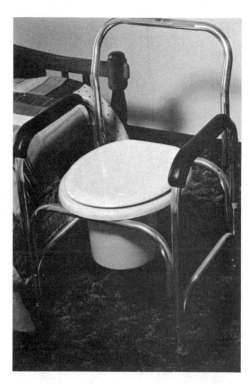

Figure 18-8
A roll of toilet paper can be tied to the arm of the commode. (Walsh J, Persons CB, Wieck L: Manual of Home Health Care Nursing, p 55. Philadelphia, JB Lippincott, 1987)

Many home health care clients have catheters, so it is likely that you will encounter them in your work. As the HM/HHA, you need to know the things you are and are not permitted to do for a client with a catheter.

1. The HM/HHA may *not* insert or remove a catheter. This must be done by the nurse or the doctor under sterile conditions.
2. The HM/HHA is *not* licensed to irrigate the catheter.

Because the catheter goes all the way into the bladder, there is a great risk of infection or damage to the internal organs if the catheter is not inserted or removed under sterile conditions. Once the catheter has been inserted by the nurse, a small balloon is inflated in the tip of the catheter. The balloon rests inside the bladder to keep the catheter in place (see Figure 18-9). It can be painful if the catheter is pulled while the balloon is inflated. The catheter tubing should be fastened to the inside of the client's thigh with tape or a garter so that the catheter is less likely to be pulled out (Figure 18-10). For example, if the client stands up and catches the tubing in his chair acci-

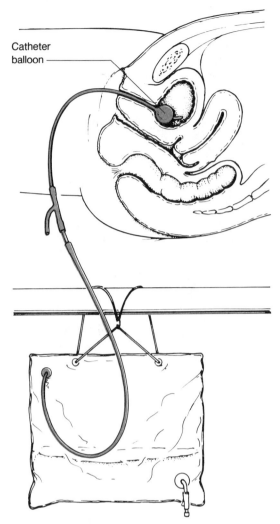

Figure 18-9
A small balloon is inflated in the bladder to keep the catheter in position. The tubing must not be pulled. (Lewis LW: Fundamental Skills in Patient Care, 3rd ed, p 292. Philadelphia, JB Lippincott, 1984)

dentally, there will be a pull on the tubing attached to his leg instead of pulling on the balloon inside the bladder.

Guidelines for Working With Catheters

1. *Keep the catheter bag lower than the bladder* (Figure 18-11). This prevents old urine, which has been sitting in the bag, from flowing back into the sterile bladder.
2. *Secure the tubing to the client's leg.* This prevents the catheter from being pulled out of the bladder. See Figure 18-10. A male client may be concerned if he has an erection while the catheter is in place. This is a normal occurrence and poses no danger.

3. *Keep the tubing free from kinks.* Do not let the client lie or sit on the tubing because this may block the drainage. Keep the tubing as straight as possible.
4. *Provide catheter care.* The genital area (where the catheter enters the body) needs to be cleaned daily to prevent germs from entering the urinary system along the outside of the catheter tubing. Many clients clean this area themselves. You should never see urine leaking from around the tubing, but it is normal for the client to have some discharge. The outside of the tubing should be cleaned with a mild soap.
5. *Observe the urine.* The urine should be clear yellow and without sediment or blood. Any blood or unusual appearances of the urine should be reported to the supervisor.
6. *Emptying the catheter bag.* Record the amount and color of the urine and the time the bag was emptied. There are many different types of catheter clasps used for emptying the catheter bag. If you are unfamiliar with a particular clasp, ask your supervisor for instruction. The measurement lines on most catheter bags are good for estimates, but if you need an exact output measurement, a urine measuring cup must be used.

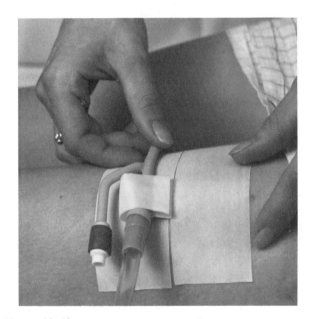

Figure 18-10
The catheter tubing must be secured. A commercial device can be used as shown in this picture, or your home health supervisor will show you the proper method for taping catheters. (Photo courtesy of the M.C. Johnson Company, Inc., Leominster, MA)

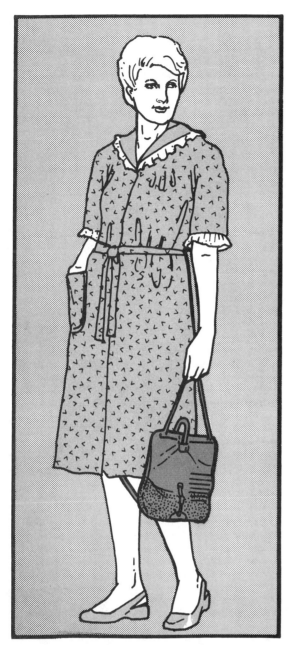

Figure 18-11
The catheter bag must always be kept lower than the hips.

7. *The leg bag.* Some clients may use a smaller collecting bag that cannot be seen under clothing. Your supervisor will show you how to attach the leg bag (Figure 18-12).

8. Notify the home care supervisor immediately if
   • The catheter bag is not filling over a period of hours or the bag suddenly fills rapidly.
   • There is blood in the tubing.
   • The client complains of pain.
   • The catheter falls out.

   • The client has a strong urge to urinate.
   • Urine is leaking from the catheter at any place.

The Client Who Is Incontinent

Incontinence is the temporary or permanent inability to control the release of waste products from either the bowel or the bladder. Urinary incontinence is more common. There are several complicated medical reasons for this problem. The client may dribble continuously, he may dribble when he coughs, or he may occasionally drain the bladder completely. In any case, incontinence is extremely embarrassing for the client and is a problem he cannot control. When you keep the client clean in a matter-of-fact, nonjudgmental manner, you will be showing respect for the client's dignity and privacy.

The home health agency may put the client on a program to help regain bladder control. Your encouragement and assistance to the client and family will be invaluable.

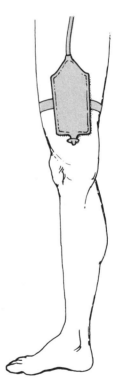

Figure 18-12
The catheter tubing can be attached to a small collecting bag known as a leg bag. With the leg bag, the client can wear a dress or trousers and the catheter will not be visible. (Lewis LW: Fundamental Skills in Patient Care, 3rd ed, p 297. Philadelphia, JB Lippincott, 1984)

Guidelines for Working With the Client Who Is Incontinent

1. *Show tact and understanding.* Let the client know that you want to help and encourage him in his efforts to overcome his incontinence.
2. *The client should maintain a normal fluid intake,* drinking up to 2000 ml per day. Some people who are incontinent try to restrict their fluid intake, but plenty of fluid is needed to stimulate the bladder to work properly.
3. Take the client to the bathroom or offer the bedpan every 2 to 3 hours. It may help to offer this after the client has had fluids.
4. Absorbent pads may need to be placed on the bed and chairs the client uses. There are several types of appliances available for both men and women that cannot be detected by others. The man may wear an external appliance over his penis that drains urine into a collection bag attached to his leg. Women often can wear absorbent pads.

Assisting With Bathing

There are several reasons for regular bathing.

1. The bath cleans the skin and refreshes the client. It promotes a sense of well-being.
2. The friction and massage of the skin encourage the blood to circulate, which refreshes and relaxes tired muscles.
3. A bath provides exercise for the client.
4. Lastly, assisting with a bath allows the HM/HHA to observe the condition of the client's skin.

Bathing Guidelines

1. *Not all clients will need a daily bath.* Your supervisor will determine how often and what type of bath your client should receive based on his condition. A client might need a daily bath if:
   - He has oily skin.
   - He perspires a lot.
   - He is incontinent.
   A client might not need a daily bath if:
   - He has dry skin.
   - He is not very active.
2. *Encourage the client's independence.* Before beginning any procedure, explain to the client what you are about to do and what he can do to assist. Whenever possible allow and encourage the client to do as much as the health care team allows. Sometimes it is easier and quicker for the caregiver to do more than necessary. Soon the client may think he is not strong enough or quick enough to take care of himself. As a

(*Bathing Guidelines continue on page 237.*)

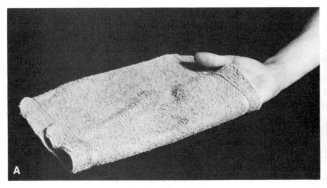
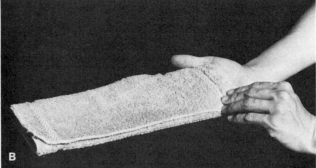
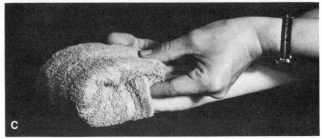

Figure 18-13
How to fold a secure bath mitt.

HM/HHA Procedure:
The Bed Bath

Purpose: To clean the skin, provide exercise, stimulate circulation, and promote a sense of well-being

Equipment:
- Washcloths (2)
- Basin filled with warm water
- Towels (2)
- Soap
- Lotion
- Bath blanket or large towel for draping
- Clean clothes for client
- Apron for the HM/HHA

Safety:
- Keep bathwater comfortably warm between 90°F and 100°F to avoid burns.
- Get fresh bathwater as often as necessary to keep it clean and warm.
- Close the windows to prevent drafts.

Steps

1. Gather your equipment, wash your hands, and tell the client what you are about to do before beginning the procedure. Offer to assist the client to the toilet or with the bedpan.

2. Assist the client to the side of the bed where you will work. Have the client remove his pajamas and cover himself with a large towel or bath blanket. Then have him lie on his back.

3. If the client needs assistance covering himself while in bed, remove all his blankets except the top sheet. Give the client the top edge of the bath blanket to hold. You pull the bottom edge of the bath blanket to cover the client while also pulling the top sheet to the bottom of the bed to remove it (Figure 18-14).

Reasons

1. Encourage the client to empty his bladder because the sound of water is likely to stimulate the bladder.

3. This method is quick and ensures warmth and privacy for the client.

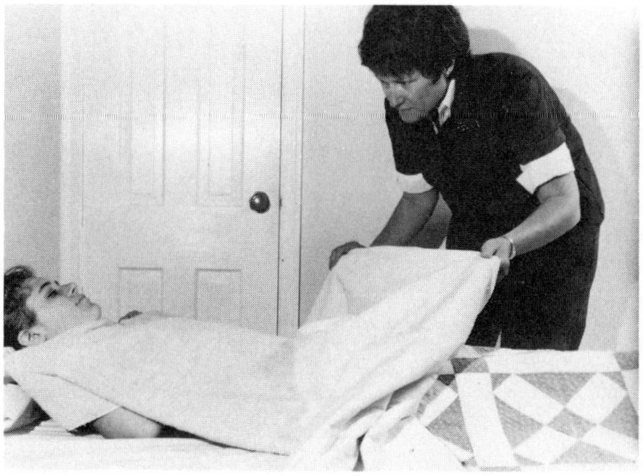

Figure 18-14
The client can cover herself with a large towel while you pull the sheets and blankets off the bed.

(continued)

HM/HHA Procedure:
The Bed Bath *(continued)*

Steps

4. *The face.* Place a towel under the head. Begin by washing the eyes. Use plain water without soap and wipe from the inner corner near the bridge of the nose outward in one gentle stroke (Figure 18-15). Repeat using a fresh part of the washcloth until the eye is clean. Pat dry. Turn to a fresh part of the washcloth and do the same for the other eye. Wash, rinse, and dry the cheeks, forehead, neck, and ears using a small amount of soap. Never insert a cotton swab into the inner ear.

Reasons

4. Wipe from the inner eye outward so that germs and dirt cannot enter the tear duct. This leads directly to the nose and could cause an infection in the nose or tear duct. A cotton swab inserted into the ear canal can injure the eardrum. Ear wax will leave the ear canal naturally. Some clients may not use soap on their faces at all because it dries the skin.

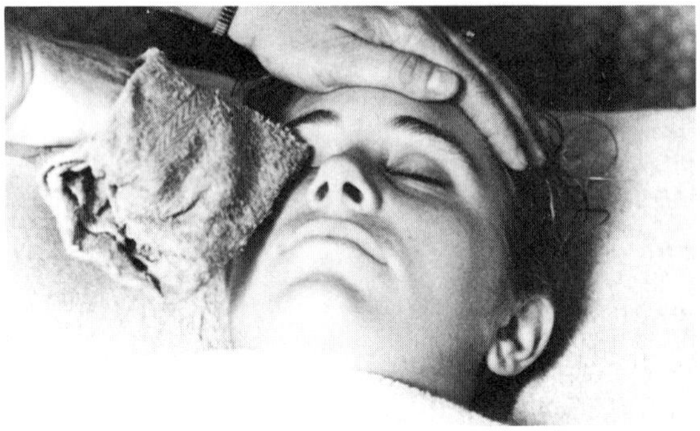

Figure 18-15
Use plain water and a clean washcloth when wiping the eyes from the inside corner to the outside corner.

Steps

5. *The arms.* Place the towel under the arm farthest from you. Use long strokes to wash, rinse, and dry the arm. Then wash the armpit. If you need to support the arm, hold the joints at the elbow, wrists, and shoulder (Figure 18-16). Move the towel and wash, rinse, and dry the arm and armpit closest to you.

Reasons

5. If you wash the arm closest to you first, you may accidentally drip on that arm when you are washing the far arm.

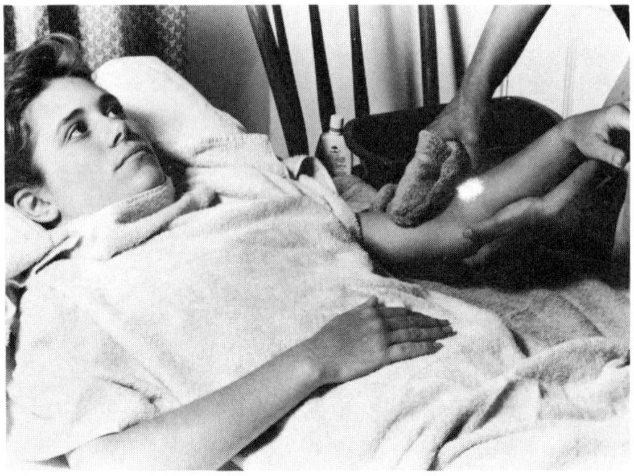

Figure 18-16
Support the main joints as you give a bedbath.

(continued)

HM/HHA Procedure:
The Bed Bath *(continued)*

Steps

6. *The hands.* Have the client soak his hands in the basin of water for a few minutes. Then he can wash his hands with soap and clean under the fingernails with an orange stick or nailbrush. Rinse, dry, and apply lotion as needed.

7. *The chest.* Place a towel over the chest area and bath blanket. Then pull the bath blanket down to waist level. Fold the towel down to wash, rinse, and dry the chest. Be sure to clean the skin folds and, for females, under breasts. Note the condition of the skin in these sensitive areas. Replace the towel over the chest area.

8. *The abdomen.* Now fold the towel up so the abdomen is exposed. Wash, rinse, and dry the abdomen using circular motions. Clean the skin folds and navel. Note the condition of the skin.

9. Empty, rinse, and refill the basin with fresh warm water. Rinse the washcloth out well, too.

10. *The legs.* Put the towel under the leg farthest from you. Wash, rinse, and dry the leg using long, firm strokes. To support the leg when lifting or moving it, hold the knee and ankle. Then wash the leg closest to you.

11. *The feet.* Put the basin on a towel at the foot of the bed. Have the client bend his knees so he can soak his feet in the basin for a few minutes. As you wash between the toes, look for sores or redness. Rinse the feet and dry them carefully, especially between the toes.

12. Empty, rinse, and refill the basin with fresh warm water. Rinse the washcloth out well too.

13. *The back.* Have the client turn on to his side with his back facing you. Tuck the towel under him lengthwise. Wash, rinse, and dry the back using long firm strokes. Apply lotion and give the back a 1-minute massage. Use a long, firm stroke from the hips to the shoulders and then make small circular motions as you go from the shoulders to the hips.

Reasons

6. Soaking is relaxing and makes it easier to remove dirt from the hands and under the nails.

7. Dry the skin carefully, especially the skin folds. Apply powder to those areas where the skin rubs to prevent irritation.

8. Apply powder to places where the skin rubs to prevent irritation.

10. Again, washing the leg farthest from you prevents water from dripping on the clean leg.

11. Report any sores to the supervisor, because they can lead to serious foot problems., Careful drying of the toes prevents foot problems. For more on foot care, see Assisting With Foot Care on pages 237–238.

13. Many clients who can do every other part of the bath will need help with the back because it is difficult to reach. This is a good time to give a 1-minute backrub to stimulate the circulation and relax the muscles. See the HM/HHA Procedure for giving a backrub later in the chapter.

(continued)

HM/HHA Procedure:
The Bed Bath *(continued)*

Steps	Reasons
14. *Between the legs.* Have the client roll onto his back. Offer the washcloth to him so he can clean his genitals and bottom. You may need to assist, especially with the bottom, because this area is hard for some clients to reach.	14. If you need to help the client wash his genitals, let him know you realize it is difficult to wash thoroughly while in bed. Some women need to be reminded to wash from front to back to prevent the stool particles around the anus from entering the vagina and urinary tract.
15. The client may wish to use lotion or powder before getting dressed. Assist the client with dressing if necessary. Most people will want to comb their own hair.	
16. Clean up the area and put away all the equipment. Wash your hands. Make a note in the client's record about how he tolerated the procedure and the condition of his skin.	

HM/HHA Procedure:
The Partial Bath

Purpose: To clean the skin, promote exercise, stimulate circulation, and promote a sense of well-being. The client may need little assistance. A partial bath is ideal for the client who does not need a full bed bath.

Equipment:
- Washcloths (2)
- Basin filled with water
- Towels (2)
- Soap
- Lotion
- Bath blanket or large towel for draping
- Clean clothes for client
- Apron for HM/HHA

Safety:
- Keep bathwater between 90°F and 100°F to avoid burns and provide comfort.
- Get fresh bathwater as often as necessary to keep it clean and warm.
- Close the windows to prevent drafts.

Steps	Reasons
1. Gather the equipment, wash your hands, and tell the client what you are about to do before beginning the procedure. Find out how much assistance he thinks he will need.	1. If medically permitted, encourage the client to do as much of his bath as possible to promote exercise and independence. Often clients can take their partial bath in the bathroom or standing at a sink.

(continued)

HM/HHA Procedure:
The Partial Bath *(continued)*

Steps

2. Put the basin and bathing supplies on a table covered with newspaper within easy reach of the client. Many clients will be able to give themselves a partial bath and may only need help with hard-to-reach areas such as the back. Provide privacy and any needed assistance. For the client who does not need a full bath, the face, hands, armpits, genitals, and bottom should be washed daily.

3. If you leave the client, make sure there is a bell or jar of marbles close by so he can call you for assistance. Offer to assist with the back and then give the 1-minute backrub.

4. When the client calls, assist with the bath and dressing as needed. Make sure the client is comfortable before cleaning up and putting away the bath supplies.

5. Wash your hands and make a note in the client's record about how he tolerated the procedure and the condition of his skin.

Reasons

2. The newspaper will protect the furniture. If the client is used to bathing alone, your supervisor may permit you to leave the room. A way to give privacy while remaining in the room is to look away occasionally. Light conversation may help you and the client feel more comfortable.

3. If you leave the room, do not go too far so that you can hear the client if he calls for help. If a client looks unsteady, never leave the room even if you normally do. See the HM/HHA Procedure for the backrub later in the chapter.

4. Try not to hurry a person who is trying to bathe or dress himself. It takes time to recover and regain former skills. See the Guidelines for Assisting With Dressing and Undressing later in the chapter.

HM/HHA Procedure:
The Tub Bath or Shower

Purpose: To clean the skin, promote exercise, stimulate circulation, promote a sense of well-being, and encourage independence

Equipment:
- Washcloths (2)
- Towels (2 or more)
- Soap
- Shampoo
- Clean clothes for client
- Stool for the tub or shower
- Nonskid mat for the tub or shower
- Apron for HM/HHA

Safety:
- Keep bathwater comfortably warm between 90°F and 100°F to avoid burns and provide comfort. Water that is too hot may lower the blood pressure, which can cause the client to become weak, dizzy, and even faint.
- If the client does faint or if he feels faint while in the tub, empty the tub, cover him with towels for warmth and have him lean back. Rub his skin to stimulate the blood flow and call for assistance.

(continued)

Personal Care and Medical Procedures

HM/HHA Procedure:
The Tub Bath or Shower *(continued)*

- Always encourage the client to sit on a shower stool in the tub. *Never* let a client immerse himself in a tub unless another family member is in the house who can help you lift the client if he is not able to get out on his own. Attempting to lift a heavy, tired client out of a tub on your own could hurt you and the client.
- To determine if your client can have a tub bath or shower, check with your home care supervisor. Do not give a tub bath or shower if your client's condition has worsened or if he seems extremely tired.
- Do not use oils or lotions in the tub because they can make the tub slippery and cause a fall.

Steps

1. *Tub bath preparation.* Tell the client you are about to prepare his bath. Gather the bath supplies and set them up near the tub before bringing the client into the bathroom.

2. Clean the bathtub or shower. If there are hand rails, check to see if they are secure. A nonskid rubber mat should be pressed firmly to the floor of the tub or shower. The tub or shower stool can be set on top of the nonskid mat.

3. Check the temperature of the room and water.

4. *When the bathroom is ready, get the client.* Explain what you are about to do. If he is in bed and needs assistance, have him sit on the edge of the bed while you put on his slippers. Help him with his robe and then assist him to the bathroom.

5. In the bathroom, ask the client if he needs to use the toilet before getting in the shower or tub.

6. Take the client's glasses and robe. Help the client remove his clothes while providing privacy.

7. *For a man*, have the client remove his pajama top and slippers. Hold a bath towel around his waist (Figure 18-17). The client can undo his bottoms and let them fall to the floor while the towel is in place.

Reasons

1. It can be very tiring and frustrating for the client if everything is not ready when he enters the bathroom to take his bath. It can also be a safety concern if you need to leave the bathroom after the client is in the tub.

2. Grab bars, a rubber mat, and a plastic shower stool are all fairly inexpensive safety items. A nonskid mat must be secured properly or it can cause a serious fall. A plastic chair or a sturdy chair covered with heavy plastic can be used as a tub or shower stool as long as the client and family do not mind if the chair gets wet.

3. Hot water can burn sensitive skin on older adults or young children. It may also cause a person to tire easily and to faint.

4. Let the client know how you are going to help him to the bathroom so he can be prepared to assist. Remember, his family may use a slightly different way of helping him out of bed. Sitting on the edge of the bed for a minute avoids dizziness and the slippers may prevent a fall.

5. The sound of running water may stimulate the bladder. It is easier if the client uses the toilet before the bath.

7. The towels ensure the client's privacy during the bath or shower.

(continued)

HM/HHA Procedure:
The Tub Bath or Shower *(continued)*

Steps   **Reasons**

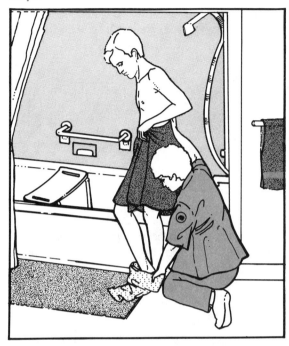

Figure 18-17
The male client can keep a towel around his waist for
privacy as he sits on the tub stool during his bath.

8. *For a woman*, wrap the towel so that her
torso is covered for privacy and warmth.
Two towels may be used after she sits
down; one in her lap and another around
her shoulders. (Figure 18-18).

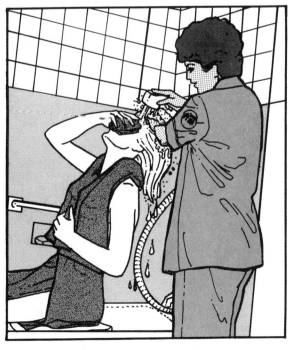

Figure 18-18
The female client can be well draped while having her
hair shampooed in the tub.

(continued)

HM/HHA Procedure:
The Tub Bath or Shower *(continued)*

Steps	Reasons
9. *Getting into the tub.* Have the client hold onto the grab bars or side of the tub while he lifts one leg at a time into the tub. To assist, stand behind the client and hold onto his waist. He can then sit on the tub stool with the privacy towel still wrapped around him.	9. Encourage the client to do as much as he can by himself. A bath can be good exercise.
10. *The shower.* Have the client sit on the shower stool to take his shower. If the client is taking a standing shower, keep the stool in a corner of the shower so it is available if needed.	10. You may need to have the shower curtain partway open so that you can assist.
11. Stay in the bathroom while the client bathes unless your supervisor says it is not necessary. If you need to assist, bathe the client using the same principles in the bed bath procedure. The client should not sit in the tub for longer than 20 minutes.	11. Never leave a weak or unsteady client alone in the bathroom. More accidents occur in this room than in any other room in the house. If the phone rings, just don't answer it. After 20 minutes, the bath may become tiring and the relaxing effect diminishes.
12. *To shampoo,* have the client tilt his head back so you can get the hair wet. Apply the shampoo, lather well by massaging with your fingertips, and rinse thoroughly. Dry with a towel in the bathroom. Never use a hairdryer while the client is in the tub or standing on a wet surface.	12. It is easier to shampoo in the tub or shower than during a bed bath. A shower attachment can make this job even easier. People do get electrocuted, so keep the hairdryer and other electrical appliances out of the bathroom and away from water.
13. Empty the water from the tub and dry the client lightly while he is still sitting in the tub. As the client stands, wrap a clean towel around his waist and let the wet one fall.	13. Most people who are ill or tired find it easier to get out of an empty tub than a full tub. While still in the tub, dry the person briefly to avoid puddles of water outside the tub.
14. Once out of the tub, the client can dry himself more thoroughly with help if needed. Apply lotion as desired. Then the client can dress. Make sure his feet are dried well as you assist him with his slippers.	14. While applying lotion, a short backrub may be appropriate. If the client is tired, do the backrub when he is in bed.
15. The client can finish his oral care, shaving, and hair care in the bathroom or, if he seems tired, in his bedroom.	15. During the bath, check to see how tired the client seems to be. A short bath is better than getting the client overtired.
16. Walk the client out of the bathroom and see that he is seated comfortably in a chair or in his bed. Clean up the bathroom and put away all the supplies.	
17. Wash your hands and record your observations about the client's tolerance to the bath.	

Bathing Guidelines (*continued*)
HM/HHA, your job is to help the client regain his independence.

3. *Provide privacy.* When assisting with a bath, provide privacy and warmth by keeping the client covered with towels. Expose only the part of the client being washed. If the client is being bathed in bed, the bed linens should be covered with a towel to prevent the linens from getting wet.

4. *Wash from clean to dirty.* Wash from the cleanest areas of the body to the most soiled areas. Use gentle friction and massage to remove the dirt and stimulate the circulation. Be sure to clean the hard-to-reach areas where germs hide, such as under the arms, between the legs, in the skin folds and navel, and behind the ears.

5. *The bath water.* The bath water should be between 90°F and 100°F. You can use a bath thermometer to test the temperature or test it on your inner wrist. That temperature will feel comfortably warm. Hotter water may burn the client or make him weak and faint. If using a basin, change the water as often as necessary to keep it clean and warm. Soap should not sit in the basin because the water will become too soapy to use as rinse water.

6. *The washcloth.* Fold the washcloth like a mitt as shown in Figure 18-13 on page 228. Wet the mitt until it is damp but not dripping, to avoid splashing the client.

7. *Use proper body mechanics to avoid injury.* Remember the rules for lifting:
   • Keep a wide base of support.
   • Keep your back straight when lifting.
   • Use your legs to lift, not your back.
   • Squat instead of bending at the waist to lift an object.

8. *Bathroom safety.* Look for and correct potential safety hazards when preparing the bathroom such as wet floors, loose grab bars, and slippery floor mats.

9. *Disposable gloves.* To prevent the spread of infection, wear gloves when you may have contact with body fluids.

Assisting With Foot Care

The feet are more prone to infection and trauma than any other part of the body. Proper foot care is not a luxury, but an essential part of daily care for all of your clients. A client who has a circulatory problem or diabetes will be more prone to infection and other foot problems due to poor circulation and a lowered ability to feel sensations. This person may not be able to feel a small sore on his foot, so he needs to look at his feet carefully every day to prevent small sores from growing into serious infections. A *podiatrist* is a medical doctor who specializes in foot care. Older clients and those with diabetes or circulatory problems should see their podiatrists regularly to have their toenails cut.

Foot Care Guidelines

1. The feet should be cleaned and checked for sores daily.
   a. Soak the feet for a few minutes in a basin of warm water to loosen the dirt, soften the nails and skin, and relax the feet (Figure 18-19).
   b. Wash between the toes well. Gently clean under the nails with a blunt orange stick.
   c. Rinse the feet well. Be sure to remove all the soap so it does not irritate the skin.
   d. Dry the feet thoroughly, especially between the toes.

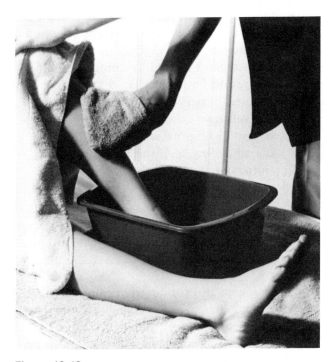

Figure 18-19
The client may want to have her legs washed while her feet are soaking.

2. For dry skin, massage the feet with lotion starting at the toes and working up to the heels and ankles. This is a good time to look for sores or reddened areas that may be the beginning of a pressure sore. If an area is red, massage around the area gently with lotion and report the condition to your home care supervisor at an appropriate time. For feet that perspire, talcum powder should be applied when the feet are well dried.

3. The HM/HHA should never cut a client's toenails. Older adults and those with health problems often need their nails cut by a podiatrist or a specially trained nurse. A small cut could lead to a serious infection.

4. HM/HHAs are sometimes instructed to file the toenails. Filing toenails is safer than cutting them. You will still need instructions on filing the toenails from the home care supervisor before doing this. The nail should be filed straight across. Do not round the edges, because this could lead to ingrown toenails.

5. A *callus* is an area of thickened skin that is caused when the foot rubs against the shoe. A callus should never be cut off because this could lead to infection. A bothersome callus should be treated by a podiatrist. Report any unusual foot problems such as calluses, ingrown toenails, sores or cuts, bunions, warts, or areas of redness to your home care supervisor so that prompt medical attention can be given.

6. Socks and shoes should be comfortable, fit properly, and be kept in good condition. Sometimes darned or mended socks can irritate sensitive skin. If this is the case, new socks should be purchased. Changing the socks daily helps keep the feet clean and dry.

7. For information on foot care for diabetic clients, see Chapter 10.

Assisting With Hair Care

The appearance and condition of our hair play an important part in the image we have of ourselves. We all tend to feel better when hair is clean and in good condition. Keeping the hair clean also promotes hair growth and prevents hair loss and scalp infections. Illness, medications, poor nutrition,

and stress can all affect the condition and appearance of the hair.

Guidelines for Grooming the Hair

1. Brush the hair daily to distribute the natural oils in the hair and to avoid tangles. An ill client may not want his hair brushed, but if it is not done, the hair will probably be very difficult to brush the next day, especially if it is long. Begin by brushing the hair slowly and gently. This stimulates the scalp better than combing.

2. The comb can be used after the brush to arrange the hair into the style that the client prefers. A wide-toothed comb is best for curly hair. If there are tangles, begin by combing a small section of the hair at the ends farthest from the scalp. Gradually work your way up until you can comb from the scalp to the ends (Figure 18-20).

3. The black client's hair is likely to be dry and curly. Use a wide-toothed comb. The client may want to use a hair-care product to treat his dry hair. Mineral oil, castor oil, or petroleum jelly can be used instead of a commercial product. Usually the client will state his preference.

4. Long hair may be more comfortable in braids if the client is confined to bed. Part the hair down the middle of the back of the head, and then make two braids. If you make one braid or a bun, the client will have

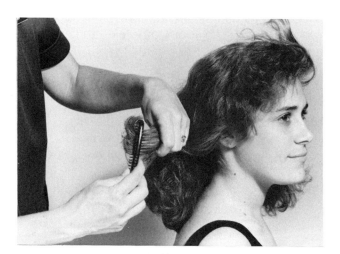

Figure 18-20
Hold tightly to the hair as shown without pulling it. Comb the ends, and work up to the scalp until you can comb from the scalp to the ends.

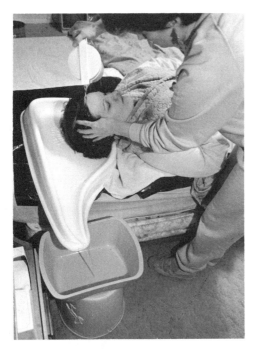

Figure 18-21
A commercial shampoo board. (Walsh J, Persons CB, Wieck L: Manual of Home Health Care Nursing, p 246. Philadelphia, JB Lippincott, 1987)

to lie on a large bump, which will be uncomfortable.

5. Never cut or color the client's hair without specific orders from your home care supervisor and from the client and family. If

you think the hair needs cutting, discuss this with your supervisor.

Guidelines for Shampooing the Hair

1. Washing the hair once or twice a week is usually adequate for a client confined to her home, but the client may want her hair washed more frequently. The comb and brush should also be washed every time the hair is washed.
2. Before washing, the hair should be brushed well to stimulate the scalp circulation.
3. If the client is able, she can then wash her hair in the shower or at the sink at the time of her bath.
4. If the client is confined to bed, she may have a shampoo board like the one shown in Figure 18-21. The client can lie back in bed and have her hair washed over the board. The board catches the water and drains it into a nearby bucket or container. These devices vary a little, so you will need to be instructed on how to use a particular shampoo board by your home care agency. If you do not have a shampoo board, you can make a shampoo trough for the client using household items as shown in Figure 18-22.

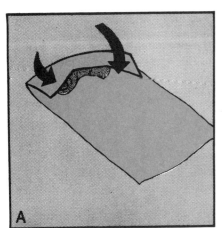
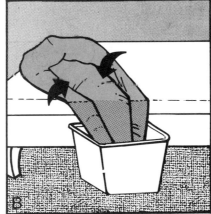
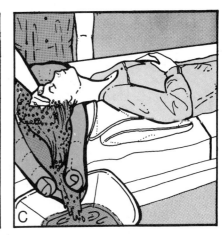

Figure 18-22
(*A*) A shampoo trough can be made by laying a piece of plastic (such as a large trash bag) on a flat surface. Put a rolled towel at one end and roll the edge of the plastic around the towel. (*B*) Roll the two sides of the plastic to make the trough. (*C*) To use, put the top of the trough under the client's head. Place the open end in a bucket at the bedside to catch the shampoo water.

HM/HHA Procedure:
Shampooing the Hair in Bed

Purpose: To clean the hair and refresh the client who cannot shampoo her own hair

Equipment:
- Shampoo board or homemade trough (You will need a piece of plastic, 60 inches by 60 inches and a bath towel to make the trough.)
- Pitcher
- Several basins of warm water
- Bucket to catch the excess water
- A chair (to set the bucket on)
- Newspaper (to protect the chair)
- Shampoo
- Several towels
- Washcloth
- Bath blanket or large towel
- Bed protector
- Comb and brush
- Apron for the HM/HHA

Safety:
- Keep the water comfortably warm to avoid burns.
- Close the windows to avoid drafts.

Steps	Reasons
1. Before beginning the procedure, gather your equipment, wash your hands, and tell the client what you are about to do and how she can help.	1. One of your primary goals is to have the client help as much as she is able.
2. Place the chair next to the bed and make sure the seat is lower than the mattress. Cover the seat with newspapers before putting the bucket on the chair.	2. Cover the seat of the chair to protect the furniture.
3. Have the client sit up, and remove the pillow. Place the bed protector over the top of the bed so that it hangs over the edges. Then place the shampoo board or the homemade trough on top of the bed protector.	3. The bed protector can be bought or made by putting newspapers on the bed and covering them with a towel or using a large sheet of plastic. It is used simply to keep the bed linens dry.
4. Put a towel around the client's shoulders and tuck it in so it is securely around her neck. Have the client lie back so her head fits into the trough. Place a rolled towel under her neck for comfort and to tilt the head back.	4. Tuck the towel into the collar of the client's shirt. You may want to cover the client with the bath blanket for warmth.
5. Make sure the end of the trough leads into the bucket. Test the temperature of the water and have the client hold the washcloth over her eyes. The client may want cotton in her ears to keep them dry.	
6. Wet the hair by pouring a small amount of water over the hair until it is ready for the shampoo.	6. Pour the water using a cup or a pitcher. Have the client turn her head to wet the hair thoroughly.

(continued)

HM/HHA Procedure:
Shampooing the Hair in Bed *(continued)*

Steps	Reasons
7. Apply the shampoo and massage the scalp with your fingertips. Rinse well by pouring water over the head and continuing to massage the scalp. Repeat the shampoo if needed.	
8. Apply conditioner or cream rinse as directed by the instructions on the container if the client uses these products.	8. Use the hair care products of the client's choice. Cream rinse and conditioner make the hair easier to comb and style.
9. Dry the hair well with a towel. See that the client is positioned comfortably and that her clothes are dry. Put a towel over her pillow to keep the linens dry.	
10. Clean up the room and put away the hair-washing supplies.	10. Clean up the room while the client's hair begins to dry. This is a good time to have the client sit in a chair if she is able while you make the bed.
11. Comb the client's hair and continue to towel-dry the hair. If the client has a hairdryer and is permitted, use the hairdryer on a low setting. Do not use the hairdryer if the client is using oxygen, and do not use it near water.	11. Oxygen is highly flammable. If you use a hairdryer, set it on a low temperature to avoid burns. The low setting is also less damaging to the hair. Comb the hair in the style the client prefers.
12. Wash your hands and make a note in the client's record regarding how she tolerated the procedure.	

Assisting With Shaving

Shaving is a normal part of the daily routine for most men. Most men will use an electric razor and will be able to shave themselves. You may only need to help clean the razor. Others will need some assistance with the electric razor, and a few may need help with a safety razor. Never shave a client unless you have been instructed to do so by the supervisor. See the procedure on page 242.

The Backrub

Learning to give a good backrub is a valuable skill. You may find some clients who do not enjoy hav-

ing a backrub, but most will find it refreshing. A backrub:

1. is relaxing,
2. stimulates the blood flow to the back muscles, and
3. gives the HM/HHA a chance to look for reddened areas on the back, which could lead to bedsores. An inactive or bedridden client is more prone to bedsores. For more on bedsores, see Chapter 20.

The backrub can be given at almost any time: after the bath, before sleeping, or after helping the client change positions in bed. The backrub procedure begins on page 243.

(Text continues on page 245.)

HM/HHA Procedure:
Shaving the Male Client With a Safety Razor

Purpose: To remove facial hair using a safety razor

Equipment:
- Safety razor
- Basin of warm water
- Shaving cream
- Washcloth
- Towel
- Good lighting

Safety:
- Never shave a client unless you have been instructed to do so by the home care supervisor. There may be a reason he should not be shaved.
- Shave in the direction of hair growth to avoid ingrown hairs.
- An electric razor should not be used if oxygen is being administered to the client.

Steps

1. Gather the equipment, wash your hands, and tell the client what you are about to do and how he can assist.

2. Have the client sit up and place the towel around the client's chest and shoulders. Adjust the light so you can see his face clearly.

3. Wipe the client's face with the warm wet washcloth to soften the facial hair. Then apply the shaving cream.

4. Hold the skin tight with one hand and carefully shave the cheeks and the chin using short downward strokes. Begin below one sideburn and work your way around to the other side of the face. Always shave in the direction of hair growth (Figure 18-23). Rinse the razor frequently in the basin.

Reasons

2. The client can either sit up in bed or sit in a chair.

3. Encourage the client to do all that he can by himself.

4. Shave in the direction of hair growth to prevent ingrown hairs.

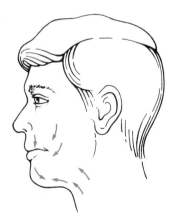

Figure 18-23
Shave the face in the direction of hair growth. (Walsh J, Persons CB, Wieck L: Manual of Home Health Care Nursing, p 275. Philadelphia, JB Lippincott, 1987)

(continued)

HM/HHA Procedure:
Shaving the Male Client With a Safety Razor *(continued)*

Steps	Reasons
5. To shave the neck, use short upward strokes because this is the direction the hair grows on the neck. Use special care when shaving near the nose, lips, and skin conditions such as warts or moles.	5. Shave around the mole, not directly over it, to avoid cutting it.
6. Remove the remaining shaving cream with the warm washcloth and pat the face dry. Apply shaving lotion if that is the client's preference.	6. Shaving lotion makes the skin feel cool and refreshed.
7. See that the client is comfortable and then clean up the room and put away the supplies.	
8. If you cut the client while shaving, report this to your home care supervisor.	
9. Wash your hands and record your observations about how the client tolerated the procedure.	

HM/HHA Procedure:
The Backrub

Purpose: To refresh the client, to increase the circulation to the back muscles, and to observe the skin condition.

Equipment:
• Lotion
• Towel

Safety: You should never give a backrub to someone who has had recent back surgery, broken ribs, or a recent heart attack without the permission of the doctor.

Steps	Reasons
1. Ask the client if he would like a backrub. Wash your hands and prepare the lotion by warming it in a basin or sink full of warm water for a few minutes (Figure 18-24). Take your supplies to the bedside.	1. Regular hand lotion is used for normal or dry skin. Rubbing alcohol may be used for oily skin.
2. Have the client move to the side of the bed where you will stand. The client can either lie down on his stomach with a pillow at his head or lie on his side so that his back faces you.	2. Use good body mechanics by keeping your back straight and bending at the hips and knees while rubbing the back.

(continued)

HM/HHA Procedure:
The Backrub *(continued)*

Steps

Reasons

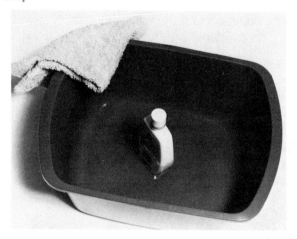

Figure 18-24
Warm the lotion in a basin of water.

3. Expose the client's back from his neck and shoulders to his hips. Look at the skin to see if he has any reddened areas that may be potential bedsores.

3. If there are any reddened areas, gently rub around the sensitive skin with lotion to increase the circulation. The potential bedsore must be reported to the home care supervisor that day. See Chapter 20 for more information on bedsores.

4. Rub a small amount of lotion into your hands to make sure it is warm. Then put your hands on both sides of the client's spine at hip level.

4. This is a systematic and relaxing method of promoting blood flow to all the back muscles.

5. Begin the backrub by moving the heels of both your hands up the client's spine to his neck using one firm stroke. When you get to the neck, continue to move along the shoulders and then down the back using a circular motion (Figure 18-25). Ideally, these movements are made in one continuous motion from the hips, to the neck and shoulders and then back down to the hips without lifting your hands.

5. You want to apply enough pressure so that you are not tickling the client, but not pressing too hard, either. Ask the client, and he will tell you how much is the right amount.

6. Try to use more pressure while moving up the spine and less pressure when making the circles and moving down the spine.

7. Repeat these motions for 3 to 6 minutes and use more lotion as necessary.

7. Your supervisor will be able to tell you how long to rub the back if you have questions.

8. When finished, dry the back with a soft towel, assist the client with his clothes, and help him into a comfortable position.

(continued)

HM/HHA Procedure:
The Backrub *(continued)*

Steps

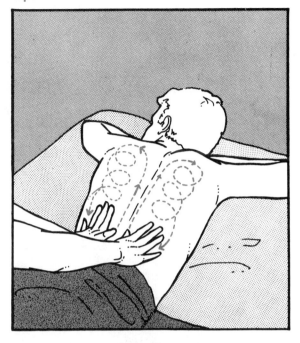

Reasons

Figure 18-25
The backrub.

9. Put away your supplies, wash your hands, and make a note in your record about how the client tolerated the procedure. Call your supervisor if there are any red or sore areas on the back.

9. The potential bedsore must be reported to the home care supervisor that day.

Assisting With Dressing and Undressing

When a person is ill or disabled, a routine habit such as getting dressed or undressed can become awkward and difficult. When you know some basic principles, you will be able to make dressing easier for your client. When a person is ill, he often may not feel like taking the trouble to get dressed in the morning, especially if he does not plan on leaving the house. Encourage your clients to dress and groom themselves as though they were going out. Getting dressed seems to make people feel better, because we tend to think that people who stay in their pajamas all day are ill.

Some clients may have developed their own method of getting dressed, and may not be interested in your suggestions. As long as the method is safe, there is no reason to interfere. You may even learn some good techniques. Other clients will welcome your suggestions.

Guidelines for Assisting With Dressing and Undressing

1. Encourage the client to do as much for himself as he is able. You could probably get the job done more quickly if you did it, but this would not help the client regain his dressing skills or his confidence in his ability to care for himself.
2. Allow for privacy and warmth by covering the client. Do not expose the client unnecessarily.
3. A weak arm or leg should always go into the sleeve or pants leg first when dressing. When undressing, the weak arm or leg

Guidelines for Assisting the Client with a One-Sided Weakness to Dress and Undress

Button Shirts

To put the button shirt on:
1. Help the client put his weaker arm into the sleeve.
2. Then, the stronger arm can reach around and slide into the sleeve.

To remove the button shirt:
1. Slide the stronger arm out before removing the weaker arm.

Trousers or Underpants

Put the weaker leg into the pants leg first. The stronger leg can follow. The client, if able, should sit on the edge of the bed and stand to pull them up to his waist. If he needs to remain in bed, he should bend his knees to lift his hips as he pulls the pants up to his waist. To remove the trousers, pull the stronger leg out of the pants before removing the weaker leg.

Shoes

A shoehorn will make putting on shoes easier. An extra-long handle may be helpful for the client who has trouble bending.

Pullover Shirts

To put the pullover on:
1. Help the client place his weaker arm in the sleeve.
2. Then slide the stronger arm into the sleeve.
3. Slide the neck over the head and pull the shirt down.

To remove the pullover:
1. Pull the shirt up and over the head.
2. Remove the weaker arm before removing the stronger arm.

Bras

Some bras fasten in the front and are easy to manage. When the clasp is in back, the client can put the bra around her waist so that the clasp is at her navel. Then she can hook the clasp, turn the bra around, and pull it up into position.

Socks or Stockings

Socks or stockings should be gathered like an accordion (Figure 18-26). Then the foot can be placed in the toe, and both hands can be used to pull up the socks.

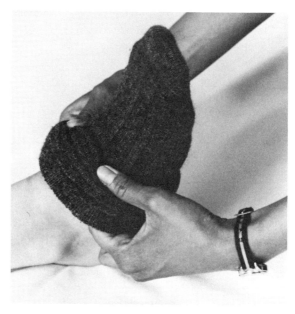

Figure 18-26
Fold socks like an accordion before putting them on.

---

should come out of the sleeve or pants leg last. See the box, Guidelines for Assisting the Client With a One-Sided Weakness to Dress and Undress.

4. Have the client look in the mirror so he can see if his shirt is tucked in or if he has missed a button. He should not have to depend on anyone else to tell him these things.

Adapting Clothes

There are a number of ways that clothes can be altered so that they are easier to use. Members of the home care team at your agency may have other suggestions.

1. Replace buttons with Velcro connectors. Sew the buttons onto the outside of the buttonholes. Sew the Velcro connectors where the buttons were to hold the article of clothing together. No one will be able to tell that the button is not being used.
2. Sew loops into socks near the top edge to make them easier to pull up.
3. Many clients find buttons are easier to manage with a device known as a *button aid*. A button aid is a hand tool with a wire end that helps pull the button through the buttonhole.
4. Elastic shoelaces stay tied better than regular shoelaces.

Review Questions

True or False

1. ____ The HM/HHA should demonstrate a procedure before a qualified health professional before doing that procedure for a client.

2. ____ Dentures only need to be brushed once a month.

3. ____ The HM/HHA should never irrigate, insert, or remove a urinary catheter.

4. ____ The client who is incontinent should drink plenty of fluids to encourage the bladder to work properly.

5. ____ If a client faints in the bathtub, drain the water, cover him with towels to keep him warm, and call for assistance.

6. ____ The HM/HHA should cut the client's toenails every week.

7. ____ A podiatrist is a doctor who specializes in foot care.

8. ____ The HM/HHA may cut or color a client's hair without orders from the supervisor or doctor.

9. ____ Facial hair should be shaved in the direction of hair growth to avoid ingrown hairs.

10. ____ Not every client will want a backrub.

11. ____ When helping a client dress, the weak arm or leg should always go into the sleeve or pant leg first.

12. ____ When undressing, the weak arm or leg should come out of the sleeve or pant leg first.

Chapter 19

Caring for the New Mother and Baby

Objectives

At the conclusion of this chapter, the homemaker/home health aide will:

1. Understand the importance of diet for a pregnant woman.

2. Be able to list three things the pregnant woman should avoid for the safety of her unborn child.

3. Be able to distinguish normal from abnormal physical and emotional reactions after a new baby arrives.

4. Explain the needs of a newborn and know what he is able to do.

5. Demonstrate how to hold a baby using the cradle, football, and shoulder holds.

6. Demonstrate and explain how to feed and bathe a newborn.

Caring for the Pregnant Woman

Although most pregnancies are normal, HM/HHA services may be needed when the pregnancy is not normal or when the pregnant woman is not able to care for herself, her family, and her home. All women are urged to see a doctor when they become pregnant to prevent problems and to detect and to treat pregnancy problems if they already exist. No one can guarantee a healthy baby, but a pregnant woman can do several things to increase the chances of having a healthy baby. The main task of the HM/HHA is to encourage the pregnant client to do those things, including the following:

1. *Follow the care plan.* Do not give advice that has not been approved by the doctor. The care plan will include instructions regarding exercise, nutrition, and medications, and any special orders for the client. For example, bedrest may be ordered for a client who has vaginal bleeding or high blood pressure.

2. *Eat a balanced diet with plenty of fluids.* Good nutrition is important for the health of both the mother and baby. The pregnant woman needs more nutrients and calories than an adult who is not pregnant. The following is

> **A pregnant woman should NOT use:**
> **Aspirin/Medications**
> **Beer/Wine/Alcohol**
> **Cigarettes**
> **Caffeine**

Figure 19-1
Things a pregnant woman should avoid.

a daily food plan that is recommended for a pregnant woman:

Milk—4 servings
Protein—3 to 4 servings
Fruit and vegetables—4 servings
Grains and breads—3 servings
Water—6 to 8 glasses

3. *Avoid smoking, alcohol, caffeine, and medications.* Smoke, alcohol, caffeine, and over-the-counter medications can all affect the growth and health of the unborn baby (Figure 19-1). No medications should be taken without the doctor's knowledge. A client may find it difficult to quit smoking or quit drinking alcohol and caffeine, but if the client understands the health of her baby may be at stake, she may be able to cut down considerably while pregnant.

4. *Bathe and brush the teeth daily.* When preparing the tub, make sure the bath water is not too hot. Because a pregnant woman may not have her usual sense of balance and a fall could be especially dangerous, use a nonskid mat in the tub or shower. Pregnant women are more likely to develop dental cavities. Encourage your client to brush and floss her teeth after meals to avoid this problem.

5. *The pregnant woman should use good body mechanics to prevent back injuries.* Stand with the hips tucked under and wear comfortable shoes with low heels. Avoid lifting whenever possible. To lift, squat and hold the object close to the body. Keep the back straight and slowly rise, using the legs to lift.

6. *Report the following symptoms to the doctor and home health agency.*
   • Bleeding from the vagina
   • Severe nausea and vomiting

- Swelling of the feet, ankles, and hands
- Fever over 100°F.

Being pregnant can be stressful and exhausting. Your client may have many worries about the health of the unborn child, her own health, reactions of other children in the family, family relationships, job, money—the list is endless. Your concern and ability to listen may make things much easier for her.

Caring for the Mother After the Baby Arrives

During the first 6 weeks after birth, the new mother has two major adjustments in her already busy life:

1. Adjustment to the physical changes as her body recovers from birth and pregnancy.
2. Adjustment to the delights and demands of caring for a new baby.

Ways to Help the Adjustment to a New Baby

Encourage the father and other family members to help take care of the baby while the mother rests. Adult family members can hold the baby when she cries or cuddle her when she's happy, change her diapers, and feed her if she is being fed with a bottle. They can also help with the housework and cooking. Young children may be able to hold the baby with adult supervision. It may be easier for family members to adjust and accept the new baby when they have helped care for her.

Baby Blues

Some women experience mild depression after the birth of a baby (postpartum depression). These low feelings may be due to hormonal changes in the body or they may be due to the change in lifestyle, especially for a first-time mother. Let the client know it is normal to go through some postpartum depression. Occasionally, postpartum depression is more serious and the new mother may not be able to care for her new baby properly. If you suspect that this is happening, let your supervisor know.

Normal Postpartum Reactions

- Mother cries easily.
- Mother may be irritable.
- Mother feels burdened and tired, but takes care of the baby's needs.

Postpartum Reactions to Report to the Agency

- Mother regularly forgets to feed the baby or to change the baby's diapers.
- Mother does not respond to the baby's cries.
- Safety needs of the baby are not met.

Caring for the New Baby

The HM/HHA may be assigned to care for a new infant or care for a parent who has a new baby. The family may use HM/HHA services when the baby is ill; the baby has had surgery; one of the parents is ill; the baby or a child in the family has been abused; or the parents need extra help caring for their newborn.

A newborn baby depends on others for everything: food, clothing, stimulation, love, and affection. The baby has little muscle control for the first few months of life and needs to be supported well when held.

Feeding and Burping the Baby

Breast-Feeding

The mother who is breast-feeding the baby may already have a routine. If the mother has sore breasts, is worried about the amount of milk she is producing, or needs any other assistance, your supervisor should be contacted. The nursing mother may need to be gently reminded:

- To wash her hands before feeding the baby. She should also wash her nipples with plain warm water before each feeding.
- To burp the baby after feeding. Have the mother hold the baby up against her shoulder or on her lap. Then gently rub or pat the baby's back. Be sure to use a small towel or diaper as a burp cloth.
- To eat a balanced diet and drink plenty of fluids in order to produce milk for the baby.

HM/HHA Procedure:
Lifting and Holding the Baby

Purpose: This section will demonstrate how to lift the baby and several ways to hold the baby securely.

Safety: Support the baby's head until he can support it well on his own, after he is about 4 to 6 months old.

Steps

Reasons

Lifting the Baby

1. Place one hand under the infant's shoulders to support the head, neck, and shoulders (Figure 19-2). Slide the other hand under the hips to support the bottom and legs. Lift the baby slowly.

1. The infant is not able to control his head and needs support when being held and lifted.

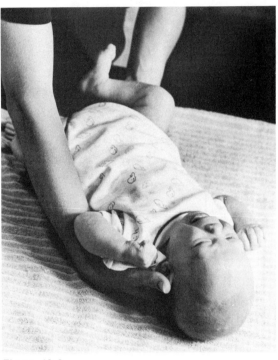

Figure 19-2
Support the baby's head when lifting him.

(continued)

HM/HHA Procedure:
Lifting and Holding the Baby *(continued)*

Steps

Reasons

The Cradle Hold

1. Lift the baby as directed at the beginning of this procedure.

2. Hold the baby securely on your forearm so the baby's head is at your elbow and you are holding his hips in the palm of your hand (Figure 19-3). If sitting, you can rest the baby's hips on your lap. This position allows the baby to look at the caregiver.

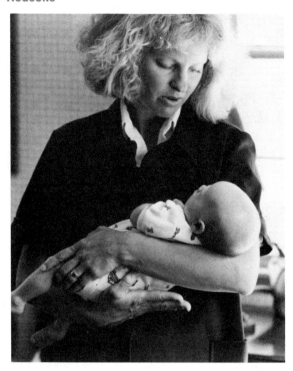

Figure 19-3
The cradle hold.

The Football Hold

1. Lift the baby as directed at the beginning of this procedure.

2. Place the baby across your arm with his head in the palm of your hand and his hips and legs supported by your elbow and waist (Figure 19-4).

2. The football hold lets you hold the baby securely with one arm and have the other hand free to straighten blankets, wash the baby's hair, etc.

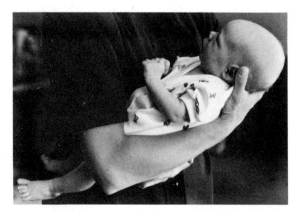

Figure 19-4
The football hold.

(continued)

HM/HHA Procedure:
Lifting and Holding the Baby *(continued)*

Steps

Reasons

The Shoulder Hold

1. Lift the baby as directed at the beginning of this procedure.

2. Place the infant's head on your shoulder, supporting his head with one hand and his hips with the other hand (Figure 19-5).

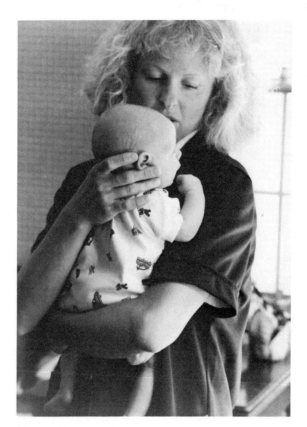

Figure 19-5
The shoulder hold.

(continued)

HM/HHA Procedure:
Lifting and Holding the Baby *(continued)*

Steps

Helping the Baby Sit With Support

1. Lift the baby as directed at the beginning of this procedure.

2. Place the baby on your lap in a sitting position (Figure 19-6). This is a good position to use when burping the baby. Lean the baby forward slightly and pat him on the back with your free hand.

Reasons

2. A young baby will need to have his head and neck supported carefully when you lift him up and carry him.

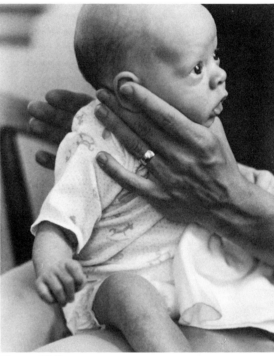

Figure 19-6
This is a good position to use when burping a baby.

HM/HHA Procedure:
Changing the Baby's Diapers

Purpose: Change the diapers whenever they are soiled to prevent skin rashes.

Equipment: • Fresh diaper
            • Container for the soiled diaper
            • Washcloth, soap, and warm water (or disposable wipes)
            • Lotion or baby cream if instructed to use
            • Waterproof changing pad to protect floor or bed if a changing table is not available

Safety: • *Never leave a baby alone on a changing table for a moment.* Even a newborn might manage to wiggle off a table, chair, or countertop if your back is turned.
            • Keep safety pins closed and out of reach of the baby.

(continued)

Steps

1. Wash your hands before the procedure. Gather your equipment and set it near the changing area. A bed, a large table, or even the floor can be used if a changing table is not available.

2. Place the infant on the changing table. Strap the baby to the table, but do not leave the baby alone on the table for an instant. A mobile above the infant's head, a toy, or a picture on the wall may help amuse the baby.

4. Undress the baby and remove the soiled diaper. Place the diaper aside and wash the baby's bottom, wiping from front to back. Pat dry. Use cream or lotion if instructed.

5. *Disposable diapers.* Unfold the fresh disposable diaper. Slide it under the baby's hips with the tabs at the back. Tape the corners together securely (Figure 19-7). There is no need to use rubber pants with disposable diapers.

6. Roll the disposable diaper up and retape it before throwing it in the trash.

7. *Cloth diapers.* See Figure 19-8 on diaper folding. Put the diaper under the baby's hips. Pin the corners together with your fingers between the baby's skin and the diaper (Figure 19-9). Put waterproof pants or a cloth diaper cover over the cloth diaper to prevent leaking.

Reasons

2. The strap helps keep the baby from wiggling, but it will not keep the baby from falling off the table.

4. To avoid diaper rash, let the skin dry completely before putting the fresh diaper on.

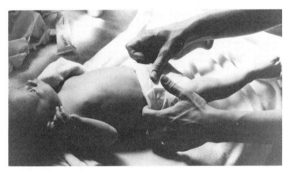

Figure 19-7
Taping the disposable diaper.

7. Fold the diaper as shown in Figure 19-8. Keep your fingers between the baby and diaper to prevent sticking the baby. Never keep open diaper pins on the changing table near the baby.

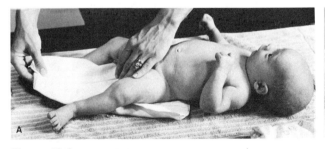
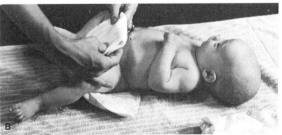

Figure 19-8
(*A*) Fold the cloth diaper in thirds lengthwise and place the baby on the diaper. (*B*) The front edge may need to be folded over before pinning.

(continued)

HM/HHA Procedure:
Changing the Baby's Diapers *(continued)*

Steps

Reasons

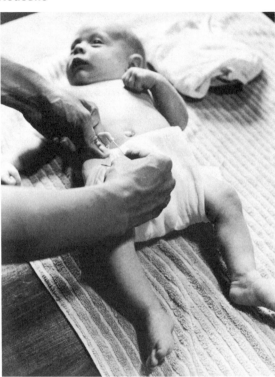

Figure 19-9
To avoid poking the baby with the diaper pin, put your finger between the diaper and the baby's skin when pinning the cloth diaper.

8. Follow the directions of your supervisor and the parents on what to do with the soiled cloth diaper. Never flush the diaper down the toilet.

9. Dress the infant and put him in a safe place, such as crib or playpen. Talk to the baby while you care for him to keep him relaxed and happy.

10. Clean the changing area and return the supplies to the proper place. Wash your hands thoroughly.

11. Record your observations in the progress notes. Note if diaper was wet or soiled; color and amount of stool; and any skin redness or irritation.

8. Usually soiled diapers are rinsed in the toilet and then soaked in a pail of water with disinfectant.

HM/HHA Procedure:
Bottle-Feeding

Purpose: The doctor will prescribe a formula suited to meet the needs of the baby. Some formulas need to be prepared, and others are ready to serve.

Equipment: • Sterile baby bottle
             • Formula

Safety: • Formula can be kept in the refrigerator for 48 hours without spoiling. If you do not know when the formula was put in the refrigerator, throw it out.
             • Formula will spoil if left at room temperature.
             • Do not reuse formula that has been warmed.

Steps

1. Wash your hands and gather the equipment. If you need to prepare the formula, make it before the baby is hungry and store it in the refrigerator.

2. Sterilize the bottle and equipment as directed by your supervisor. Usually this involves boiling the bottle, nipple, and formula in water for 5 minutes (Figure 19-10).

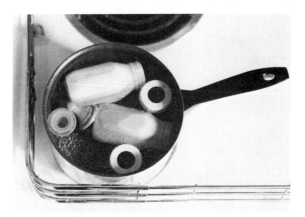

Figure 19-10
Boil baby bottles to sterilize them.

3. Prepare the formula as instructed by the label and your supervisor. Some liquid formulas need to be diluted with boiled water and others do not. Label and refrigerate the formula.

4. Check to see that the baby's diapers are dry before feeding.

5. If the formula has been in the refrigerator, set the bottle in a bowl of hot tap water to warm the formula. The bottle is ready when the formula feels lukewarm when tested on your inner wrist.

Reasons

1. Babies must have their needs met quickly. A hungry baby will cry and may be difficult to calm. If the baby cries too hard, he may have trouble eating when the formula is ready.

2. An unsterile bottle can cause the baby to become ill.

3. The baby may become ill if the formula is not prepared according to the directions.

(continued)

HM/HHA Procedure:
Bottle-Feeding *(continued)*

Steps	**Reasons**
6. Cradle the baby and talk to him while you feed him (Figure 19-11). Encourage the mother and father to hold and feed the baby if possible.	6. If you are helping to teach the new parents how to care for an infant, you must give them time to practice the new skills they are learning.

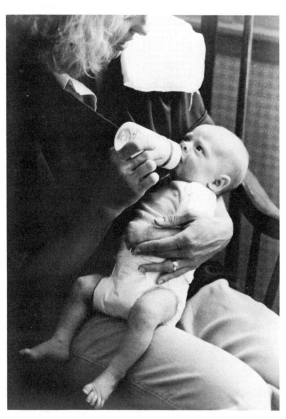

Figure 19-11
Cradle the baby as you feed him.

7. Burp the baby.	7. Burping the baby gets rid of extra air in the stomach. Excess air causes discomfort for the baby.
8. Note the amount of formula taken and how well the baby took the formula. Record your observations in the progress notes.	

Bathing the Baby

HM/HHA Procedure:
The Infant Sponge Bath

Purpose: A sponge bath is given in the first few weeks until the baby's navel and circumcision have healed.

(continued)

HM/HHA Procedure:
The Infant Sponge Bath *(continued)*

Equipment:
- Basin
- Two large soft bath towels and washcloth
- Cotton balls
- Clean clothing and diaper
- Mild soap

Safety:
- *Never leave the baby alone on a table.*
- Do not bathe the baby right after feeding because it may upset her stomach.
- When giving a bath, be quick enough so the baby does not get too cold, but relaxed enough so the baby enjoys it.
- The water temperature should be 90°F to 100°F and the room should be warm.

Steps	Reasons
1. Gather your supplies. Remove your jewelry and watch. Wash your hands, and make sure your fingernails are trimmed and smooth. Take supplies to the bathing area.	1. Check to make sure that all your equipment is within reach before you start the baby's bath. If you forget something, take the baby with you while you get it. Even newborns may roll off a table.
2. Half fill the basin with comfortably warm water and bring the baby to the bathing area. You can either remove the baby's clothes now (except for the diaper) and wrap the baby in a towel or leave the clothes on while you wash the face and hair.	
3. *The eyes.* Use a clean, wet cotton ball and no soap to wipe from the inner corner of the eye outward in one gentle stroke (Figure 19-12). Use a fresh cotton ball and wipe again. Pat dry. Use a new cotton ball to clean the baby's other eye in the same way.	

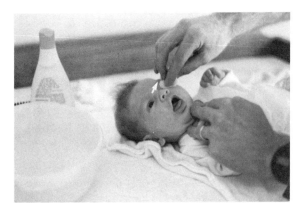

Figure 19-12
Use a cotton ball dipped in clean water to wipe the baby's eye from the inside corner to the outside corner.

Steps	Reasons
4. *The face.* Wash the baby's face with the soft washcloth using plain water. Gently pat dry.	
5. *The ears.* Use a clean, damp cotton ball to clean the outside of the ear and behind the ear. *Do not put anything into the baby's ear canal.*	5. A cotton swab can seriously damage the eardrum and inner ear. The ear canal does not need to be cleaned because the ear expels wax and dirt naturally.

(continued)

Steps

6. *The hair and scalp.* Use the football hold when washing the hair. Hold the head over the basin and use your free hand to pour warm water over the baby's head (Figure 19-13). Wash the baby's head with mild soap using a circular motion. Rinse well and towel dry.

Reasons

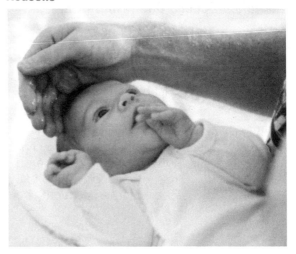

Figure 19-13
The football hold allows this homemaker/home health aide to hold the baby with one arm and wash the baby's scalp with the other.

7. *The body.* Set the baby down on a towel or soft surface by the basin. Lather, rinse, and dry the rest of the baby, paying particular attention to the skin folds. Do not get the navel wet until the cord has fallen off and the area has healed.

7. Dry the skin well to prevent skin rashes. The umbilical cord will fall off 1 to 3 weeks after birth. Follow your supervisor's instructions for keeping the cord clean and dry.

8. *The bottom.* Remove the diaper to wash the baby's bottom and genitals. Wash, rinse, and dry the bottom. Consult your supervisor for care of the boy's circumcision. For girls, use a cotton ball to gently wipe from front to back.

9. Dress the baby. Slide your hand through the arm of the baby's shirt and hold her hand as you pull the shirt up her arm.

10. Put the baby in the crib or playpen while you clean up the bathing area and put away all the equipment. Record your observations about the baby's skin and tolerance to the bath in your progress notes.

HM/HHA Procedure:
The Infant Tub Bath

Purpose: A tub bath can be given when baby's navel and circumcision have healed.

Equipment: • Infant tub, basin, or sink
             • Two large soft bath towels and washcloth

(continued)

- Cotton balls
- Clean clothing and diaper
- Mild soap

Safety:
- *Never leave the baby alone in a tub or on a table.*
- Do not bathe the baby right after feeding because it may upset his stomach.
- When giving a bath, be quick enough so the baby does not get too cold, but relaxed enough so the baby enjoys it.
- The water temperature should be 90°F to 100°F and the room should be warm.

Steps

1. Gather your supplies. Remove your jewelry and watch. Wash your hands, and make sure your fingernails are trimmed and smooth. Take supplies to the bathing area.

2. Fill the tub with about 4 inches of comfortably warm water. A washcloth or large sponge on the bottom of the tub will help keep the baby from slipping. Wash the baby's face and hair before placing him in the tub.

3. *The eyes.* Use a clean, damp cotton ball and no soap to wipe from the inner corner of the eye outward in one gentle stroke. Use a fresh cotton ball and wipe again. Pat dry. Use a new cotton ball to clean the baby's other eye in the same way.

4. *The face.* Wash the baby's face with the soft washcloth using plain water. Gently pat dry.

5. *The ears.* Use a clean, damp cotton ball to clean the outside of the ear and behind the ear. *Do not put anything into the baby's ear canal.*

6. *The hair and scalp.* Use the football hold when washing the hair. Hold the head over the basin and use your free hand to pour warm water over the baby's head. Wash the baby's head with mild soap using a circular motion. Rinse well and towel dry.

7. Undress the baby and place him into the tub feet first using the safety hold. Keep the baby in a sitting position and do not let go of him during the bath. Use your free hand to wash and rinse the baby's front, making sure to get all the skin folds (Figure 19-14). Reverse the safety hold to wash the baby's back (Figure 19-15). Never leave the baby in the bath alone for even an instant.

Reasons

1. Check to make sure that all your equipment is within reach before you start the baby's bath. If you forget something, take the baby with you while you get it. Even newborns may roll off a table.

3. Do not reuse any part of the cotton ball because you do not want to put the dirt particles or germs back into the eye after you have wiped them away.

5. A cotton swab can seriously damage the eardrum and inner ear. The ear canal does not need to be cleaned because the ear expels wax and dirt naturally.

7. Always use the safety hold to prevent the baby from slipping out of your hands. Reversing the safety hold allows you to wash the baby's back and hold the baby securely without turning the baby over.

(continued)

HM/HHA Procedure:
The Infant Tube Bath *(continued)*

Steps

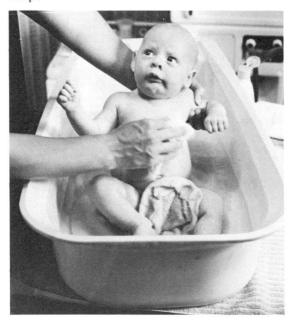

Figure 19-14
Use the safety hold to wash the baby's front.

Reasons

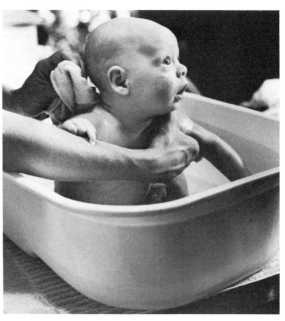

Figure 19-15
Use the safety hold to wash the baby's back.

8. Use the safety hold to lift the baby out of the tub and onto a warm, dry surface. Wrap the baby in a soft towel, pat dry, and then dress him.

9. Put the baby in the crib or playpen while you clean up the bathing area and put away all the equipment. Record your observations about the baby's skin and tolerance to the bath in your progress notes.

Review Questions

True or False

1. ___ An infant should not have a tub bath until his umbilical cord has fallen off and healed.

2. ___ A pregnant woman should not take medication unless advised to by her doctor.

3. ___ A newborn must always have his head supported when being lifted and carried.

4. ___ A pregnant woman who has a fever of 101°F does not need to report this to her doctor.

Multiple Choice

5. Pregnant women should avoid:
   a. smoking, calcium, and alcohol
   b. smoking, caffeine, and alcohol
   c. exercise, calcium, and protein
   d. aspirin, caffeine, and protein

Questions for Discussion

You are caring for a client who has a 5-week-old baby. The client often lays the baby on a chair or on the couch for his nap and leaves the room. Is this a problem? Why or why not? How would you deal with this situation?

Chapter 20

Common Procedures and Treatments

Objectives

At the conclusion of this chapter, the homemaker/home health aide will:

1. Be able to explain the purpose of deep breathing exercises.

2. Be able to state two early signs of a pressure sore and describe two ways to help prevent pressure sores.

3. Be able to list the six common cast problems and explain how to deal with them.

4. Understand why hot and cold treatments may be used for a client, and describe three safety precautions to consider when using an electric heating pad.

5. Know how to measure fluid intake and output.

6. Be able to change a nonsterile dressing and chart the dressing change in detail in the client's progress notes.

7. Understand the role of the HM/HHA in assisting the client with an ostomy, know when to call the supervisor for assistance, and be able to demonstrate how to help the client clean the skin around the ostomy or help the client empty the contents of the ostomy bag.

8. Be able to demonstrate the correct procedure for collecting a clean-catch midstream urine specimen and a stool specimen.

9. Know how to teach a client the relaxation exercise upon a supervisor's approval.

This chapter covers treatments and procedures you may perform in your job as a HM/HHA. Your home health agency may have you do the procedure in a different manner than the way you are instructed in this text. This may be due to a client's particular needs, or because there may be several ways to do a procedure correctly and safely.

Guidelines for All Procedures

1. Before performing any procedure for a client, a nurse or other qualified professional should watch you successfully demonstrate the procedure. This is for your protection and the protection of your clients. Be aware that some home health agencies and some state laws may not allow the HM/HHA to perform some of the procedures described in this book without further training and testing.

2. In a friendly manner, tell the client what you are about to do and why. Let the client know how he can help. Allow the client to make some decisions about the procedures whenever possible, such as when the procedure will take place. The client is more likely to cooperate when he has some understanding and control over the situation. Treat the client as you would want to be treated if you were in his position.

3. To prevent the spread of disease and infection, wash your hands before and after giving care to the client, using the toilet, or preparing food. Remember to give your client the opportunity to wash his hands, too.

4. Think about the supplies you will need for the procedure and make sure you have them all together *before* starting the procedure. Always consider safety precautions before starting a procedure.

5. Allow the client privacy. Talk to the client before the procedure begins and find out if he might want others in the room to leave.

6. Finish the procedure as quickly and efficiently as you can for the comfort of the client. Sometimes, you may need to ignore the telephone or doorbell.

7. Clean and put away all the equipment. Record your observations about the client and his tolerance to the procedure.

8. If your client has an unexpected reaction, phone your home health agency to report the situation.

Deep Breathing Exercises

HM/HHA Procedure:
Deep Breathing Exercises

Purpose: Clients with lung disorders may be required to do deep breathing exercises. These exercises help expand the lungs, allow the client to take in more air with less effort, and help the client to relax. These exercises may be uncomfortable because they often will make the client cough. Coughing helps clear the lungs by bringing up mucus.

Equipment:
- Box of tissues
- Wastebasket or bag
- Mouth care supplies to use after the procedure

Safety: Do not assist with deep breathing exercises unless you have been instructed to do so. Every client has individual needs, and the procedure must be done carefully considering their needs.

Steps	Reasons
1. Gather your equipment, wash your hands, and tell the client about the procedure before beginning. Tell the client what he is to do.	
2. Ask any visitor to leave the room if this is the client's wish.	2. Clients often do not want others in the room when they are doing the deep breathing exercises.
3. To breathe in: Have the client breathe through his nose very slowly and deeply until you can see his abdomen expand. His chest and shoulders should not move.	
4. To breathe out: Have the client purse his lips as though he were blowing out a candle, and slowly release the air through his mouth.	
5. It is normal for the client to cough and spit up mucus during the procedure. Note the color and amount.	5. Assure the client that it is good to bring up mucus from congested lungs. The description of the mucus should be recorded in your progress notes later.
6. Repeat this exercise ten times, or as many times as you have been instructed by the home care supervisor.	
7. Offer the client a chance to wash his hands and brush his teeth.	7. Handwashing prevents the spread of infection, and oral care will leave a pleasant taste in the client's mouth.
8. When the client is comfortable, put the supplies away, throw away the tissues, wash your hands, and record your observations about the mucus and about the client's tolerance of the procedure.	

Care and Prevention of Pressure Sores (Decubitus Ulcers)

What Are Pressure Sores?

Pressure sores, which are also known as *decubitus ulcers (decubiti)* or *bedsores*, are painful, deep wounds that occur from pressure. An ill or disabled person who is unable to change positions is likely to get decubti when he lies or sits in one position for long periods of time. The constant pressure on the skin does not allow the blood to bring oxygen and nutrients to that area, and the skin becomes tender, red, and sore. Eventually an open wound may form. Decubitus ulcers are most likely to form on areas where the bone is near the skin surface. These areas of the body are called *bony prominences* (Figure 20-1).

Which Clients Are Likely to Get Pressure Sores?

- Clients who remain in a bed or a wheelchair most of the time.

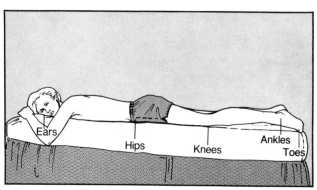

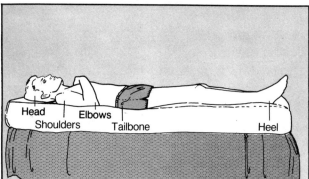

Figure 20-1
Pressure sores often occur on clients who cannot reposition themselves. They are most likely to develop on the bony areas of the body shown here.

- Older adults who have trouble changing positions.
- Clients with diabetes, loss of sensation, or poor circulation.
- Thin or undernourished clients.
- Clients who are incontinent.
- Clients who wear braces or other appliances.

Early Signs of Pressure Sores

1. An area of skin looks pale because blood cannot get to that area.
2. Skin becomes red, tender and sore.
3. A break in the skin and a visible wound is a late sign.

What to Do if You See a Bedsore Forming

1. Keep pressure off that area of the body. Continue to turn and reposition the client at least every 2 hours.
2. Gently massage the area around the bedsore to bring blood to the area. Do not rub the sensitive sore or the skin may break.
3. Report the problem to your supervisor at the first sign of a bedsore.

Guidelines for Preventing Pressure Sores

1. Turn and reposition the immobile client at least every 2 hours. Some may need to be turned more frequently.
2. Do not slide the client when moving him in the bed or the chair. This causes a shearing force, which can burn and tear the skin (Figure 20-2).
3. Keep the skin clean and dry. Rinse soap off completely after a bath and use a moisturizer if the skin tends to be dry.
4. Check the skin where pressure sores are likely to develop and massage those areas carefully.
5. Keep the bed linens clean, dry, and free from wrinkles or loose objects that the client could sit on accidentally.
6. Protect the client's heels, lower back, elbows, and other areas prone to bedsores. Your supervisor can suggest ways to do this.
7. Nutritious foods, plenty of rest and sleep, and exercise activities approved by the doctor are all ways of promoting health. Healthy cells are less likely to be damaged.

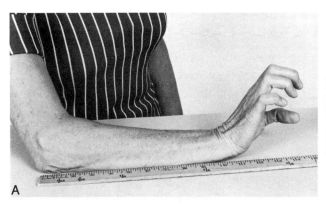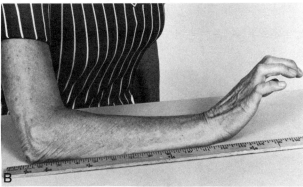

Figure 20-2
Shearing force occurs when the skin and underlying tissues are pulled. (*A*) The woman's arm is placed so that her elbow is at the end of the ruler. (*B*) Without lifting her arm off the table, the woman slid her arm more than an inch. (Wolff L, Weitzel MH, Zornow RA et al: Fundamentals of Nursing, 7th ed, p 409. Philadelphia, JB Lippincott, 1983)

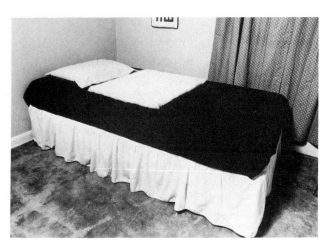

Figure 20-3
The sheepskin pad can be placed on top of or under the bottom sheet.

Devices That Can Help Prevent Pressure Sores

- Sheepskin or synthetic pads (Figure 20-3)
- Foam mattress pad (Figure 20-4)
- Elbow, ankle, and heel protectors (Figure 20-5)
- Bed cradle (Figure 20-6)

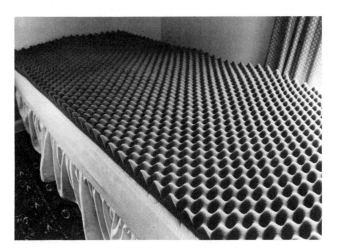

Figure 20-4
The foam or egg-crate mattress is placed under the bottom sheet.

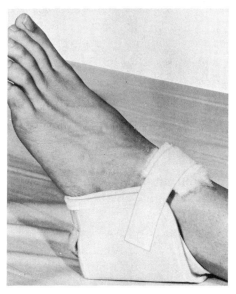

Figure 20-5
The heel and ankle protector. (Courtesy of J.T. Posey Company, Arcadia, CA 91006-0021)

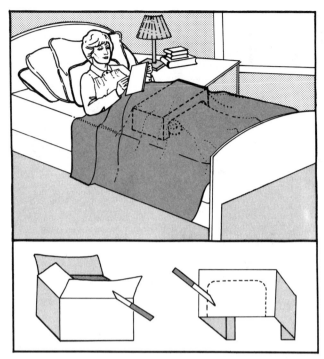

Figure 20-6
The bed cradle.

Care of the Client With a Cast

Casts keep broken bones or strained muscles in the proper position while they heal. Casts can be placed on arms, legs, hips, and abdomens. Let the doctor or nurse answer the client's questions about whether the cast fits properly or the amount of movement he will have after the cast has been removed.

Cast Care Guidelines

1. Keep the cast dry and clean. Cover the cast with plastic before baths and showers.
2. If the client complains of itching under the cast, do not let him stick anything under the cast to scratch.
3. Keep the skin around the cast clean. Massage the area around the cast with alcohol for comfort. Do not use lotion near the cast edge because it can leave a sticky film.
4. A small amount of white shoe polish will brighten a dirty spot on a cast. Do not use too much or the cast will soften.

Six Common Cast Problems and What to Do About Them

1. *Swelling of the hands or feet.* This may happen after activity. Have the client elevate the limb. Report the condition to your supervisor.
2. *Poor circulation.* Test circulation in the fingers and toes by squeezing the nails. They should become white when squeezed and quickly turn pink when released. In clients with dark skin, the color change is not as great, but you can still see it. Call your home health agency if you cannot see a color change. Nail polish must be removed to do this test.
3. *Numbness or pain.* The cast should not cause pain and the client should have a normal sense of feeling in the leg or arm with the cast. Any loss of sensation should be reported to the supervisor right away.
4. *Odors.* A foul odor coming from a cast may mean infection. Report odors right away.
5. *Discharge or spotting on the cast.* Circle the spot with a pen and label the circle with the date, the time, and your initials (Figure 20-7). If the spot gets bigger, circle it and label it again. Report the spot right away.
6. *Loss of movement.* If the client has lost some of the ability to move his fingers or toes on the casted limb, report this to your supervisor.

If you suspect that something is wrong with

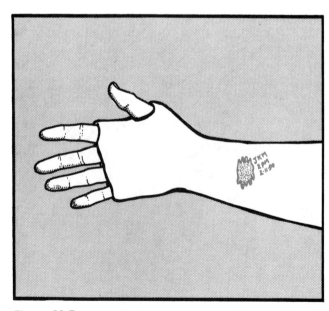

Figure 20-7
Write the date, the time, and your initials next to spot marks on the cast.

the cast, report the situation to the supervisor. The supervisor can check the cast carefully and tell the client if there is a problem. You should not alarm the client by telling him something might be wrong when you are not certain.

Hot and Cold Applications

The Body's Reaction to Hot and Cold Applications

The Effects of Heat

- The blood vessels get larger and more blood flows to the warm area.
- The muscles relax.
- Food is converted into energy by the cells at a faster rate.
- The body adjusts to the higher temperature and the benefits of the heat treatment are not as effective after 20 minutes.

The Effects of Cold

- The blood vessels become smaller and less blood is brought to the cold area.
- The muscles become tense.
- Food is converted into energy by the cells at a slower rate.
- The body adjusts to the lower temperature and the benefits of the cold application will not be as effective after 20 minutes.

Hot Applications

Why Heat Is Used

1. Heat helps wounds heal by bringing blood and nutrients to the area where heat is applied.
2. Heat relaxes muscles, relieves discomfort, and promotes rest.

When Heat Should not Be Used

Do not apply heat unless you are instructed to do so by your supervisor. There are several situations when heat may do more harm than good. The doctor and your supervisor will determine when it is safe to use hot applications. Some home health agencies and some state laws do not allow the HM/HHA to apply hot applications without further training and testing.

Heat tends to increase swelling. The doctor may not want to use heat on a client's swollen joint, limb, or jaw.

Heat should be used very carefully for all clients and especially those who may not be able to judge temperatures well. A client with a stroke, circulatory problems, or paralysis may not be able to tell when his skin is getting burned.

The Electric Heating Pad

The electric heating pad is another method of applying dry heat. The heating pad keeps its temperature better than a hot water bottle, but if the hot water bottle is a little too hot, it cools down. The heating pad does not. The skin becomes used to temperatures after a period of time even if the temperatures are at dangerous levels. If the heating pad is not used properly, people with poor circulation can be seriously burned without being aware of it at the time.

Safety and the Electric Heating Pad. The electric heating pad has so many potential problems that many home health agencies do not allow them to be used. If they are used, the client may need to sign a form to release the agency and home care staff from all responsibility should something go wrong.

1. The electric heating pad, including the cord, must be in good repair.
2. Do not fold or crease a heating pad because the electric wires in the pad can be damaged and cause the pad to malfunction.
3. Put a loose-fitting waterproof cover on the heating pad. The waterproofing prevents an electrical shock and the loose covering allows air to circulate around the pad so heat can be released. Most covers can be washed between uses, but must be absolutely dry when used.
4. Use tape or strips of cloth to secure the pad around the client's leg or arm. Do not use safety pins because they can hit the electric wires inside the pad and cause a shock.
5. Do not allow the client to lie on the heating pad. This could cause the pad to overheat and burn the client or his bedclothes.
6. Set the temperature on *low* and do not permit the client to raise the setting. Some agencies use pads where the temperature setting cannot be changed. Let the client

(*Text continues on page 272.*)

HM/HHA Procedure:
Using the Hot Water Bottle

Purpose: To relieve discomfort and encourage relaxation

Equipment: • Hot water bottle and cloth cover
             • Bath thermometer

Safety: Check the water temperature with the bath thermometer using the guide in Step 2
             of this procedure.

Steps

1. Gather your equipment, wash your hands, and explain to the client what you are about to do.

2. Use the water temperature guide below when preparing the hot water bottle.
   98° to 110°F
     Young children
     Older adults
     Those who cannot tell you if temperature is too hot
   105° to 115°F
     Healthy adults
     Older children

3. After checking the temperature with the bath thermometer, fill the hot water bottle half full. Release the excess air before closing the lid.

4. Dry the bottle and turn it upside down to make sure it does not leak. A soft cloth cover should be placed over the bottle to make the bag more comfortable and to protect the client from burns.

5. Apply the hot water bottle. Check the client's skin after a few minutes to make sure the bottle is not too hot.

6. Keep the hot water bottle in place for as long as you have been instructed by your supervisor.

7. After removing the hot water bottle, put away your supplies, wash your hands, and record the client's tolerance to the procedure.

Reasons

2. Some clients may feel these temperatures are too cool. Explain that these temperatures promote safe healing.

3. Releasing the extra air allows the bottle to mold to the body.

6. Hot applications are usually left on for 20 minutes and then removed. The treatment can be repeated in another hour or two to get the most benefit from the heat therapy.

Hot Wet Applications

HM/HHA Procedure:
Warm Soaks

Purpose: Warm soaks promote wound healing, relieve discomfort, and encourage relaxation.

Equipment:
- Basin or tub filled with warm water
- Bath thermometer
- Towels

Safety: Check the water temperature with the bath thermometer to prevent burns.

Steps

1. Gather your equipment, wash your hands, and explain to the client what you are about to do.

2. Fill the basin with warm water that has been checked with the bath thermometer. Water temperature should be between 100° and 110°F.

3. Assist the client so he is comfortable and time the soak as instructed by your supervisor. Soaks usually take 15 to 20 minutes.

Reasons

1. A styrofoam ice chest is an ideal basin for soaks because it holds the water temperature fairly well. A clean plastic basin, bathtub, or sink can also be used.

2. Regulate the water temperature according to your supervisor's instructions.

3. For example, rest a rolled washcloth on the edge of the basin to support the client's forearm while he soaks his hand (Figure 20-8).

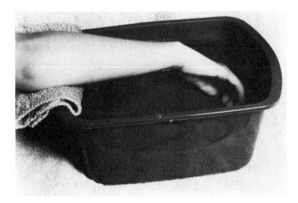

Figure 20-8
Pad the basin to make the soak more comfortable for the client.

4. To maintain the temperature, the water should be checked every 5 to 8 minutes with a bath thermometer.

5. After the soak, put away your supplies, wash your hands, and record the client's tolerance to the procedure.

4. If warm water needs to be added, have the client remove his foot or hand and stir in the hot water thoroughly to avoid discomfort or burns to the client.

Cold Dry Applications

HM/HHA Procedure:
Using the Ice Bag

Purpose: Dry cold is used to reduce pain and swelling.

Equipment: • Ice bag or a zip-lock plastic bag
            • Crushed ice
            • Cotton towel or cover for the ice bag

Safety: Do not leave the ice bag on the skin for more than 20 minutes unless instructed otherwise.

Steps

1. Gather your equipment, wash your hands, and explain to the client what you are about to do.

2. Fill the ice bag half full with crushed ice. Add cold water to the bag for 2 to 3 minutes. Then pour the water out, leaving the crushed ice in the bag.

3. Squeeze the extra air out of the bag, tightly close the top, and dry the outside of the bag with a towel.

4. Cover the bag with a soft thin cloth and apply it to the client. If the client says the bag is too cold, put another cloth around the ice bag.

5. Remove the ice bag as instructed by your supervisor.

6. After removing the ice bag, put away your supplies, wash your hands, and record the client's tolerance to the procedure.

Reasons

3. Removing the excess air allows the bag to mold to the body.

4. The ice bag has been on too long or is too cold if the skin becomes pale or numb.

5. Ice bags are usually left in place for 20 minutes and removed for at least an hour before being replaced. This gives the skin time to adjust to its normal temperature so the cold treatment can be effective when started again.

know that even though the pad will feel cooler after a while, the temperature will remain constant and at a safe level for tissue healing. Many people are seriously burned every year when they turn their heating pads up too high.

Cold Applications

Why Cold Is Used

1. Cold packs reduce swelling (edema) and inflammation by slowing the blood circulation and slowing the growth of germs and bacteria.
2. Cold packs can be used to relieve the pain of a strained or sprained joint, such as a wrist or ankle.
3. Cold applications can also be used to lower the body temperature.

When Cold Should not Be Used

Do not apply cold unless you are instructed to do so by your supervisor. There are several situations when cold may do more harm than good. The doctor

Cold Wet Applications

> *HM/HHA Procedure:*
> **Using the Cold Wet Compress**
>
> Purpose: Cold compresses relieve pain and swelling.
>
> Equipment: • Basin filled with water and ice cubes
>   • Two washcloths
>   • Waterproof pad to protect bed linens
>   • Towels

Steps	**Reasons**
1. Gather your equipment, wash your hands, and explain to the client what you are about to do.	
2. Soak the washcloths in the basin of ice water. If the client is in bed, use the waterproof pad or a towel to protect the linens.	
3. When the client is ready, wring out one washcloth and place it on the affected area. Change the washcloths frequently to keep the compresses cold.	
4. Remove the cold compresses as instructed by your supervisor.	4. Cold compresses are usually left in place for 20 minutes and removed for at least an hour before being replaced. This gives the skin time to adjust to its normal temperature so the cold treatment can be effective when started again.
5. After removing the cold compresses, put away your supplies, wash your hands, and record the client's tolerance to the procedure.	

and your supervisor will determine when it is safe to use cold applications.

Changing a Nonsterile Dressing

A bandage or *dressing* has several purposes.

• It protects the wound from infection.
• It absorbs drainage.
• It covers an unsightly sore.

A *nonsterile dressing change* means that the HM/HHA uses clean, but not sterile, technique. If medication needs to be applied to a wound, this must be done by the client or a family member. The HM/HHA is not licensed to apply medications or to change dressings that require sterile technique. After changing a dressing for a client, you will need to describe the color and amount of drainage on the old dressing. Your observations will go in the written progress notes for the client. For more details on progress notes, see Chapter 11.

Charting Example for a Nonsterile Dressing Change

Mrs. Smith's bandage removed from her left ankle at 11 AM. Dry, dark red drainage on bandage is 5-cent size. Wound is 10-cent size.

(*Example continues on page 275.*)

HM/HHA Procedure:
Changing a Nonsterile Dressing

Purpose: Cleaning the wound and applying a fresh dressing reduces the chance of contamination and infection. Changing the dressing also allows you to observe the wound so the home care team can note the progress of the treatment.

Equipment:
- A fresh bandage
- Dressing tape
- Cleansing solution and gauze pads
- A paper or plastic bag for the old dressings

Safety:
- Never change a dressing unless instructed to do so by your supervisor.
- The frequency of dressing changes will be ordered by the doctor depending on the client's medical condition.

Steps

1. Gather your equipment, wash your hands, and let the client know what you are about to do and how he can assist.

2. Ask any visitor to leave the room if this is the client's wish.

3. Prepare your equipment. Open the trash bag. Cut some pieces of tape and place them in easy reach. Open the clean dressing without touching the center.

4. To remove the old dressing, hold the skin above the tape and grasp the tape close to the skin. Using short, quick motions, pull the tape straight back toward the dressing. Try to pull the tape so it is parallel to the skin (Figure 20-9).

Reasons

1. Do not change a dressing either before or after a meal, because it may be unappetizing to the client. If possible, let the client help decide when the dressing will be changed.

2. Clients often do not want others in the room when this procedure is being done. They may also not wish to watch you changing the dressing.

4. Pull the tape toward the wound and in the direction of hair growth to avoid unnecessary discomfort of the client.

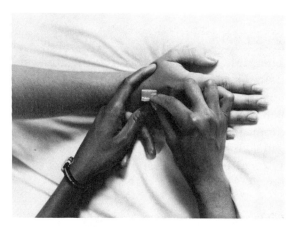

Figure 20-9
Hold the skin tight and pull the tape straight back to remove an old bandage.

(continued)

HM/HHA Procedure:
Changing a Nonsterile Dressing *(continued)*

Steps

5. Note the color and amount of drainage on the bandage for your progress notes. Also observe any changes in the wound and the surrounding skin since you last saw it. Discard the old dressing in the plastic bag.

6. Clean the wound as you have been instructed by your supervisor. Usually one stroke is used to clean from the center of the wound to the skin surrounding it. Then the gauze pad is discarded. A new gauze pad is used with each cleaning stroke.

7. Let the wound air dry. Or, gently pat the wound dry with a fresh gauze pad, and discard the pad.

8. Place the new bandage over the wound and secure it with tape. Do not put tape around the entire bandage.

9. When the client is comfortable, put the supplies away and throw away the closed trash bag of discarded dressings. Wash your hands carefully.

10. Record your observations about the client's wound and his tolerance to the procedure in your progress notes.

Reasons

5. Your observations should be specific so others will clearly understand what you have seen. See Charting Example for a Nonsterile Dressing Change on page 273.

6. The wound is considered cleaner than the surrounding skin. So you are following the basic principle of cleaning: going from the least soiled area to the most soiled area.

7. A moist wound is more likely to become irritated. Rubbing the wound instead of patting it or letting it air dry is likely to irritate it, too. Use gauze instead of cotton because cotton fibers may stick to the wound.

8. The new dressing should not be covered with tape so the wound can get air circulation.

9. All the old dressings and gauze pads used to clean the wound should be put into a closed plastic or paper bag before putting it in the trash to reduce the chance of spreading infection.

(Continued)

Skin red where tape from old dressing was secured. Mrs. Smith states, "That new tape bothers my skin." Wound cleaned with soap and water and new dressing applied with non-allergenic tape that client said she used last week with no problem. Tape not applied to reddened skin.———*Sandy Holmes, HM/HHA*

Measuring Fluid Intake and Output

For some health problems, the doctor may have your client keep track of the amount of fluids that go in and out of his body. This is known as *intake and output* or *I and O*. Generally, the amount of fluid taken into the body should equal the amount that leaves the body in a 24-hour period.

Measuring Fluid Intake

The doctor may have written orders that say the client must *force fluids*. You will be told how much the client should drink each day. A few clients may need to restrict their fluid intake, but you will find that you need to encourage clients to drink fluids more often than not. A client who is restricting fluids will only be able to drink a measured amount of fluids. The client who needs to force fluids can drink liquids or choose from several foods that are considered fluids. Foods that are sources of fluids are listed below.

Milk

Fruit juice

Vegetable juice

Coffee

Tea

Soft drinks

Gelatin

Custard/pudding

Ice cream/sherbet

Soup

Water

Water with a slice of lemon or lime

Whether the client is supposed to force or restrict fluids, you may be asked to help him keep track of the amount he is drinking by measuring and recording his fluid intake. Figure 20-10 shows an intake and output record. Common liquid measurement equivalents are listed in Table 20-1.

How to Measure Fluids in Everyday Glassware or Dishes

1. Fill the client's glass with water as he normally fills it.
2. Then pour the water into a measuring cup to see how much the glass holds (Figure

Table 20-1
Measuring Equivalents*

Cups	Ounces	Cubic Centimeters
	1	30
½	4	120
1	8	240
2	16	480

*cc, cubic centimeter; mm, millimeter; oz, ounce.
1 cc = 1 mm
2 cups = 1 pint
2 pints = 1 quart
4 quarts = 1 gallon

20-11). Use the same kind of measurement (cubic centimeters or cups) for each container.
3. Write down how much each glass or dish holds so you can refer to it later.
4. Intake should be recorded each time the client finishes a glass of water or fluid substitute. Write it down immediately or you will forget.

Measuring Output

Output can be urine, feces, drainage from wounds, or vomit. If you are asked to measure the urinary output, all the urine must be collected and measured. If one voiding is not measured, the supervisor should be told so the results are not misleading. Usually the client will know how to

Fluid Intake and Output Record	Name _____ Date _____			
Time	Intake	Total Fluid Intake	Output	Total Fluid Output
			Urine, 400 cc	400 cc
7 AM	1 cup tea (240 cc) ½ cup juice (120 cc) 1 cup milk (240 cc)	600 cc		
9 AM	½ cup water (120 cc)	720 cc		
11 AM			Urine, 550 cc Vomit, 50 cc	950 cc 1000 cc
1 PM	½ cup broth (120 cc) ½ cup Jello (120 cc)	960 cc		
3 PM				
5 PM				
7 PM				
9 PM				
11 PM				

Figure 20-10
How to keep track of fluid intake and output.

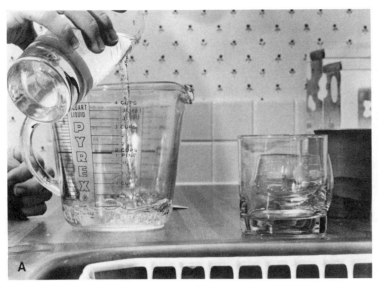

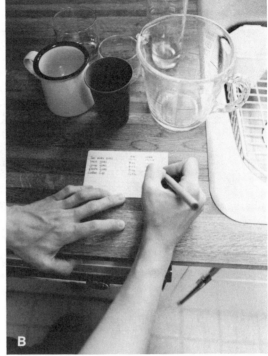

Figure 20-11
(*A*) After filling the glass with water, pour it into the measuring cup to determine how much the glass holds. (*B*) Keep a record of the amounts of fluid that commonly used glasses and cups hold.

measure his own urine, but you may need to assist or to help teach some clients how to measure or how to keep output records.

How to Measure the Urinary Output

If your client can use the toilet, he may have a measuring container that fits under the toilet seat. This container is easy to use because it allows the client to use the toilet normally and is easy to read.

How to Measure Output With a Bedpan or Urinal

1. After the client has voided in the bedpan, cover the bedpan with a paper towel and take it to the bathroom.
2. Pour the contents into a container that is meant for measuring urine. These containers are often marked in milliliters and should be used only for urine.
3. Place the measuring container on a flat surface and read the measurement at eye level for accuracy. Record the amount.
4. Dispose of the waste in the toilet. Clean the bedpan and measuring containers as directed by your agency.
5. Most urinals are marked with measuring lines, so you will not need a separate measuring container.

Ostomy Care

What Is an Ostomy?

Ostomy means "opening into." The general term *ostomy* refers to the surgical procedure where a part of the intestine is attached to an opening in the abdomen. The new opening on the abdomen is called a *stoma*. The stoma becomes the new exit for urinary or fecal wastes, depending on the kind of ostomy the client has.

A client may have an ostomy because of an accident, an illness, or a disease. There are various kinds of ostomies. They can be temporary or permanent, depending upon the client's condition.

1. The *colostomy* is an opening into the colon or large intestine. The client with a colostomy will have solid or liquid stools, depending on the location of the surgery. Some clients wear a collection bag over the stoma at all times to catch leaks, while others only need to wear a small patch.
2. The *ileostomy* is an opening into the ileum, which is a part of the small intestine. The client with an ileostomy will have liquid stools that drain continuously, so he will need to wear a collection bag all of the time.
3. The *ureterostomy* is an opening into the

HM/HHA Procedure:
Changing a Colostomy Bag

Purpose: To assist a client in changing an ostomy appliance

Equipment:
- Bedpan
- Disposable bed protector
- Large towel or blanket
- Ostomy collection bag
- Skin cream if used
- Toilet tissue
- Basin of water
- Soap
- Washcloth and two towels
- Disposable gloves
- Plastic trash bag or old newspaper

Safety:
- Do not attempt to help a client change an ostomy appliance unless you have had further training and instructions from your supervisor.
- Do not hesitate to call the home health agency if you have a question or there is a problem.
- Use disposable gloves whenever you work with a client's body wastes.

Steps

1. Gather your equipment, wash your hands, and tell the client what you are about to do. Find out how he can help.

2. Ask any visitor to leave the room if this is the client's wish.

3. If the client is in bed, help him put the bed protector under his waist and hips. Have the client remove his trousers and cover himself with a towel. The client may prefer to sit in a chair and lift his shirt to expose the ostomy instead of removing his clothes. Make sure all the ostomy supplies are within the client's reach.

4. Carefully remove the collection bag from the ostomy belt. Place the collection bag in the bedpan if it is to be reused or in the plastic trash bag or newspaper if it is to be thrown away. The stoma should be dark pink. Call the agency if the stoma looks very red or bluish, if it looks swollen, or if it is bleeding.

5. Gently clean the skin around the stoma with toilet tissue. Wash with a mild soap and washcloth. Rinse well and pat dry with a towel. Let the area dry thoroughly before applying the ostomy bag or dressing.

Reasons

1. Listen to the client's suggestions and encourage him to assist as much as he can with this procedure.

2. A family member may want to stay in the room to assist. The nurse, not the HM/HHA, should teach family members this procedure.

3. All the supplies should be within easy each because stopping in the middle of this procedure can be especially unpleasant for the client.

5. Some clients may not use soap around the stoma if soap irritates their skin.

(continued)

HM/HHA Procedure:
Changing a Colostomy Bag *(continued)*

Steps

6. Place the clean ostomy collection bag on as directed by your supervisor (Figure 20-12).

Figure 20-12
Applying a clean ostomy bag for the client. This procedure can be performed only after you have had extra training from your home health nurse supervisor. (Walsh J, Persons CB: Wieck L: Manual of Home Health Care Nursing, p 108. Philadelphia, JB Lippincott, 1987)

7. Remove the bed protector from the bed and make sure the client is comfortable.

8. Take the used ostomy equipment to the bathroom for cleaning and disposal. The contents of the collection bag can be emptied into the toilet, and the bag should either be cleaned or thrown away in a plastic bag. An ostomy belt is usually washed and reused.

9. Put all the ostomy supplies away and wash your hands thoroughly. Then record your observations and the client's tolerance to the procedure.

Reasons

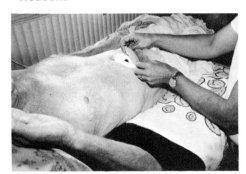

ureter and allows urine to leave the body through the stoma instead of the urethra. This client also needs to wear a collection bag at all times because the ureterostomy drains urine continuously.

An *ostomy appliance* is a device worn over the stoma to collect the waste products, to protect the skin, and to control odors.

You may be asked to help a client clean the skin around the ostomy appliance or to help the client empty the ostomy bag. Your supervisor will explain how to work the particular kind of appliance that your client is using. You will appreciate having individual instructions because there are so many different types of appliances.

Notify your supervisor if you see any of the following:

1. The skin around the stoma is red or irritated.
2. The stoma is very red, bluish, or swollen.
3. The appliance does not fit correctly.
4. The client has abdominal cramps.
5. The ileostomy has not drained for 2 hours.

Irrigation of the Colostomy

Some clients need to infuse water into the colostomy stoma to stimulate the bowel movement. This is known as *irrigation* and is similar to giving an enema. Most clients do this procedure alone or with the assistance of a nurse or family member. HM/HHAs do not irrigate colostomies.

Diet

A balanced diet is an important part of any treatment plan. The client with an ostomy may be more comfortable if he avoids gas-producing foods, such as beans, cabbage, broccoli, onions, and spicy foods.

Supporting the Client With an Ostomy

Your client will need emotional and physical support, especially if his ostomy is fairly new. It takes time and understanding to deal with the loss of a

(Text continues on page 283.)

Collecting Specimens

HM/HHA Procedure:
Collecting a Midstream Clean-Catch Urine Specimen

Purpose: A clean urine sample may be needed to detect illness or infection.

Equipment:
- A clean-catch urine kit *or*
- Several cotton balls moistened with soap and water, or three towelettes moistened with an antiseptic solution recommended by the home health agency
- A wide-mouth sterile specimen cup
- Bedpan (if client is unable to get to the toilet)
- Disposable gloves
- Hand washing supplies

Safety:
- Do not touch the inside of the sterile specimen container or lid.
- Use disposable gloves whenever you are working with body fluids to prevent the spread of infection and disease.
- A voided specimen does not stay fresh very long. Follow your supervisor's directions for storing the specimen before taking it to the lab for testing.

Steps

1. Gather your equipment, wash your hands, and explain to the client that you need a urine specimen. Label the specimen container with the client's name and address, the doctor's name, the date (write the time after the specimen has been collected), how the specimen was collected (midstream clean-catch), and your initials (Figure 20-13).

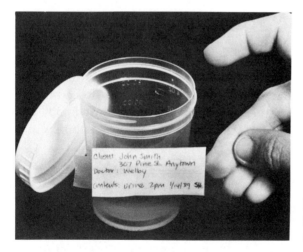

2. Explain the procedure to the client. If he is able, he may get the specimen without your assistance. The female client can sit on the bedpan if she is unable to get to the toilet.

Reasons

1. If you do not have a sterile container, boil a small glass jar for 5 minutes if a sterile container is needed.

Figure 20-13
Label the specimen container with the client's name and address, the doctor's name, the date and time the sample was taken, and your initials.

(continued)

HM/HHA Procedure:

Collecting a Midstream Clean-Catch Urine Specimen *(continued)*

Steps	Reasons

3. *For a female client:*
   a. Have the client separate the folds of her labia and wipe one side of the labia from front to back using one stroke. Dispose of the used towelette.
   b. Clean the other side of the labia in one stroke with a fresh towelette and then dispose of it.
   c. Use the third towelette to wipe down the middle. Dispose of the used towelette.
	3. Keeping the labia separated and clean prevents getting germs from outside the body into the urine specimen.

4. Instruct the female client to begin voiding into the bedpan or toilet while the labia are still separated. Then she should catch a specimen midstream and fill the container one-third full. Remove the cup to finish voiding. Encourage her to make sure the specimen container does not touch her genitals.	4. The first part of the stream rinses out the urinary tract and should not be used in a specimen collection.
5. *For a male client:* Instruct the man to clean the tip of the penis in three circular strokes. Use a separate towelette for each stroke. If the man is uncircumcised, he will need to pull the foreskin back before cleaning the penis.	
6. The man should begin to void into the bedpan or toilet and then fill the specimen container one-third full using the midstream urine. Do not let the sterile container touch the penis.	6. The first portion of the urine stream rinses out the urinary tract and should not be used for urine specimens.
7. Cover the container without touching the lid and write the correct time on the label of the container.	
8. Wash your hands thoroughly and allow the client to wash his hands.	
9. Make a note on the client's record: what kind of specimen was collected; the date and time the specimen was collected; the method of storage; and reactions of the client to the procedure. If records of the client's intake and output are being kept, note the amount of urine in the sterile container and record that on the client's record.	
10. Clean up and put away the equipment. Wash your hands thoroughly.	

HM/HHA Procedure:
Collecting a Stool Sample

Purpose: A stool sample may be needed for examination to detect disease, infection, or parasites.

Equipment: • A clean bedpan
             • Tongue depressor
             • A specimen container
             • A paper towel
             • Disposable gloves
             • Handwashing supplies

Safety: • Do not touch the inside of the sterile specimen container or lid.
             • Use disposable gloves whenever you are working with body fluids to prevent the spread of infection and disease.
             • A stool specimen does not stay fresh very long. Follow your supervisor's directions for storing the specimen before taking it to the lab for testing.

Steps

1. Prepare the equipment. Label the specimen container with the client's name and address, the doctor's name, the date and time (write in time after the specimen has been collected), and the kind of specimen —stool specimen, and your initials.

2. Explain to the client that you need a stool specimen. He will need to urinate before collecting the stool so the urine does not mix with the stool. The client will need to have his bowel movement in the bedpan.

3. When the client is ready, wash your hands and get your equipment. Help the client onto the bedpan and allow him privacy. When he is done, remove the bedpan, cover it with a paper towel and allow the client to wash his hands.

4. Take the bedpan to the bathroom. Use the tongue depressor to put one or two teaspoonfuls of the stool into the clean specimen container. Make sure the outside of the specimen container is clean. Discard the remaining stool into the toilet and clean the bedpan as instructed by your agency.

5. Label container with the correct date and time.

6. Your supervisor will instruct you on the method of storage and tell you how soon the specimen needs to be taken to the lab for testing.

Reasons

2. The client's urine cannot mix with the stool for an accurate test. The specimen cannot be collected from the toilet because water may destroy the specimen.

3. See Chapter 18 for the procedure on helping the client onto the bedpan.

6. The method of storage depends on the tests being done. Most stool specimens need to get to the lab within an hour.

(continued)

HM/HHA Procedure:
Collecting a Stool Sample *(continued)*

Steps

7. Make a note on the client's record: what kind of specimen was collected; the date and time the specimen was collected; the method of storage; and reactions of the client to the procedure.

8. Clean up and put away the equipment. Wash your hands thoroughly.

Reasons

---

major body part. The client will also need time to adjust to the new method of eliminating waste products and the special care his new ostomy will need. It is not unusual for a person to think that he will need to change his lifestyle, or that others will be able to tell that he has an ostomy. One cannot tell that a fully clothed person has an ostomy. The appliances are small and odor-free, and allow people to live active, normal lives. Women are able to have children, and several well-known actors, politicians, and sports figures have continued their normal lives without difficulty after recovering from surgery. The client may or may not wish to discuss his fears or concerns with you. If the client or family asks you questions you cannot answer, tell them you will find out the answer by asking your supervisor.

Assisting With Relaxation

Stress is a part of all our lives. Learning to relax can help people sleep better and help them to cope with illness and everyday living. This 30-minute exercise promotes relaxation by contracting and relaxing groups of muscles. You, your clients, and your client's family may find this relaxation method helpful.

1. Find a comfortable place for the client to do the relaxation exercises. They can be done in a chair, or in a bed if the client intends to sleep afterwards.

2. Explain to the client that she will be tensing specific groups of muscles for 5 to 10 seconds. She can keep track of the time by slowly counting 1001, 1002, 1003, and so on. When the time is up, she will relax all the muscles in her body for 10 seconds. The client should contract and relax each muscle group twice before moving on to the next muscle group.

3. The order for contracting and relaxing the muscles is:
   • right hand and arm
   • left hand and arm
   • forehead (raise and lower eyebrows)
   • eyes
   • mouth
   • neck and shoulders (forward, back, up, and down)
   • chest
   • stomach
   • bottom
   • thighs
   • calves (point feet up and down)
   • feet (up and down, in and out)

4. When all the muscle groups have been through the exercise, have the client go back and contract and relax any muscles that still feel tense.

Review Questions

True or False

1. ____ It is not necessary to let the client know what you are about to do each time you begin a procedure.

2. ____ It is the HM/HHA's responsibility to clean and put away any equipment used during a procedure.

3. ____ Deep breathing exercises do not help the lungs expand.

4. ____ Two early signs of a pressure sore are redness and pain.

5. ____ A person who uses knitting needles to scratch under his leg cast cannot hurt himself.

6. ____ A spot on a cast should be circled and labeled with the date, time, and your initials.

7. ____ A cold application is used to reduce swelling.

8. ____ A hot application is used to reduce swelling.

9. ____ Heating pads and electric blankets are always safe.

10. ____ Another name for a *bandage* is a *dressing*.

11. ____ The HM/HHA should never remove a sterile dressing.

12. ____ An *ostomy* is the surgical procedure where an opening is made from the abdomen into the intestines and is used for removing body wastes.

13. ____ The *stoma* is the opening on the surface of the abdomen for an ostomy.

14. ____ A specimen of urine or feces may need to be collected and examined by the medical lab to detect disease.

15. ____ Relaxation exercises may help a client who is in pain.

Multiple Choice

16. What would *not* be a good thing to do before beginning a procedure?
    a. Wash your hands.
    b. Find out if the client would like anyone else in the room to leave.
    c. Make sure the client knows exactly what you are going to do before you start in order to prepare him. Find out how he usually helps.
    d. Tell everyone else in the room to leave.

17. You have been asked to do a procedure that you have not done in a long time. You get to the client's house and realize that you really are not sure how to do it. What would you do?
    a. Call another HM/HHA from your agency.
    b. Start the procedure hoping that you'll remember how to do it.
    c. Avoid calling your supervisor for fear of being fired.
    d. Call your supervisor for directions before you start the procedure.

Fill in the Blank

18. List three things you can do to help prevent bedsores for a client who is on bedrest.
    1. _____
    2. _____
    3. _____

Chapter 21
Assisting With Medications

Objectives

At the conclusion of this chapter, the homemaker/home health aide will:

1. Be able to describe the HM/HHA's responsibilities and limitations regarding medications.

2. Understand how to assist the client with self-medication.

3. Know what to observe and how to report on clients who take medications.

4. Know how to store medications safely.

5. Understand basic safety precautions for oxygen and other medications.

Trusting Pharmacy

212 Elm Street
Anytown, USA
(000) 000-0000

R 99887766   Dr. M. Welby

John Smith
Take one tablet by mouth after breakfast and supper. Do not take with alcohol.

GRISPEG 250 mg Tablets
Griseofulvin
12/19/89   No Refills

Figure 21-1
Label from a prescription medication.

Medications are used to prevent illness, to help a client recover from an illness, or to reduce the symptoms of an illness. While medications can be helpful, they can also be dangerous if not used properly. The two basic kinds of medications are prescription and over-the-counter medications.

Prescription and Over-the-Counter Medications

Prescription medications are drugs that can be obtained only with a doctor's order. After a doctor has examined the client, he will write a prescription. A *prescription* is a note from the doctor that tells the pharmacist what medicine to sell to the client. When the client gets the medication, no one else should take the medication. And the medication should only be taken by that client for the purpose indicated by the doctor. Penicillin is an example of a prescription medication. Figure 21-1 shows what a label from a prescription medication looks like.

Over-the-counter (OTC) medications are drugs that can be bought without a prescription. Aspirin is an example of an over-the-counter medication. Many people think nonprescription drugs cannot do any harm because they are so easily available. This is not true.

Both prescription and nonprescription medications can cause serious health problems and even death when they are not used correctly. For example, some people are allergic to some medi-

cations and can have a serious reaction from drugs as common as penicillin or aspirin. Sometimes, foods or other medications can interfere with or can help medications to work. Because of this, the doctor should be aware of all the prescription and over-the-counter medications being taken by the client. Both prescription and nonprescription medications must be taken according to the directions given by the doctor.

Assisting With Medications

The HM/HHA is not permitted or licensed to give medications to the client. Medications can be given only by the family, or by nurses or doctor's because they are licensed by the state to give medications. Nurses and doctors learn about medications when they are trained, and take responsibility for any problems when they give medications to the client.

The HM/HHA may only help a client to take his own medications. When you assist a client with his medications, the client is taking the responsibility. Assisting means that you may bring the client his medicine and open the bottle, but you may *not* take the medication out of the bottle. This is the responsibility of the client, family member, or nurse.

Responsibilities of the Home Health Care Team

As the HM/HHA, you must understand your own responsibilities as well as those of the home health nurse.

*Responsibilities of the Home
Health Nurse*

1. It is the nurse or doctor's role to make sure the client understands the name of the medicine and why he needs it, when and how to take the medicine, the amount to take, and how to store the medicine. The nurse may make a medication chart (Figure 21-2) for the client to help him keep track of his medications.
2. The nurse updates the medication schedule and tells the HM/HHA whenever the doctor changes the medication orders.
3. The nurse administers medications that the client cannot take himself.

*Responsibilities of the Homemaker/
Home Health Aide*

1. The HM/HHA is not licensed to give medications. This is the responsibility of the client, the family, or the nurse. The HM/HHA may assist the client by opening a pill container or by bringing the client a glass of water.
2. Know the client's medications and any special directions regarding time and dose so you can tell your supervisor if the medications are not taken correctly.
3. Report any unusual reactions such as nausea, diarrhea, abdominal pains, confusion, itching, rashes, or comments the client makes about taking the medications. The supervisor should be notified if the client does not take a medication or if he vomits soon after taking the medication.
4. See that medications are stored according to the directions given by your supervisor.
5. If the client refuses to take his medication, try to find out why. The client may have a good reason. Often the medication can be changed if there is a problem. It is the client's right to refuse his medications, but if he does, tell your supervisor promptly so the doctor can be informed.
6. In the unusual case where a client has an allergic reaction and has trouble breathing, the emergency squad should be called immediately. The home health agency can be called as soon as it is safe to do so.

Emergency phone numbers, such as those for the emergency squad, poison control center, doctor, home care agency, fire department, and police should all be kept next to the telephone. In an emergency it is very easy to forget a simple phone number.

7. Tell your supervisor if the client is taking either prescription or nonprescription medications that are not written on the medication schedule. The doctor needs to know about all medications the client is taking so medication reactions can be prevented.
8. Report drug abuse or suspected abuse. This includes taking an incorrect amount, not taking the medications on time, or sharing the medication with a friend or relative who "seems to have the same problem."
9. When more than one person in the house is taking medicine, try to keep the containers on separate trays so they are not mixed up.
10. When you bring a client his pills, always return the bottles to the exact place where you found them. Many people with perfect eyesight will reach for a pill, take it, and then look at the bottle. If you think the medicine is not stored properly, ask your supervisor for advice.
11. If you have not been told about the client's medication schedule in advance, ask the nurse or your agency supervisor about it. Your supervisor may simply have forgotten to discuss this matter with you.

Medication Storage Guidelines

Every year there are hundreds of accidents due to improper storage of medications. This happens not only to children and infants, but also to confused, disoriented, or careless adults. If you think medicines are not stored properly, ask your supervisor how to handle the situation. Because medicines are expensive, many people want to save them "in case they need them again." Saving old medications can be dangerous for several reasons. The client may take his old medicine for a new problem that has similar symptoms as the old problem without consulting a doctor. Or the client may use old medications that have expired and are no longer effective.

(*Text continues on page 290.*)

A four-week medication calendar

Sample

In this chart, the patient has taken all his medicine through the first dose on Wednesday.

Name of medicine	Color/shape	Take with	Do not take with
Amaston	Yellow capsule	with meals	no alcohol
Somaston	Peach tablet	ok either way	—
Tarupt	Blue capsule	always with meals	no alcohol

Week 1

Name of medicine	Color/shape of medicine	Note whether to take on empty stomach or with food or milk	Note foods or oth medicines NOT t take with this dru

Week 2

Name of medicine	Color/shape	Take with	Do not take with

Week 3

Name of medicine	Color/shape	Take with	Do not take with

Week 4

Name of medicine	Color/shape	Take with	Do not take with

Figure 21-2 An example of a medication chart. (Printed with permission from Merck, Sharp & Dohme, Division . . .

w much	Times to take	S	M	T	W	T	F	S
One	8 am, 1 pm, 6 pm, 11 pm	✓✓✓	✓✓✓	✓✓✓	✓			
one	8 am, 6 pm	✓✓	✓✓	✓✓	✓			
One	8 am	✓	✓	✓	✓			

w much to ke each time	Times to take (List specific times, not just "2 or 3 times daily")	Place a check in the correct box after you take each dose of medicine						
		S	M	T	W	T	F	S

w much	Times to take	S	M	T	W	T	F	S

w much	Times to take	S	M	T	W	T	F	S

w much	Times to take	S	M	T	W	T	F	S

. of Merck & Co., Inc., West Point, PA, 19486)

Medication Guidelines (*continued*)

1. *Keep all medicine out of reach of children and confused or disoriented adults.* Older people often have friends and relatives visit with children, so even a childless home may need to be childproof. It is safest to keep medicines and poisonous substances in a locked cupboard.

2. *Store medications according to the directions on the original container.* Most should be kept away from light, heat, and humidity. Others need refrigeration, but cannot be frozen. If kept in the refrigerator, label the container clearly and keep it out of reach of children.

3. *Keep medications in their original containers.* The label identifies the drug, the dose, special directions on how to take the medication, where it was purchased, and how it should be stored. This makes it less likely that the client will take the wrong pill when there are a number of pills to take or when the client's drugs are changed frequently. This information could be crucial in an emergency. Let your supervisor know if the medications are not kept in the original container.

4. *Notify your supervisor if medications are out of date or unlabeled.* It is the responsibility of the client, the family, or the nurse to dispose of medications that cannot be used. Medications should not be put in trash cans where children or animals can get them. It is safest to flush them down the toilet, burn them in an incinerator, or put them down a garbage disposal.

5. *Safety caps can be replaced with easy-open tops for households with no children.* Many older or disabled adults have trouble opening childproof containers. A pharmacist will provide an easy-to-open top if asked. The client may have to sign a form stating that he requested this top, because government regulations require safety caps for many medications. The client then needs to be extra careful when children visit.

Oxygen Therapy

Oxygen is a medication prescribed by the doctor to help a person breathe. Because it is a medication, it may not be given by the HM/HHA. The

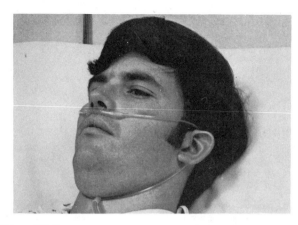

Figure 21-3
The nasal cannula. (Lewis LW: Fundamental Skills in Patient Care, 3rd ed, p 514. Philadelphia, JB Lippincott, 1984)

HM/HHA's responsibility is to observe the way the client uses oxygen and to let the supervisor know if you think it is not being used safely.

Oxygen comes in a tank. Because oxygen is very drying to the nasal membranes, it is humidified before it gets to the client. It is commonly administered to the client through a long plastic tube that leads from the tank to a *nasal cannula* or *mask*. The nasal cannula has two small prongs that fit into the nose. The tubing is wrapped around the head and ears, as shown in Figure 21-3, to hold the cannula in place. The mask fits over the nose and mouth and is kept in place with an elastic band that fits over the head, as shown in Figure 21-4. The client who uses a nasal cannula can eat, drink, or talk normally. The client who uses a mask cannot.

Safety Guidelines for Oxygen Use

1. NO SMOKING signs should be placed on the door and in the room where oxygen is being used. The client, family members, and visitors should have a clear understanding that this rule must be followed strictly. Oxygen is highly flammable, which means that a lighted cigarette or match could easily cause an explosion.

2. Nylon clothing, bed linens, or rugs can produce static electricity, which could cause a fire if oxygen is being used in the same room. Some agencies require their staff members to wear cotton clothing and

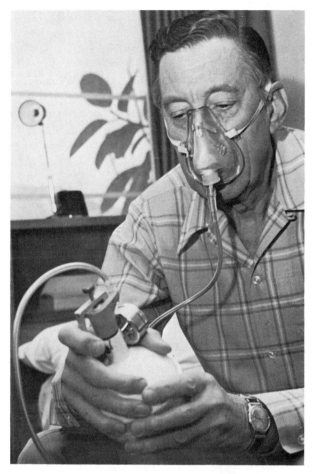

Figure 21-4
The face mask. This client is using a portable oxygen container that can be used for short periods of time. (Lewis LW: Fundamental Skills in Patient Care, 3rd ed, p 518. Philadelphia, JB Lippincott, 1984)

undergarments when caring for a client who uses oxygen.

3. Do not use hairdryers or electric appliances when oxygen is being administered. Electric appliances often give off small sparks when they are unplugged, and this may cause an explosion.

4. Due to fire hazards, oil and alcohol should not be used for backrubs and petroleum products should not be used for lip balm. A water-based lotion can be used instead.

5. No open flames such as candles for birthday cakes or religious ceremonies can be used.

6. When the oxygen is stored in a tank, the stand must be sturdy and secure. The pressure inside a full tank that is partially

opened is tremendous. A leak can cause the tank to move as quickly as a fully inflated balloon moves when the end is untied. Unfortunately, the oxygen tank will have much more force and is much heavier, so it will be very dangerous.

7. Keep a fire extinguisher in the room where oxygen is used and make sure you, the family, and the client know how to use it.

Review Questions

True or False

1. ____ When a nurse takes a pill out of a container and hands it to a client, she is administering medication.

2. ____ A HM/HHA is not licensed to administer medication.

3. ____ Over-the-counter (OTC) medications are always safe.

4. ____ If a client forgets to take his medication, the HM/HHA should remind him.

5. ____ Oxygen is not a medication.

6. ____ "No smoking" rules must be strictly followed when oxygen is being used by the client.

Multiple Choice

7. You are caring for Mr. Brown, a client who is in severe pain. He took a pain pill 5 minutes ago and tells you that he is "going to take a few more because one pill just doesn't help at all." You read the prescription label and find that it says the client should take only one pill every 4 hours for pain. How would you respond?
   a. Do nothing and let the client take as much medication as he thinks he needs.
   b. "I would prefer it if you would wait to see how the pill will work. The label says you should only take one pill every 4 hours. I just don't want you to take too many. Let me call my supervisor to see if she has any suggestions."
   c. "Mr. Brown, I know that pain pills usually take some time to work. I think it might help if you would take a few deep breaths and try to relax a little."
   d. *b* or *c*

8. Mrs. Olsen is an 85-year-old client who is bedridden. Her daughter Jane stops on her way to work each morning to give Mrs. Olsen her medicine. This morning Jane phones as soon as you arrive and tells you that she cannot come to the house this morning. She asks you to give her mother the medicine. What do you say to Jane?

   a. "Sure, I'll be glad to do that for you."

   b. "I really shouldn't, but I guess it won't hurt just this once."

   c. "I better call my supervisor to see if she will let me give the medicine."

   d. "I'm sorry. I am not allowed to give medication. I will call my agency for you to see if a nurse can come out to give the medication this morning."

Part Seven

Emergency Care

Chapter 22

First Aid and
Emergency Care

Objectives

At the conclusion of this chapter, the homemaker/home health aide will:

1. Be able to explain the guidelines for dealing with any emergency and list the three problems that must be checked and treated immediately.

2. Demonstrate and explain first aid techniques for bleeding.

3. Demonstrate and explain first aid techniques for restoring breathing and controlling choking.

4. Demonstrate and explain first aid techniques for burns.

5. Demonstrate and explain first aid techniques for chest pain (angina) or a possible heart attack.

6. Demonstrate and explain first aid techniques for hypothermia or low body temperature.

7. Demonstrate and explain first aid techniques for poisoning.

8. Demonstrate and explain first aid techniques for seizures.

9. Demonstrate and explain first aid techniques for shock.

10. Demonstrate and explain first aid techniques for a possible stroke.

Accidents and Emergencies

Accidents happen very quickly. Read this chapter carefully so you will know what to do before an accident happens. Then you can act quickly when you need to.

Cardiopulmonary resuscitation (CPR) is a lifesaving skill that is used when someone has stopped breathing. It is an important skill to know, but cannot be learned from a book. You must complete a course in order to practice CPR. Your local Red Cross and American Heart Association both offer CPR courses that will teach you how to allow you to handle emergency situations such as resuscitating adults and infants. Some information on lifesaving techniques is provided in this book, but a full course in CPR training and first aid is highly recommended for HM/HHAs.

General Guidelines for Accidents and Emergencies

1. *Check responsiveness and shout for help.* First, shake the victim gently and loudly say "Are you OK?" If there is no response, shout to someone by name for help: "Martha, phone for help." Have the other person phone for medical help while you take care of the victim. If you are alone, you should phone for help after following steps 2 to 4.

2. *Look for dangers.* You cannot help a victim if you become a victim too. If there is smoke, gas, an electrical hazard, or if the person is violent, call for help instead of putting yourself at unreasonable risk.

3. *Do not move the victim unless you absolutely must.* Moving an injured person can cause more damage. This is especially true if the person has a neck or back injury. A victim may have to be moved before you give treatment if he is in immediate danger, for example, if he is in a burning house.

4. *Know what injury must be treated first.*
   FIRST—Check breathing.
   - If the victim stops breathing and you are trained in CPR, open the airway and begin mouth-to-mouth resuscitation.
   - See page 299 for more on restoring breathing.
   SECOND—Check pulse (heartbeat).
   - A person who is breathing will always have a pulse.
   - If there is no pulse, start CPR chest compressions if you have had CPR training.
   THIRD—Control bleeding.
   - Apply direct pressure to wounds after breathing and the pulse are restored.
   - See page 297 for more on controlling bleeding.

5. *Phone for help if you are alone.* After you have given the initial first aid you can take a minute to phone the emergency services or operator for help. See the box, When to Call Emergency Services. The emergency services operator may keep you on the phone and give you further instructions until the ambulance arrives.

6. *Treat for shock and any other conditions as soon as possible.* If a victim has other medical problems, you may need to judge which needs to be treated first. For more about shock, see page 309.

7. *Do not give a seriously injured person any fluids or food.*

First Aid Procedures

First aid procedures are listed here alphabetically.

Bleeding

A person can bleed to death from a severe loss of blood in 1 minute. Bleeding must be stopped as soon as possible. It is normal to feel queasy when you see a person bleeding, but if you follow this simple procedure, you may save a life. A doctor should see anyone with a large wound.

What You Should Do

1. Apply a clean bandage directly over the wound. If a bandage is not available, use a clean sheet or towel, clothing, or your clean bare hand.
2. Press firmly on the wound for at least 10 minutes without stopping. This may hurt the victim, but it will stop the bleeding.
3. While applying pressure, raise the arm or

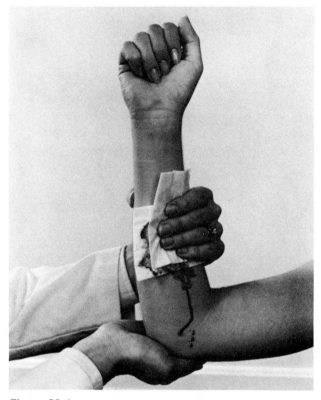

Figure 22-1
If the bandage becomes soaked, apply another pad over the first. Do not remove the first pad.

leg so the wound is above the client's heart (Figure 22-1).
4. If bleeding does not stop, press harder. Call supervisor for advice if possible.
5. When bleeding stops, tie a long strip of cloth (gauze, a tie, or a scarf) over the bandage to keep it in place (Figure 22-2). Check the pulse in that arm or leg. If there is no pulse, loosen the cloth holding the bandage.
6. Treat the client for shock by having him lie down with his legs up. Then cover him with a blanket (Figure 22-3). If the wound is on the arm, raise it above heart level by putting it on blankets or pillows. If you think the arm may be broken, apply pressure but do not raise the arm.
7. *Pressure points.* When you cannot stop a bleeding wound on an arm, hand, leg, or foot wound, use the pressure point. *Do not use a pressure point unless you cannot stop bleeding by direct pressure and raising the limb.* When a pressure point is used, blood cannot get to the entire arm or leg. A pressure point should be held for less than 5 minutes and used only when absolutely necessary.

8. How to find the pressure point.
   - The pressure point for a wound on the arm or hand is in the middle of the upper arm (halfway between the elbow and the shoulder). Place your four fingers flat against the client's inner forearm and press firmly (Figure 22-4).
   - The pressure point for a wound on the foot or leg is located on the bend in the leg where the thigh joins the body. Place the heel of your hand on the bend where the leg joins the hip and press hard (Figure 22-5).
9. How to use the pressure point.
   - Keep pressure on the wound.
   - Raise the arm or leg.
   - Apply pressure to the pressure point on the arm or leg for a short time (less than 5 minutes). Check to see if the bleeding has stopped every minute.
   - When bleeding stops, do not use the pressure point anymore.
10. Notes on controlling bleeding.
   - Do not remove a blood-soaked bandage.

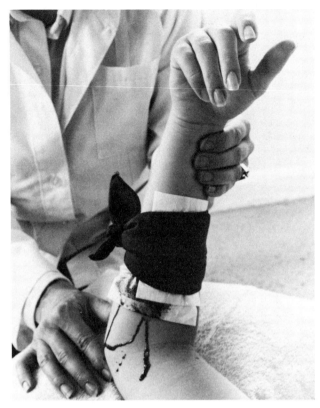

Figure 22-2
Do not tie the scarf too tightly or the circulation will be cut off. Check the radial (wrist) pulse after securing the bandage to make sure the scarf is not too tight.

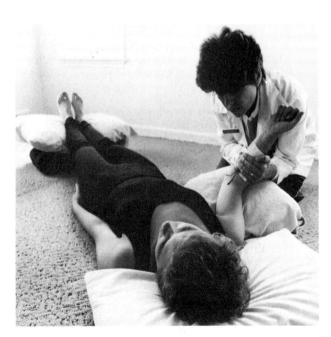

Figure 22-3
Elevate the feet and elevate the bleeding limb.

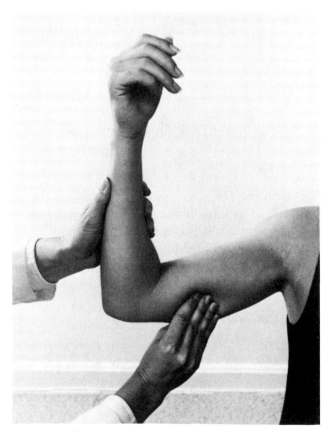

Figure 22-4
The pressure point for the arm.

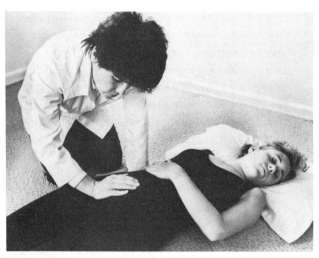

Figure 22-5
The pressure point for the leg.

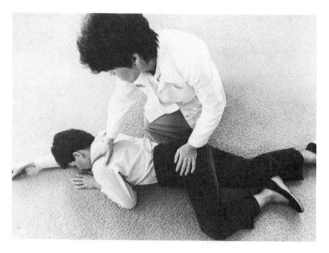

Figure 22-6
Roll the client onto her back and find out if she needs help.

Instead, put another pad over the first one. Removing the first bandage may make the wound start bleeding again by removing a clot that is forming.
- Do not remove an object caught in a deep wound. Have a doctor do that.
- Small cuts should be washed with soap and water and covered with a bandage.
- Large wounds need prompt medical attention.
11. Call the home health agency as soon as possible to report the incident.

Care of the Person Who Stops Breathing

Resuscitation means reviving a person who is not breathing. A person who stops breathing may suffer permanent brain damage in 4 to 6 minutes and can die soon afterwards. When breathing stops, you must act quickly. If you find a person who is not breathing, always assume that breathing has just stopped and start emergency procedures. It is always worth starting mouth-to-mouth resuscitation when a person stops breathing. Resuscitation must be continued until the person starts breathing again, medical help arrives, or you are too tired to continue.

What You Should Do

1. *Check responsiveness, roll client on back, and call for help.* First check to make sure the client is in need of help and not simply

asleep. Speak to the client by name: "Anne, are you all right?" Roll the client onto her back on a hard surface. If the client does not respond, shout to someone else in the house to call for help, "Emergency—call 911" (Figure 22-6).
2. *Open the airway.* Tilt the head back by putting one hand on client's forehead and the other under the back of her neck. This position opens the airway and makes it easier to breathe (Figure 22-7).
3. *Lift the chin to open the airway further.* Keep one hand on the client's forehead to maintain the open airway and use the other

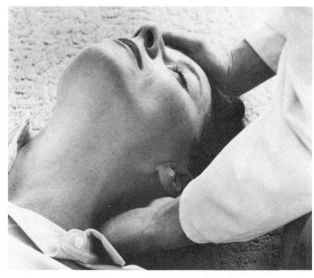

Figure 22-7
Open the airway by tilting the head.

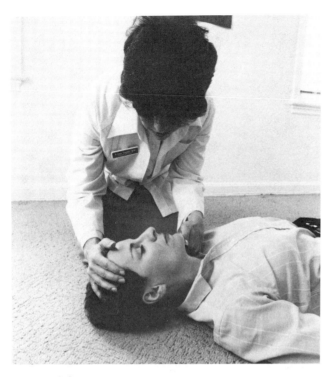

Figure 22-8
Open the airway by lifting the chin.

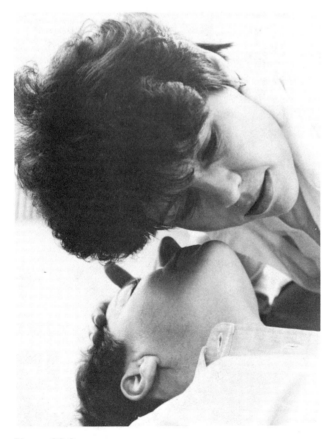

Figure 22-9
Look, listen, and feel for breaths.

hand to lift the chin. Hook fingers on the side of the jaw closest to you. Gently lift the jaw up and forward until the teeth are nearly closed (Figure 22-8).

4. *Look, listen, and feel.* With the head tilted back and the chin lifted, lean over client and place your ear over the client's nose and mouth and look towards the client's chest. In this position you can *listen* and *feel* for breaths on your ear and *look* to see if the chest is rising and falling. Keep checking breathing for 5 to 10 seconds (Figure 22-9).

5. *If the victim is not breathing, give mouth-to-mouth resuscitation immediately.*
   • Tilt head back and lift chin.
   • Pinch the nose shut.
   • Take a deep breath, open your mouth, and make a tight seal over the victim's mouth (Figure 22-10).
   • Give two full breaths. Did the chest rise? If not, open the airway again and try again.

6. *Check the carotid pulse.* Place your fingertips on the side of the victim's neck for 5 to 10 seconds as shown in Figure 22-11 to see if the heart is pumping blood.
   • If there is no pulse, start chest compressions if you are trained in CPR.
   • If there is a pulse, but the victim is not breathing, continue mouth-to-mouth resuscitation as described in step 5.

7. *When the victim starts breathing again:*
   • Treat for shock.
   • Call the emergency services if you haven't already called.
   • Continue to keep checking breathing.

Choking

Before you try to help a person who seems to be choking, make sure he needs it. A person who can breathe, talk, or cough loudly does not have his airway blocked and does not need help. A baby who can cry does not have a blocked airway. Stand by and be prepared to help.

The Conscious *Adult or Child Over 1 Year Who Is Choking*

A person needs help when:

• He cannot talk.
• He holds his neck with his hands in the universal choking sign (Figure 22-12).

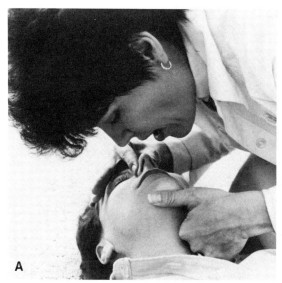
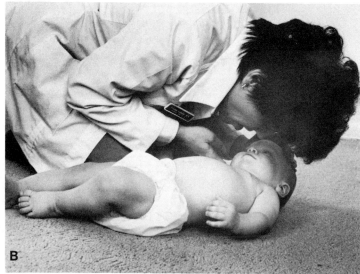

Figure 22-10
(*A*) Pinch the nose and make a tight seal over the mouth to deliver two full breaths.
(*B*) For an infant under 1 year old, make a tight seal over the mouth and nose when giving mouth-to-mouth resuscitation.

- He breathes loudly with difficulty and can barely cough. He may make a crowing sound or even turn blue.

What You Should Do

1. When a victim is choking, always ask, "Can you speak?" Do not give first aid if the victim can talk. If he cannot talk, go to step 2.
2. *Give five to ten abdominal thrusts* (as described below).
   A. Stand behind the victim who is either sitting or standing.

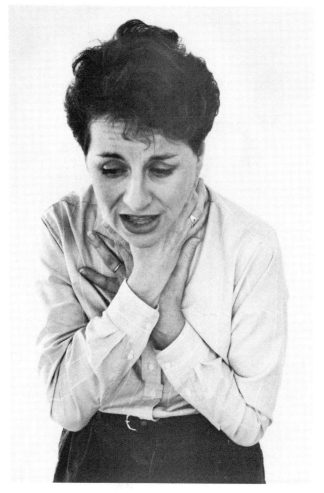

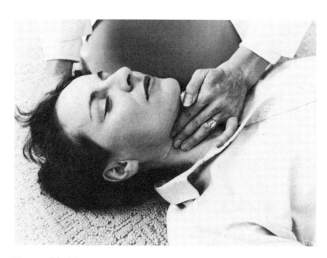

Figure 22-11
Check the carotid pulse.

Figure 22-12
The universal choking sign.

B. Make a fist with your hand.
C. Place your fist against the victim's abdomen. Your fist should be above the navel (belly button) and below the ribs (Figure 22-13).
D. Grasp your fist with your other hand and give five to ten quick sharp upward thrusts (Figure 22-14).

3. *Stop and check to see if the victim can talk, breathe, or cough.* If not, deliver five to ten more abdominal thrusts. Continue with the abdominal thrusts until:
   - The client begins to cough. Let him cough the foreign object out himself.
   - The object falls out of his mouth and the client breathes normally.
   - The client becomes unconscious. If this happens, see choking procedure for the unconscious victim.
   - Medical help arrives.

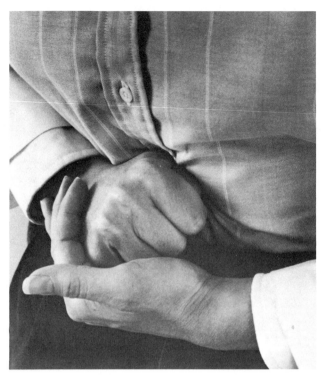

Figure 22-14
Close-up view of hand position for the abdominal thrust.

6. Report incident to the home health agency as soon as possible.

The Unconscious *Adult or Child Over 1 Year Who Is Choking*

You must act quickly if a choking client becomes unresponsive.

1. Roll the client onto her back on a hard surface.
2. Straddle the client and deliver five to ten abdominal thrusts using the heel of your hand as shown in Figure 22-15.
3. Check the client's mouth for a foreign object and clear out the mouth as shown in Figure 22-16.
4. If the client is not breathing, open the airway and attempt to ventilate as described under The Person Who Stops Breathing on pages 299 and 300.

The Baby Under 1 Year Who Is Choking

If the baby can breathe, cry, or cough strongly, do not give first aid. Stand by and be prepared to help if needed. The baby's own cough will remove a foreign object quicker than back blows or ab-

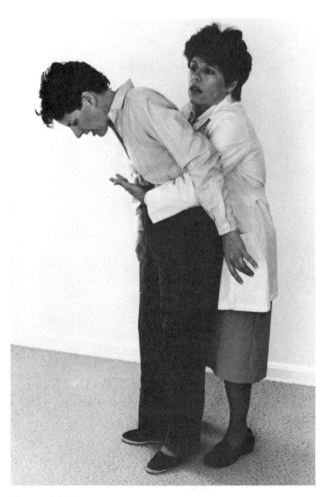

Figure 22-13
The abdominal thrust.

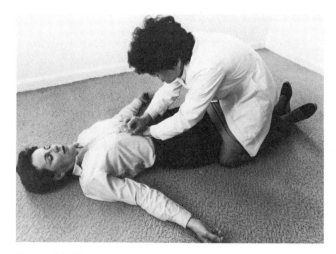

Figure 22-15
The abdominal thrust for the unconscious victim.

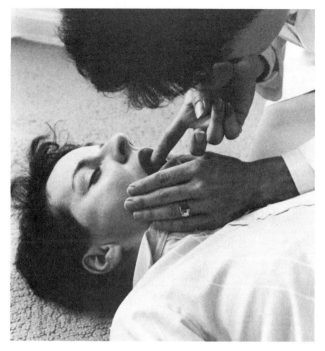

Figure 22-16
Sweep foreign objects out of the mouth.

dominal thrusts. A baby who is having difficulty breathing, is crowing, or is turning blue should be assisted right away.

Special note: The procedures in this section will only help a baby who is choking on an object. You should know that the child is choking on a toy or other object (such as a piece of food) before you begin these emergency procedures. A baby who is choking because his airway is swollen from an allergic reaction or a medical problem (such as croup) needs immediate emergency medical attention.

What You Should Do

1. Lay the baby face down against your forearm and thigh so his head is lower than his chest.
2. Deliver four quick back blows between the shoulder blades with the heel of your hand (Figure 22-17).
3. Turn the baby over and place him on a hard surface.
4. Place two fingertips at the center of the chest, one finger width below the baby's nipple line. Press four times firmly on the chest to a depth of about 1 inch (Figure 22-18).
5. If the baby keeps choking, continue the four back blows and four chest presses until:
   - The baby begins to cough loudly. Let him cough the object out himself.
   - The object falls out of his mouth and the baby breathes normally.
   - Medical help arrives.

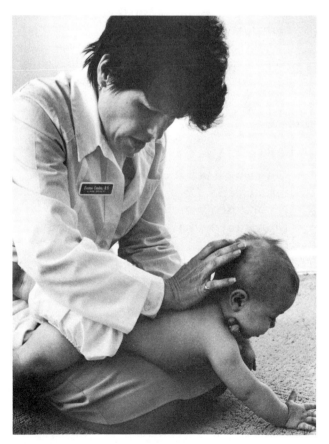

Figure 22-17
Back blows for a baby under 1 year old.

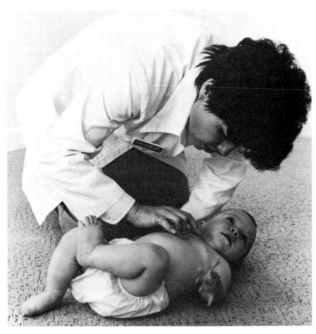

Figure 22-18
Chest presses for a baby under 1 year old.

6. If breathing is not restored after the object is removed from the mouth, begin mouth-to-mouth resuscitation as shown on page 299.
7. Report incident to the home health agency by phone as soon as possible.

Burns

Notes on Burns

- Get medical attention for all burns that form blisters. Do not open the blisters.
- Do not use ice on burns.
- Do not use butter, ointments, or other remedies.
- Remove constricting clothing, but not clothes that stick to the burn. Take rings off if the hand is burned.

A Superficial Burn

A superficial burn will have the following characteristics:

- The skin will be red in a person with light skin, but may not be for a person with dark skin.
- You may see small blisters, but not large or broken blisters.

What You Should Do

1. Cool the burned area (Figure 22-19) for 5 minutes in one of the following ways:
   - Gently run cool water over it.
   - Hold it in a basin or sink filled with cool water. Do not use ice.
   - Put cold, clean, wet towels on the burn.
2. Gently pat dry with clean towel or cloth. Most minor burns do not need to be covered. If there are small blisters, cover the burn with a bandage or clean cloth. Do not use fluffy cotton balls that will stick to the burn.

A Deep Burn

A deep burn will have the following characteristics:

- Large blisters (open or broken)
- The skin may be charred, white, and tough.
- The client may not have pain if nerves are burned.
- Any burn on the face, hands, feet, or genitals is a potential deep burn.
- Any electrical burn is a deep burn.
- Deep burns occur any time smoke or fire is inhaled.
- Burns around the mouth or nose need immediate medical attention. They may indicate that smoke or flames were inhaled.

What You Should Do

All deep burns are serious. A client with a deep burn must be seen by a doctor.

1. Remove clothing and jewelry that might become tight with swelling. Do not remove clothes that stick to the burn.
2. Cool the burned area with cool water. Do not use ice.
3. Gently pat dry and cover with a sterile or clean bandage or cloth. Do not use fluffy cotton balls that will stick to the burn.

Chest Pain (Angina) or a Possible Heart Attack

When a client has chest pains similar to the description below, it may mean the heart is not getting the oxygen it needs to keep working. The client should get prompt medical treatment if he experiences the following:

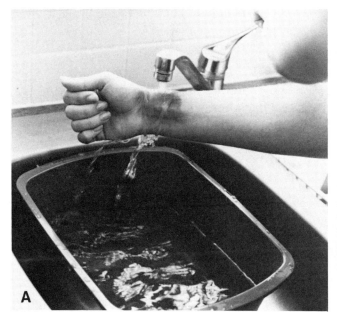
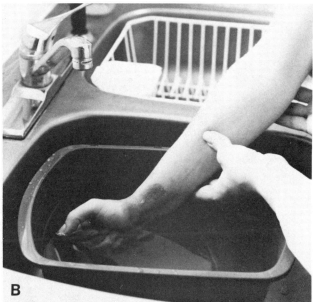
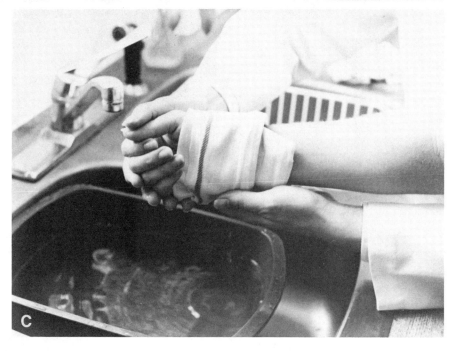

Figure 22-19
(A) Place burned area under cool running water. (B) Soak the burned arm in cool water. (C) Wrap burned area in a cool, wet, clean towel.

1. Chest pain
   - Located in the center of the chest or spreading to the abdomen, shoulder, arm (left), neck, or jaw (Figure 22-20)
   - Lasting more than 2 minutes
   - Described as crushing
2. Trouble breathing
3. May pass out (become unconscious)

What To Do

1. Call for medical help first. (Dial 911 or emergency number in your area.)

2. If client stops breathing and you are trained, start CPR.
3. Let the client decide if he wants to sit up or lie down with pillows under his shoulders. Treat for shock, keep him calm and comfortable, and stay with him until help arrives.
4. Do not let the client move around and do not give him anything to drink or eat.
5. A client who is awake and alert, and has medication for chest pain, should take it. If the pain is relieved, he has probably not suffered a heart attack.

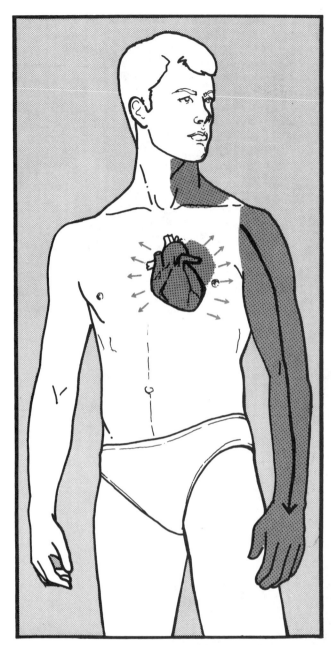

Figure 22-20
Areas where a client may feel pain during a suspected heart attack are shaded. The pain may travel in the directions shown by the arrows.

6. Report the incident to the home health agency as soon as possible.

Hypothermia (Low Body Temperature)

A client who spends too much time in a cold room or outside can lower his body temperature and cause a life-threatening situation. Infants, older adults, clients who are not fed well, clients who have lung or heart disease, or those who cannot move are less able to keep body temperature normal when in the cold.

The client with hypothermia may have the following characteristics:

1. Body temperature falls below the normal reading when you take the client's temperature.
2. May not shiver or "feel cold."
3. May be sleepy, weak, and confused, and have slurred speech.
4. The skin is pale, puffy and bluish, or bright pink.

What You Should Do

1. Take the client to a warm room if possible.
2. Warm the client slowly:
   - Take off the client's wet or cold clothing.
   - Warm him slowly by wrapping him in blankets and towels (Figure 22-21). The client must be warmed slowly.
   - Use your body warmth to help keep the client warm.

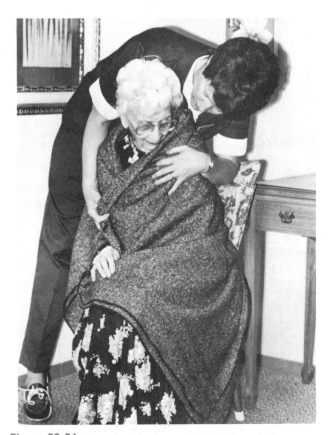

Figure 22-21
To treat hypothermia, warm the client slowly by wrapping her in a wool blanket.

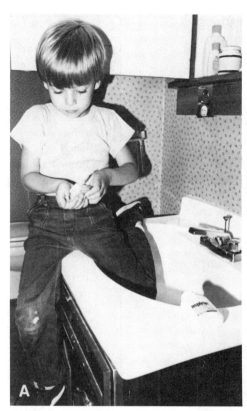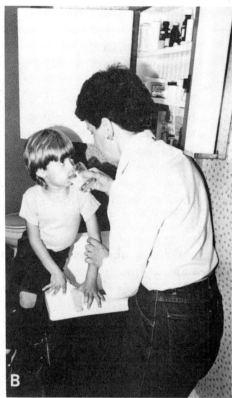

Figure 22-22
(*A*) Medicine cabinets should be locked so that small children cannot get into the medicines. (*B*) Have the client drink a full glass of milk to dilute the poison.

• Give a warm drink if the client is awake and alert.
3. Do not use hot water bottles, electric blankets, or heat lamps.
4. Call for medical help right away.
5. Report the incident to the home health agency as soon as possible.

Poisoning

Act quickly if you suspect poisoning. The phone number of the Poison Control Center can be found in the front of most telephone books. Write it by the phone. Poison Control Centers have better information on all kinds of poisonings than most doctors or emergency rooms. Suggested treatments on product labels are often wrong. If there is not a Poison Control Center number in your community, call the local hospital or doctor's office for advice.

What You Should Do

1. Have the client drink a full glass of water or milk to dilute the poison (Figure 22-22). This makes it harder for the poison to work and gives you more time.
   • Do *not* give fluids if the client has convulsions, is unconscious, or is very weak and sleepy. In that case, call 911 or the local emergency services number before doing anything.
2. Quickly find out what kind of poison was taken. Do not spend too much time with this if you cannot find out quickly.
3. Call Poison Control, report information about the poisoning, and do not hang up the phone. See the box titled, What to Tell Poison Control. They will give you step-by-step directions to follow, and will often alert emergency services if you have not already done so.

What to Tell Poison Control

• The name of the poison. Read the contents on product label (if available).
• How much was taken (if you know).
• When it was taken.
• Reactions of victim (conscious, vomiting, sleepy, slurred speech, or other reactions).
• Victim's age and medical condition.
• Your name, location, and phone number where you can be reached.

4. Continue to watch the client's breathing carefully. If breathing stops and you are trained, start CPR.

5. Position the client on his side to prevent choking on vomit or saliva.

6. Treat for shock by covering with a blanket and loosening tight clothing.

7. Do not have the client vomit unless directed to by Poison Control. If the client is vomiting, have him bend way over to make sure he doesn't breathe any fluid into his lungs. Position the adult and child as shown in Figure 22-23.

8. If you cannot reach anyone for help, you must know when not to make the client vomit. Do *not* have the client vomit if:

   • You are not sure what was swallowed.

   • He swallowed a strong acid or petroleum product, unless instructed to do so by the Poison Control Center. What burns going down will also burn coming up. Examples of acids and petroleum products are listed in the box.

9. Save the poison swallowed (leaves, berries, pills, or an empty container) and any vomit. The doctor will use them to help identify the poison and decide on the treatment.

10. Report the incident to the home health agency as soon as possible.

Do not induce vomiting if the client has swallowed strong acids or petroleum products.

Examples of Strong Acids

Ammonia
Bleach
Clinitest tablets
Dishwasher soap
Drain cleaner
Oven cleaner
Toilet bowl cleaner

Examples of Petroleum Products

Charcoal lighter fluid
Furniture polish/wax
Floor wax
Gasoline
Kerosene
Turpentine

Seizures

Any time a client has a seizure, it should be promptly reported to the home health agency. Most of the time the actual seizure is not an emergency, but the doctor needs to know when they

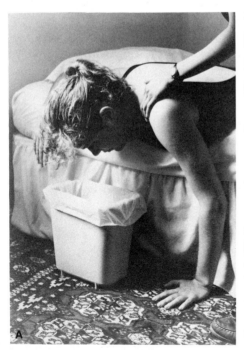
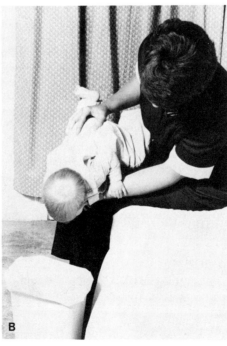

Figure 22-23
(*A*) Help the client keep her head lower than her chest when vomiting. (*B*) Keep the baby's head lower than his chest when vomiting.

occur. A seizure might be an important sign of a health problem that needs attention.

What happens when a client has a seizure:

1. The client may know when he is about to have a seizure. He may see lights or say he "feels different."
2. Muscles become stiff and begin to twitch or jerk.
3. The client may lose control of the bowels or bladder.
4. After a seizure, the client will be tired and may be confused.

What You Should Do

1. Things you should do.
   - Move furniture and objects to keep the client from hurting himself (Figure 22-24).
   - Put a pillow, a blanket, or even a coat under his head to protect him.
   - Loosen the client's tie and tight clothing.
   - Let the client move freely without restraint.
2. Stay with the client, but do not try to restrain him and do not put anything into his mouth. You are likely to hurt him if you do.
3. After the seizure, the client may not remember the seizure at all. Tell him where he is and who you are.
4. Place the client on his side to rest. This prevents choking. Check to see if the client needs clean clothes. His clothes may have become soiled during the seizure.

5. Call the home health agency promptly to report the seizure. Report the time of the seizure, how long the seizure lasted, and the client's reaction.

Shock

Shock occurs when the heart is not pumping enough blood through the body. It may be caused by severe bleeding, burns, bee stings, or any trauma to the body. A person can die from shock. Whenever there has been an accident or a client has been badly hurt, treat for shock. You may not be able to tell if a person is hurt when he is in shock.

You cannot always tell if a person is in shock. He may have some of the following signs:

1. Rapid, weak pulse
2. Shallow, fast breathing
3. Cold, clammy skin
4. Thirst

What You Should Do

1. Have the client lie down as shown in Figure 22-25. If the client is bleeding from the mouth or may vomit, lay her on her side, as shown in Figure 22-26.
2. Put the client's legs up on pillows or blankets. Do not raise a leg that might be broken.
3. Cover the client to keep her warm. You may need to put a blanket under her, too. Keep her comfortable until help arrives.

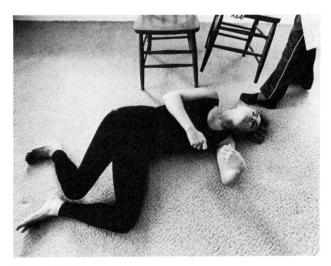

Figure 22-24
If a client has a seizure, clear the area so that she will not burn herself. *Never* put anything into the client's mouth.

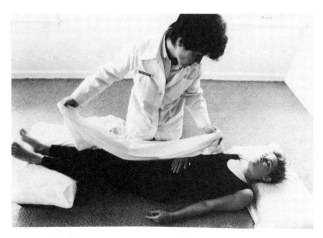

Figure 22-25
Treating for shock with the client on her back.

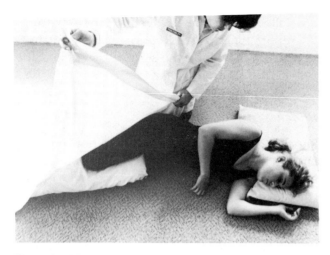

Figure 22-26
Treating for shock with the client lying on her side.

Possible Stroke

When a blood vessel in the brain breaks or is clogged, blood and oxygen cannot nourish the brain. When this happens, a part of the brain may die. This is known as a stroke. (For more on strokes, see Chapter 10.)

The characteristics of a stroke include:

1. Loss of feeling on one side of the body
2. Slurred speech or may not be able to talk
3. Loss of consciousness
4. Trouble walking

What You Should Do

1. Check breathing.
2. Call for help.
3. Help the client turn his head to the side to avoid choking while lying down.
4. Stay with him and reassure him.
5. Report the incident to the home health agency as soon as possible.

Review Questions

True or False

1. ____ It is highly recommended that all HM/HHAs take a course in Basic First Aid and CRP because you cannot master first aid techniques from a book.

2. ____ A person with a severe wound can bleed to death in 1 minute.

3. ____ The first thing you should do if a client is bleeding badly is to apply firm pressure over the wound.

4. ____ Ice should never be applied to a burn because it can make the burn worse.

5. ____ A client who lives in a house or apartment and rarely goes outside can never get hypothermia (low body temperature)

6. ____ The best place to get immediate help in the case of a poisoning is your local Poison Control Center, because they have the latest information on treating all kinds of poisonings and they will often call the emergency squad for you if it is necessary.

7. ____ Anyone who needs first aid should be treated for shock even if they say they "feel fine."

Multiple Choice

8. You arrive at your client's house and enter through the back door as you always do. As you enter the kitchen, you see your client lying on the kitchen floor. She appears unconscious. What should you do?
   a. Quickly shake the client's shoulder gently and call her name to see if she responds.
   b. Phone your supervisor right away.
   c. Roll the client on her back and clear out her mouth. Tilt her head back to open her airway and put your ear to her mouth as you check to see if she is breathing. If not, begin mouth-to-mouth resuscitation.
   d. *a* and *c*.

9. In an emergency situation where there could be several health problems, what is the correct order for treating first aid problems?
   a. Bleeding, breathing, and heartbeat (pulse)
   b. Burns, bleeding, and paralysis
   c. Breathing, heartbeat (pulse), and bleeding
   d. Shock, breathing, and bleeding

Questions for Discussion

10. Your client begins coughing loudly in the middle of eating his lunch. He tells you he is choking. Should you begin abdominal thrusts? Why or why not?

The Homemaker/Home Health Aide Evaluation

Each skill on the list should be initialed by the homemaker/home health aide's supervisor or classroom instructor when the homemaker/home health aide has demonstrated ability and understanding for the individual areas of training.

Homemaker/Home Health Aide's Name————————————————

Class Location————————————————

Class Dates———————————————— Number of Hours of Training————

Names of Class Instructors   Instructors Who Observed HM/HHA's
                                              Skill Demonstrations.

————————————————   ————————————————

————————————————   ————————————————

Skills and Knowledge	Date HM/HHA Displayed Understanding of Material	Date HM/HHA Demonstrated Procedure for Supervisor	Comments
1. Shows understanding of homemaker/home health aide role in relation to clients, supervisor, and home care team (Chapter 1).			
2. Shows willingness to follow care plan as written by agency and report changes in client's condition promptly.			
3. Can identify verbal and nonverbal communication (Chapter 2).			

(continued)

Skills and Knowledge	Date HM/HHA Displayed Understanding of Material	Date HM/HHA Demonstrated Procedure for Supervisor	Comments
4. Can instruct clients or family members using proper teaching techniques (Chapters 2, 5, and 14).			
5. Can define human needs, explain how people react to unmet needs, and the role of the family in meeting needs (Chapter 3).			
6. Shows appreciation and respect for people from other cultures (Chapter 3).			
7. Has a basic understanding of the growth and development of children (Chapter 4)			
8. Can identify some of the physical, social, emotional, and intellectual changes associated with aging (Chapter 5).			
9. Is able to understand some of the reactions a family or client may have to a serious illness or disability (Chapter 6).			
10. Can identify some of the characteristics of good mental health (Chapter 7).			
11. Is able to understand and explain the emotional and physical needs of the dying client (Chapter 8).			
12. Has a basic understanding of the human body (Chapter 9).			
13. Has basic understanding of common health problems (Chapter 10).			

Skills and Knowledge	Date HM/HHA Displayed Understanding of Material	Date HM/HHA Demonstrated Procedure for Supervisor	Comments
14. Is able to document accurately care provided to clients on written progress notes (Chapter 11).			
15. Is alert to safety hazards when visiting clients (Chapter 12).			
16. HM/HHA Procedure: Handwashing (Chapter 13)			
17. Shows understanding of home management procedures (Chapters 13 and 14). Cleaning the house Using appliances Washing laundry			
18. Demonstrates ability to use time efficiently (Chapter 14).			
19. Can plan and prepare nutritious meals using the Four Food Groups (Chapter 15).			
20. Can demonstrate the lifting rules (Chapter 16).			
21. HM/HHA Procedure: Positioning the Client on his Side (Chapter 16).			
22. HM/HHA Procedure: Positioning the Client on his Back (Chapter 16).			
23. HM/HHA Procedure: Moving the Client to the Side of the Bed (Chapter 16).			
24. HM/HHA Procedure: Turning the Client From his Back to his Side (Chapter 16).			

(continued)

Skills and Knowledge	Date HM/HHA Displayed Understanding of Material	Date HM/HHA Demonstrated Procedure for Supervisor	Comments
25. HM/HHA Procedure: Assisting the Client With a One-Sided Weakness to Move to One Side of the Bed (Chapter 16).			
26. HM/HHA Procedure: Assisting the Client Who Can Help to Move to the Head of the Bed (Chapter 16).			
27. HM/HHA Procedure: Sliding the Client to the Head of the Bed With a Drawsheet— One Person (Chapter 16).			
28. HM/HHA Procedure: Sliding the Client to the Head of the Bed With a Drawsheet— Two Persons (Chapter 16)			
29. HM/HHA Procedure: Assisting the Client to Sit up in Bed Using the Arm Lock (Chapter 16)			
30. HM/HHA Procedure: Assisting the Client to Move From the Bed to a Chair (Chapter 16)			
31. Assisting With Walking (Chapter 16)			
32. HM/HHA Procedure: Using a Walker (Chapter 16)			
33. HM/HHA Procedure: Using a Cane (Chapter 16)			
34. HM/HHA Procedure: Rising From a Chair With a Walker or Cane (Chapter 16)			

Skills and Knowledge	Date HM/HHA Displayed Understanding of Material	Date HM/HHA Demonstrated Procedure for Supervisor	Comments
35. HM/HHA Procedure: Sitting With a Walker or Cane (Chapter 16)			
36. HM/HHA Procedure: Range-of-Motion Exercises (Chapter 16)			
37. HM/HHA Procedure: Cleaning the Glass Thermometer (Chapter 17)			
38. HM/HHA Procedure: Taking the Temperature Orally (Chapter 17)			
39. HM/HHA Procedure: Taking the Axillary Temperature (Chapter 17)			
41. HM/HHA Procedure: Taking the Rectal Temperature (Chapter 17)			
42. HM/HHA Procedure: Measuring the Radial Pulse (Chapter 17)			
43. HM/HHA Procedure: Measuring the Apical Pulse (Chapter 17)			
44. HM/HHA Procedure: Measuring the Respirations With the Pulse (Chapter 17)			
45. HM/HHA Procedure: Estimating the Blood Pressure (Chapter 17)			
46. HM/HHA Procedure: Measuring the Blood Pressure (Chapter 17)			
47. How to Make the Sounds of Blood Pressure Louder (Chapter 17)			

(continued)

Skills and Knowledge	Date HM/HHA Displayed Understanding of Material	Date HM/HHA Demonstrated Procedure for Supervisor	Comments
48. HM/HHA Procedure: Flossing the Teeth (Chapter 18)			
49. HM/HHA Procedure: Assisting the Client With Mouth Care (Chapter 18)			
50. HM/HHA Procedure: Care of Dentures (Chapter 18)			
51. HM/HHA Procedure: Assisting With the Bedpan (Chapter 18)			
52. Assisting With the Commode (Chapter 18)			
53. Guidelines for Working With Catheters (Chapter 18)			
54. HM/HHA Procedure: The Bed Bath (Chapter 18)			
55. HM/HHA Procedure: The Partial Bath (Chapter 18)			
56. HM/HHA Procedure: The Tub Bath or Shower (Chapter 18)			
57. Foot Care (Chapter 18)			
58. Guidelines for Grooming the Hair (Chapter 18)			
59. Guidelines for Shampooing the Hair (Chapter 18)			
60. HM/HHA Procedure: Shaving the Male Client With a Safety Razor (Chapter 18)			
61. HM/HHA Procedure: The Backrub (Chapter 18)			

Skills and Knowledge	Date HM/HHA Displayed Understanding of Material	Date HM/HHA Demonstrated Procedure for Supervisor	Comments
62. Guidelines For Assisting the Client With a One-Sided Weakness to Dress and Undress (Chapter 18)			
63. HM/HHA Procedure: Lifting and Holding the Baby (Chapter 19) Lifting the Baby The Cradle Hold The Football Hold The Shoulder Hold Helping the Baby Sit With Support			
64. HM/HHA Procedure: Changing the Baby's Diapers (Chapter 19)			
65. HM/HHA Procedure: Bottle-Feeding (Chapter 19)			
66. HM/HHA Procedure: The Infant Sponge Bath (Chapter 19)			
67. HM/HHA Procedure: The Infant Tub Bath (Chapter 19)			
68. HM/HHA Procedure: Deep Breathing Exercises (Chapter 20)			
69. Care and Prevention of Pressure Sores (Decubitus Ulcers) (Chapter 20)			
70. IIM/IIIA Procedure: Using the Hot Water Bottle (Chapter 20)			
71. HM/HHA Procedure: Warm Soaks (Chapter 20)			
72. HM/HHA Procedure: Using the Ice Bag (Chapter 20)			

(continued)

Skills and Knowledge	Date HM/HHA Displayed Understanding of Material	Date HM/HHA Demonstrated Procedure for Supervisor	Comments
73. HM/HHA Procedure: Using the Cold Wet Compress (Chapter 20)			
74. HM/HHA Procedure: Changing a Nonsterile Dressing (Chapter 20)			
75. Measuring Fluid Intake and Output (Chapter 20)			
76. HM/HHA Procedure: Changing a Colostomy Bag (Chapter 20)			
77. HM/HHA Procedure: Collecting a Midstream Clean-Catch Urine Specimen (Chapter 20)			
78. HM/HHA Procedure: Collecting a Stool Sample (Chapter 20)			
79. Assisting with Medications (Chapter 21)			
80. Safety Guidelines for Oxygen Use (Chapter 21)			
81. First Aid for Bleeding (Chapter 22)			
82. First Aid for a Conscious Adult or Child Over 1 Year Who Is Choking (Chapter 22)			
83. First Aid for a Baby Under 1 Year Who Is Choking (Chapter 22)			
84. First Aid for Burns (Chapter 22)			
85. First Aid for Chest Pain (Angina) or a Possible Heart Attack (Chapter 22)			

Skills and Knowledge	Date HM/HHA Displayed Understanding of Material	Date HM/HHA Demonstrated Procedure for Supervisor	Comments
86. First Aid for Hypothermia (Low Body Temperature) (Chapter 22)			
87. First Aid for Poisoning (Chapter 22)			
88. First Aid for Seizures (Chapter 22)			
89. First Aid for Shock (Chapter 22)			
90. First Aid for Possible Stroke (Chapter 22)			

Additional Comments:

_____

_____

_____

_____

_____

_____

_____

_____

_____

_____

_____

_____

_____

_____

_____

_____

_____

_____

_____

_____

Instructor/Supervisor's Signature   Date

Homemaker/Home Health Aide's Signature   Date

Glossary

Abdomen The area on the body below the ribs and above the pelvis

Abduction The act of moving an arm or leg away from the center of the body

Abuse Physical or mental harm or neglect; mistreatment

Active exercise An exercise that is performed by a person without help from others

Activities of daily living (ADLs) Activities that are carried out in the normal course of daily life—bathing, dressing, meal preparation, and so on

Acute illness A sudden, short-term illness that needs immediate medical care

Addiction A physical or psychological dependence on a substance such as alcohol, caffeine, cigarettes, or cocaine

Additive A substance added to food or medications, usually to preserve or improve the color, flavor, or consistency of the food or medication

Adduction The act of moving an arm or leg toward the center of the body

Advocate To work on behalf of another person's rights. HM/HHAs should be advocates for their clients.

Alignment To have the body lined up in the proper anatomical position

Allergy An abnormal reaction that occurs when the body is overly sensitive to a particular substance

Amputation The surgical removal of an arm, leg, or other body part

Anemia A reduction in the number of red blood cells or in the amount of hemoglobin in the blood

Anorexia Loss of appetite, or a lack of interest in eating

Anticipatory grief Grief that begins before a loss occurs, such as when a woman mourns the loss of her terminally ill husband

Antiseptic A cleaning agent that can be used on living things to destroy or slow the growth of pathogens and infection

Anxiety A feeling of uneasiness

Aphasia The inability to communicate through speech, writing, or signs, or the inability to understand written or verbal communication due to a disease or brain injury

Apical pulse The pulse rate obtained by placing a stethoscope directly over the heart. An apical pulse should be taken for a full minute.

Apnea The absence of breathing

Arrhythmia An irregular or unsteady pulse

Asepsis The absence of disease-causing organisms

Assignment sheet Lists the daily jobs the HM/HHA is assigned to complete

Atrophy The wasting away of muscle tissue from lack of use

Autopsy The examination of organs and tissues of the human body after death to determine the cause of death

Axilla Armpit

Axillary temperature A way to measure body heat. Obtained by placing a thermometer under the arm for 10 minutes.

Balance A steady position

Bandage A dressing for a wound or body part

Base of support The area on which an object rests

Bedsore A deep wound caused by pressure and poor circulation to the skin. Also called *pressure sore* and *decubitus ulcer*.

Biopsy A test where tissue is removed from the body and examined

Blood pressure The force or pressure that blood exerts against an artery wall when the heart is pumping

Body mechanics   The efficient and safe use of the body as a machine

Bony prominences   Areas on the body where there is little padding and bones protrude, such as the hips and elbows. Bedsores form easily on bony prominences.

Bounding pulse   A full, strong pulse that is not very easy to stop with mild pressure. Also called *full pulse*.

Callus   A place where the skin becomes thick. A callus may form on the feet when shoes are too tight.

Calorie   The amount of heat needed to raise the temperature of 1 gram of water 1 degree centigrade

Cannula   A tube

Cardiopulmonary resuscitation (CPR)   First aid techniques to open and maintain a good airway and to provide artificial ventilation and circulation. You must be trained and certified to perform CPR.

Cardiovascular   Relating to the heart and blood vessels

Care plan   A written record of services that will be provided by the home health agency. The care plan includes a written record of the client's needs, the goals of treatment, and plans for how the home health agency will meet those goals.

Caries   The decay of teeth and formation of cavities

Cast   A bandage made to immobilize a body part. A cast is usually made from plaster of Paris.

Catheter   A tube for instilling or removing fluids

Cell   The smallest living unit in the body

Celsius scale   Water boils at 100 degrees and freezes at 0 degrees on the Celsius scale. Also called *centigrade scale*.

Celsius thermometer   A thermometer that measures temperature using the Celsius scale. Also called *centigrade thermometer*.

Center of gravity   The point where an equal amount of weight is above, below, and to each side of a single point

Centigrade thermometer   A thermometer that measures temperature using the centigrade scale. See *Celsius thermometer*.

Cervical   Refers to the neck

Chart   A confidential document that contains doctor's orders, lab reports, progress notes, and other information about a client's health. Also called *medical record* and *health-care record*.

Chronic illness   A long-term illness

Clean-catch midstream specimen   A urine specimen that has been collected in a sterile container after the genitals have been cleaned carefully

Clean technique   Practices (such as handwashing) that help reduce the number of microorganisms and the spread of infection. Also called *medical asepsis*.

Client   Any person receiving services from a home health agency

Colostomy   A surgical opening made through the abdomen and into the large intestine for the removal of waste products

Commode   A chair with an opening in the seat and a container under the seat to collect urine and feces. Used for a client who cannot walk to the toilet.

Communication   A verbal or nonverbal exchange of information

Constipation   The difficult passage of dry, hard stools

Contagious disease   A disease or illness that is easily spread from person to person. Also called *communicable disease*.

Continence   The ability to control the elimination of body wastes

Contracture   Shortening of a muscle due to inactivity resulting in the inability to contract or relax that muscle

Culture   Everything a person learns from the family and people who surround him

Cyanosis   A bluish coloring of skin, lips, nailbeds, and mucous membranes

Dangling   The position in which a person sits on the edge of a bed with his legs and feet over the side of the bed. Dangling after a nap or a night's sleep avoids dizziness on standing up.

Decubitus ulcer   A deep skin wound caused by pressure and poor circulation. Also called *pressure sore* and *bedsore*. Plural is *decubiti*.

Defecate   To have a bowel movement

Dehydration   A lack of fluid in the body

Denial   Refusal to admit that a disturbing situation is occurring

Denture   Artificial teeth that replace any or all of a person's own teeth

Deodorant   A preparation to cover or lessen body odors

Depression   A feeling of loss; an emotional state commonly associated with feelings of sadness and guilt

Diarrhea   The passage of loose, watery, unformed stools

Diastolic blood pressure   Occurs when the least amount of pressure is exerted on the artery walls during a heartbeat. It is the bottom number when the blood pressure is written as a fraction. Also called *diastole*.

Disability   A physical or mental limitation caused by injury or disease, for example, the loss of a body part, or the loss of use of a body part

Discipline   Guidance that teaches children reasonable and responsible ways of behaving

Disinfectant   A cleaning agent used on objects to destroy or slow the growth of pathogens. Not meant to be used on people

Document   To make written entries on a progress note

Dressing   A bandage or protective covering for a wound

Dyspnea   Difficult and labored breathing

Ecchymosis   A purplish mark on the skin caused by the collection of blood under the skin. Also called *bruise* or *black and blue mark*.

Embolus   A blood clot that travels. May lodge in a smaller vessel and block the blood flow. Plural is *emboli*.

Emesis   Expelling of stomach contents. Also called *vomiting*.

Emotion   A feeling, such as love, hate, or fear

Encouraging fluids   Encouraging a client to drink more fluids. Also called *forcing fluids*.

Enema   The introduction of a solution into the lower intestinal tract. HM/HHAs are not permitted to give enemas in many states. An enema is never given without orders from the home health agency supervisor.

Enuresis   Involuntary urination during the night

Erect position   Standing with good body alignment

Ethics   A moral code or standard of behavior

Evaluation   The process of measuring how well a goal or objective has been reached. The care the HM/HHA provides will be evaluated by the clients and supervisor.

Exhalation   The act of breathing out. Also called *expiration*.

Expiration   The act of breathing out. Also called *exhalation*.

Extension   Straightening or increasing an angle. When you open your fist, you are extending your fingers.

Fahrenheit scale   Water boils at 212 degrees and freezes at 32 degrees on the fahrenheit scale.

Fahrenheit thermometer   An instrument used to measure temperature

Febrile   Having a fever or a temperature that is higher than normal

Fecal impaction   A hardened mass of feces in the rectum

Feeble pulse   A pulse that feels weak to the touch and is easy to stop with pressure. May also be called a *weak* or *thready pulse*.

Fever   The body temperature is above normal. Also called *febrile*.

Flexion   Bending or decreasing the angle between bones. When you make a fist, you are flexing your fingers.

Foot drop   A condition where the foot falls forward and the toes point outward. Foot drop may occur if the feet are not supported while a client is on bedrest.

Forcing fluids   Encouraging a client to drink more fluids. Also called *forcing fluids*.

Fowler's position   The semi-sitting position

Genitalia   The external organs of reproduction

Germ   A disease-causing microorganism. Also called *pathogen*.

Gerontology   The study of aging

Goal   Something one is trying to achieve. Also called *objective*.

Grief   Emotional suffering associated with a loss

Health   Physical, mental, and social well-being, and the absence of disease

Health care   Services offered to well or ill people by health care professionals

Heimlich maneuver   A technique used to remove food caught in the throat when a person is choking

Helping relationship   A relationship of understanding between the client and HM/HHA that allows the client to move toward his goals

Hemorrhoids   Swollen rectal veins

Home care team   Members of the home health agency who provide a variety of health-related services in a client's home

Home health agency   The company that employs most members of the home care team and organizes their work

Homemaker/home health aide (HM/HHA)   People who are trained in home health care and employed by a home health agency to provide care to clients. HM/HHAs are supervised by a registered nurse or another professional member of the home care team. Duties may include providing personal care, meal planning and preparation, and light housekeeping. May also be called *homemaker, home health aide, personal care attendant, home care aide,* and *home nursing assistant*.

Hospice   Refers to the philosophy of care that allows a dying person to be cared for with dignity and comfort either in his own home or a hospice center

Hygiene   The practice of cleanliness to maintain health and prevent disease

Hyper-   A prefix meaning *above* or *excessive*

Hypertension   An abnormally high blood pressure as diagnosed by a doctor

Hypo-   A prefix meaning *under, below,* or *low*

Hypothermia   A body temperature that is below the average normal range

Ileostomy   A surgical opening through the abdomen and into the small intestine for the removal of wastes

Ill   Being sick or having a disease

Incoherent   A person who has unclear or disconnected thoughts or speech

Indwelling catheter   A sterile tube placed in the bladder by a nurse and secured so urine can drain continuously. Also called *urinary catheter* or *retention catheter*.

Infant A child less than 1 year old

Infection Invasion and growth of pathogens in the body. Causes disease, injury, inflammation, and discomfort.

Inflammation The defensive response of the body to injury, which protects the injured area

Inhalation The act of breathing in. Also called *inspiration*.

Insomnia Difficulty in falling asleep or staying asleep

Inspiration The act of breathing in. Also called *inhalation*.

Intake The amount of fluid taken into the body in a given period of time

Integument The skin

Intermittent pain Pain or discomfort that comes and goes

Irrigation To clean by flushing water over an area

Jaundice A condition where the skin, eyes, and mucous membranes turn yellowish

Korotkoff's sounds The sounds of blood pressure heard through the stethoscope

Lesion A change in tissue caused by disease or injury, such as a scab, scale, ulcer, or pimple

Malnutrition A condition caused by a lack of proper nutrients in the diet

Medical asepsis Practices such as handwashing that help reduce the number and spread of germs. Also called *clean technique*.

Meniscus The curved surface at the top of a column of liquid in a tube, such as a mercury manometer, used to measure the blood pressure. The reading should be taken from the top of the meniscus when viewed at eye level.

Microorganism A tiny living animal or plant. Most are visible only with a microscope. Also called *organism*.

Mucus A watery or slimy secretion produced by mucous membranes in the body

Nausea An unpleasant feeling of sickness that may or may not be accompanied by vomiting

Need A necessity or requirement. Everyone has basic human needs that must be met for survival. See Chapter 3.

Nonverbal communication The exchange of information without using words

Nutrient The parts of food that nourish the body cells

Nutrition The process of using foods and fluids for the growth, maintenance, and health of the body

Objective Something one is trying to achieve. Also called *goal*.

Objective report Report based on information gained by direct observation

Open wound A cut or break in the skin or mucous membrane

Oral temperature A measurement of body heat obtained by placing the thermometer in the mouth under the tongue for 8 minutes

Oriented A person who demonstrates an awareness of self, time, date, and surroundings

Orthostatic hypotension A sudden drop in blood pressure that causes dizziness or light-headedness. It occurs when a person rises quickly after a period of lying down or sitting.

Ostomy A surgical opening through the abdomen into the large or small intestines for the removal of waste products

OTC The abbreviation for *over-the-counter* medications. OTC medications are those that can be bought without a prescription.

Overdependence Occurs when a person becomes too reliant on someone else

Pain The sensation of physical and/or mental discomfort

Pallor A pale color to the skin

Passive exercise An exercise where one person moves the body parts of another person

Pathogen A disease-causing microorganisms. Also called *germ*.

Phantom limb pain A real sensation of pain or discomfort felt in a limb or body part that has been amputated.

Policy A rule. The policies of the home health agency are the agency's rules.

Posture The natural position of the body in healthy persons

Prescription The doctor's order for a medication

Pressure sore A deep wound in the skin caused by pressure and lack of circulation. Also called *decubitus ulcer* and *bedsore*.

Problem Something difficult that must be dealt with

Procedure A method for doing something

Projectile vomiting Vomiting with great force

Prosthesis An artificial part used in place of a body part that has been removed; or, a device to improve the function of a natural part

Psychology The study of the way the mind functions in relation to human behavior

Psychosocial   Relating to the way people behave in groups

Pulse   A rhythmic sensation felt in an artery that corresponds to the beats of the heart

Purulent drainage   Discharge from a wound that contains pus

Range of motion (ROM)   The normal amount of movement in a joint. Range-of-motion exercises may be prescribed by a doctor to improve circulation, to improve muscle tone, and to prevent contractures.

Rash   An eruption on the skin

Reaction time   The amount of time that it takes for a message to travel to the brain and for the body to respond to that message

Rectal temperature   A measure of body heat obtained by placing a thermometer in the rectum for 3 minutes

Referral   The process of sending or guiding someone to another place for help. Referrals are made by the doctor or home health agency supervisor.

Rehabilitation   To restore to a state of physical and mental health through treatment and therapy

Relationship   An association between people

Relax   To become less tense

Residual urine   Urine that stays in the bladder after voiding

Respiration   The act of breathing in and breathing out

Rest   To slow or stop work and activity for a period of time to become refreshed

Restricting fluids   Limiting the amount of fluid that a client drinks

Scar   A mark left by a cut, sore, or injury that has healed.

Shock   The reaction of the body when there is poor blood circulation or circulatory collapse. May be caused by physical or emotional trauma.

Sick   Means the same as *ill*

Sign   A change in a client's condition that can be observed or measured by another person

Sitz bath   A bath where the client sits in a tub with enough warm water to cover his hips

Soak   Placement of a part of the body in water or in a medicated solution

Sociology   The study of relationships between people

Sphygmomanometer   The instrument used to measure blood pressure within an artery

Sputum   Substance released from the mouth by coughing or clearing the throat

Sterile   Free from all living microorganisms, including spores

Sterilization   A process that destroys all microorganisms and spores on an object

Stethoscope   An instrument used by an examiner to listen to sounds within the client's body. Used by the HM/HHA when measuring the blood pressure.

Stoma   A surgical opening into a body wall or body cavity

Stool   Wastes discharged from the bowels. Also called *bowel movement* or *feces.*

Stress incontinence   The involuntary release of urine from the bladder due to straining or pressure such as laughing or coughing

Subjective   Information that is an opinion and cannot be measured. When a client tells you how he feels, he is giving you subjective information.

Supervisor   The home health care professional who plans, directs, and evaluates care

Symptom   Any condition, such as pain, that is felt and described by the client, but may not be observable by others

Syndrome   A predictable set of signs and symptoms that occur together

Systolic pressure   The period when the greatest amount of pressure is put upon the artery walls during a heartbeat. It is the top number when the blood pressure is written as a fraction. Also called *systole.*

Terminal illness   An illness where there is little hope of recovery

Therapeutic diet   A diet used to help treat a disease or disorder

Therapist   A professional member of the home care team trained in the treatment of disease, disability, and injury

Thermometer   An instrument used to measure the amount of heat in something. The HM/HHA uses a thermometer to measure body temperature.

Thrombus   A clot of blood that may block a blood vessel. Plural is *thrombi.*

Total incontinence   The inability of the bladder to store any urine. The client will dribble constantly.

Tracheostomy   A surgical opening made in the neck that allows a person to breathe when he cannot breathe through his mouth or nose

Transfer   The act of moving a person from one place to another

Trapeze   A triangular piece of metal that is hung by a chain on a frame over a bed or chair and is used to help a client move and reposition himself

Trauma   An injury

Tumor   An abnormal growth of cells

Ulcer   An open sore on the skin or mucous membrane

Umbilicus   Means the same as *navel* or *belly button*

Unconscious   The lack of awareness of, and the inability to respond to, one's surroundings

Unresponsive   Not able to answer when spoken to

Urinalysis   A laboratory test of the urine

Urinary incontinence   The loss of voluntary control over the discharge of urine from the bladder

Urination   The process of emptying the urinary bladder. Also called *micturition, passing water*, and *voiding*.

Urine   Liquid waste that is discharged from the body by the urinary system

Verbal communication   The exchange of information through the use of words

Virus   A microorganism that causes disease. It feeds on living cells to live and grow.

Vital signs   Measurements of body temperature, pulse and respiratory rates, and blood pressure. Abbreviated VS, or TPR and BP.

Voiding   The process of emptying the urinary bladder. Also called *micturition, urination,* or *passing water*.

Vomiting   The forceful release of the stomach contents out through the mouth. Also called *emesis*.

Vomitus   Material expelled by vomiting

Well-being   The state in which one experiences health and happiness

Worry   A mild form of anxiety characterized by preoccupation with a problem

Wound   A break in the skin. Sometimes called *lesion*.

Wound and skin precautions   Practices to limit cross-infection by pathogens from wounds and the skin

Answers to Review Questions

Chapter 1:
Introduction to Home Health Care

1. care plan
2. your supervisor
3. see Members of the Home Care Team

Chapter 2:
Communication Skills

1. F	4. e
2. T	5. b
3. F	6. e

Chapter 3:
Basic Human Needs, the Family, and Cultural Practices

1. T	9. prejudice, a stereotype
2. F	10. culture
3. T	11. C
4. F	12. D
5. F	13. B
6. T	14. A
7. T	15. A
8. F	16. B

Chapter 4:
Caring for Children

1. F	6. T
2. T	7. F
3. F	8. T
4. T	9. T
5. T	

Chapter 5:
Caring for Older Adults

1. T	4. T
2. F	5. T
3. F	6. T

Chapter 6:
Working With the Client Who Is Ill or Disabled

1. F	4. T
2. T	5. F
3. T	

Chapter 7:
*Promoting Mental Health and Understanding
Mental Illness*

1. F	5. T
2. T	6. T
3. T	7. T
4. F	

Chapter 8:
Caring for the Client Who Is Dying

1. T	4. F
2. T	5. T
3. T	

Chapter 9:
How the Body Works

1. T	9. A
2. F	10. G
3. T	11. C
4. T	12. E
5. T	13. J
6. B	14. F
7. D	15. I
8. H	

Chapter 10:
Common Health Problems

1. T	4. T
2. T	5. T
3. T	6. T

Chapter 11:
Recording and Sharing Information

Answers to the progress note exercise in Chapter 11. Compare your answers with answers given below. There are many ways of writing a good progress note. Your progress note will not look exactly like the example, but see if your note has most of the details that are mentioned below. Have your class instructor read your answers and see how your report compares.

Complete Report

Arrived at 8:30. Assisted Mrs. Brown into the tub for her bath. Needed help with her back. Small, red, tender area at center of lower back. Washed gently and applied lotion around the red area. Told Mrs. Brown not to lie on her back to relieve pressure on tender area. Reported red area to Barb Johnston, R.N., by phone at 10:35 AM. Client asked HM/HHA to cut toenails. HM/HHA refused and will notify agency so it can be arranged. While preparing breakfast, a small juice glass broken by HM/HHA. Mrs. Brown said, "Oh, that happens. It's no problem." Incident report filed with agency today. Mrs. Brown ate two fried eggs, toast, juice, and one cup of coffee. Left Mrs. Brown in easy chair by telephone at 10 AM.

Incomplete Report

Ate breakfast. Bedsore on back noticed during bath. A good day.

Reasons Answers Are Complete

1. The type of bath and Mrs. Brown's ability to assist are clear. The HM/HHA did this without going into too many details.
2. Gives a good description of the probable bedsore. It tells size, color, location, and what the HM/HHA did about it, including the telephone report to the agency.

3. A note is made about Mrs. Brown's request for cutting the toenails. In addition, the HM/HHA should make a verbal report.
4. This HM/HHA realized that even though Mrs. Brown did not seem to be bothered by the broken juice glass, she was only protecting herself by reporting the accident in a formal incident report.
5. The HM/HHA may or may not need to write out the entire menu that the client eats. It depends on the agency policy and the particular client.

Reasons Answers Are Incomplete

1. Report does not tell what kind of bath was given or if Mrs. Brown needed assistance.

2. This report talks about "a bedsore." Is there a small open wound or is it simply tender and red? The location is not described. You need to give enough information so the nurse can tell if the wound is getting worse. Another problem is that the HM/HHA did not say she called the agency about the bedsore. We must assume that she did not.

3. This HM/HHA neglected to record that the client wanted her toenails cut.

4. This report did not mention the incident where the juice glass was broken. All incidents should be reported to protect the HM/HHA, the client, and the agency.

5. Stating that the client ate all her breakfast may be fine for most clients. Some clients may need to have the amount and type of food recorded. Your home health supervisor will let you know how specific to be.

6. A comment such as "a good day" is often seen on charting but it does not tell us anything. It is better to be more specific.

1. T	5. T
2. T	6. T
3. T	7. e
4. F	

Chapter 12:
Safety for You and Your Client

1. F	4. F
2. T	5. b
3. T	

Chapter 13:
Infection Control: Preventing the Spread of Disease

1. F
2. T
3. T

Chapter 14:
Keeping the Home and Laundry Clean

1. F	4. F
2. T	5. F
3. T	6. T

Chapter 15:
Planning, Purchasing, and Serving Food

1. T	6. F
2. F	7. F
3. T	8. T
4. F	9. T
5. T	

An adult needs the following each day to complete a well-balanced diet:
2 servings Milk Group
2 servings Meat Group
4 servings Fruit–vegetable Group
4 servings Grain Group

Chapter 16:
Lifting, Positioning, and Exercise

1. T	6. T
2. T	7. F
3. F	8. d
4. F	9. c
5. F	

Chapter 17:
Measuring the Vital Signs

1. F	9. B
2. T	10. D
3. F	11. D
4. T	12. E
5. F	13. F
6. T	14. C
7. C	15. B
8. A	16. A

Chapter 18:
Personal Care Skills

1. T	7. T
2. F	8. F
3. T	9. T
4. T	10. T
5. T	11. T
6. F	12. T

Chapter 19:
Caring for the New Mother and Baby

1. T	4. F
2. T	5. b
3. T	

Chapter 20:
Common Procedures and Treatments

1. F	10. T
2. T	11. T
3. F	12. T
4. T	13. T
5. F	14. T
6. T	15. T
7. T	16. d
8. F	17. d
9. F	

18. 1. Turn and reposition a bedridden client every 2 hours.
    2. Keep the client's skin clean and dry.
    3. Check the skin daily, especially areas where pressure sores commonly occur.
    4. Protect the bony areas on the body where pressure sores are likely to occur. Use padding or heel, elbow, and ankle protectors as directed by your supervisor.
    5. Encourage the client to eat a well-balanced diet.

Chapter 21:
Assisting With Medications

1. T	5. F
2. T	6. T
3. F	7. d
4. T	8. d

Chapter 22:
First Aid and Emergency Care

1. T	6. T
2. T	7. T
3. T	8. d
4. T	9. c
5. F	

Index

Page numbers in italics indicate figures; page numbers followed by *t* indicate tables.

C

D

Fluid output measurement, 276–277
Foam mattress pads, 267, *268*
Food, 139–153. *See also* Diet(s); Nutrition
  Alzheimer's disease and, 89
  buying, 148–150
  food groups and, 139, 140, 147
  infants and, 27
  kosher, 24
  need for water and, 144–145
  nutrients and, 139, 141–144
  planning meals and, 145, 147–148
  preparation and storage of, 150–151
    saving time and, 153
  serving, 151–152
  special diets and, 145, 146
Football hold, 252, *252*
Footboard, 160, *161*
Foot care, 237–238
  diabetes and, 92–93
  guidelines for, *237*, 237–238
  washing and, 231
Footdrop, *160*, 160–161
Forearms, range-of-motion exercises for, 180, *180*
Foreign language, communication and, 17, 24
Fracture(s), 98
Fracture pan, 221, *221*
Fraternal twins, 82
Fraud, protecting older adults against, 46
Friends
  extended family, 21
  of teenagers, 31
Full liquid diet, 146

G

Gallbladder, 76
Genitals, washing, 232
  babies and, 260
Geriatrics, 37. *See also* Older adults
Germs. *See* Infection control
Gerontology, 37. *See also* Older adults
Gifts, 9
Glands
  endocrine, 83, 85
  sweat, 67
Glaucoma, 98

Goose bumps/flesh, 67
Gravity, center of, 159
Grease fires, how to stop quickly, 114
Grieving, after death, 62
Grooming, 8

H

Hair
  aging and, 38
  function of, 67
Hair care, 238–241
  babies and, 260, *260*, 261
  guidelines for, *238*, 238–239
  shampooing and, 239, *239*, 240–241
Hand(s), range-of-motion exercises for, 181–183, *181–183*
"Handicapped" people, 49
Handwashing, 8, 124, 231
  procedure for, 122–124, *122–124*
Health, 48
Health problems, 95–100
  of older persons, 38
Health services, 6
Hearing, aging and, 40
  dying client and, 61
Hearing-impaired clients, communicating with, 16, 40, 61, 97
Heart, 73
  aging and, 39
Heart attack, 74, 98
  first aid procedures for, 304–306, *306*
Heart disease, 98–99
Heating pad, 269, 272
  safety with, 269, 272
Heel protectors, 267, *268*
Hemorrhage, 74
High blood pressure, 99, 203
High chairs, 30
High-fiber diet, 146
Hips, range-of-motion exercises for, 185, *185*
Hoarseness, 75
Home care team, 4, 6
  members of, 6
Home economist, 6
Home health administrator, 6
Home health agency, 4

Home health nurse, medications and, 287
Homemaker/home health aide, 6, 7
  responsibilities of, 8–9
    medications and, 287
  supervisor and, 7–8
Homemaker/home health aide bag, 112
Home management. *See also* House cleaning
  Alzheimer's disease and, 89
Home safety checklist, 114–117
Home visit, safety and, 112–113
Hospice care, 58
Hot applications, 269–272
  body's reaction to, 269
  electric heating pad for, 269, 272
  hot water bottle for, 270
  reasons for using, 269
  warm soaks for, 271, *271*
  when not to use, 269
House cleaning, 127–131
  of bathroom, 131, *131*
  of bedroom, 131, *132*
  dying clients and, 60
  extent of, 127
  homemaker/home health aide's role and, 127
  of kitchen, 130
  organizing work time and, 129
  preparing for, 129, *129*, 130, 130t
  reasons for, 127
  teaching clients and, 127, 128t, 129, 129t
Human body, makeup of, 66
Human needs, 20–21
  meeting, 20–21
  understanding, 20
  unmet, 20
Hyperglycemia, 89
Hypertension, 99, 203
Hypotension, orthostatic or postural, 203
Hypothermia, first aid procedures for, *306*, 306–307

I

I and O. *See* Input and output
Ice bag, 272
Identical twins, 82

J

K

L

M

depression and, 42, 50, 60
promotion of, 54
homemaker/home health aide's role and, 56
Mental illness, understanding, 54–55
Mercury, 189
safety precautions and, 190
Message ring, 17, *18*
Microorganism, 120
Minerals, 142
Minister, 24
Money
buying food and, 148, *148, 149,* 149–150
carrying, 112
Mood, 54
Mouth, 74
Mouth care. *See* Dentures; Oral hygiene; Teeth
Mouth sores, serving food and, 152
Movement, loss of, stroke and, 95
Muscle(s)
aging and, 38–39
voluntary and involuntary, 72
Muscle tissue, 66
Muscle tone, 72
Muscular system, *70–72,* 72–73, 84
common problems of, 73
observations to make about, 72
Myocardial infarction, 74

N

Nails, aging and, 38
Nasal congestion, 75
Nausea, 77
serving food and, 152
Neck, range-of-motion exercises for, 178, *178*
Needs
of children, dying clients and, 61
emotional, of dying client, 60–61
human. *See* Human needs
safety
of preschoolers, 29
of school-age children, 31
of teenagers, 31
of toddlers, 29
spiritual, 23–24
of dying clients, 61

Nerve(s), 78
Nerve tissue, 66
Nervous system, *77,* 77–78, 84
observations to make about, 78
senses and, 78, *79*
Neuropathy, diabetes and, 92
New mother, 250
Noninsulin-dependent diabetes, 90
Nonverbal communication, 14–15
Nose, 74
Nurse
home health, medications and, 287
licensed practical (LPN), 6
licensed vocational (LVN), 6
public health (PHN), 6
registered (RN), 6
Nutrients, 139, 141–144
Nutrition, 139. *See also* Diet(s); Food
aging and, 39
children and, 27, 33–34
pregnancy and, 249

O

Objective report, 106
Occupational therapist (OT), 6
Oil glands, of skin, 67
Older adults, 37–46
aging and, 37–38
changes associated with, 38–44
confused, guidelines for working with, 43
homemaker/home health aide's role and, 44–46
protecting, 45–46
respecting self-worth and dignity of, 44–45
teaching guidelines for, 43
working with, 44–46
Oral hygiene, 215–221
assisting with, 217–219, *218–219*
denture care and, 219–221, *220*
dying client and, 61
flossing and, *216,* 216–217, *217*
need for, 215
Oral hypoglycemic agents, 93
Oral thermometer, 190, *190*

Organ(s), 66. *See also specific organs*
Organ systems, 66, 67–85, 84
Orthostatic hypotension, 203
Ostomy, 277, 279
care of, 277–279, 283
changing colostomy bag and, 278–279, *279*
irrigation of colostomy and, 279
diet and, 279
supporting client with, 279, 283
Ostomy appliance, 279
OT. *See* Occupational therapist
OTC. *See* Over-the-counter medications
Ovaries, 81
Overdependence, disability and illness and, 50
Over-the-counter (OTC) medications, 286
Ovulation, 82
Ovum, 81
Oxygen therapy, *290,* 290–291, *291*
safety guidelines for, 290–291

P

Pain, 99
in chest, first aid procedures for, 304–306, *306*
in children, 33t
dying client and, 61–62
Pancreas, 76, 85
Paralysis, stroke and, 94
Parathyroid gland, 85
Parents, working with, 32
Parkinson's disease, 99–100
Partial bath, 232–233
Passive range-of-motion exercises, 178
Pastor, 24
Pathogens, 120
Penis, 81
Personal care
Alzheimer's disease and, 88
dying clients and, 60
skills for, 215–247
Pets, home visits and, 113
PHN. *See* Public health nurse
Physical changes
of aging, 38–39, 41
in Alzheimer's disease, 88

Q

R

S

T